IAN Reviews in Neurology 2024

Dementia

IAN Reviews in
Neurology 2024
Dementia

Editors

Sita Jayalakshmi MD DM
Senior Consultant Neurologist
Department of Neurology
Krishna Institute of Medical Sciences
Secunderabad, Telangana, India

Sangeeta Ravat MD DM
Dean, Professor and Head
Department of Neurology
Seth GS Medical College and KEM Hospital
Mumbai, Maharashtra, India

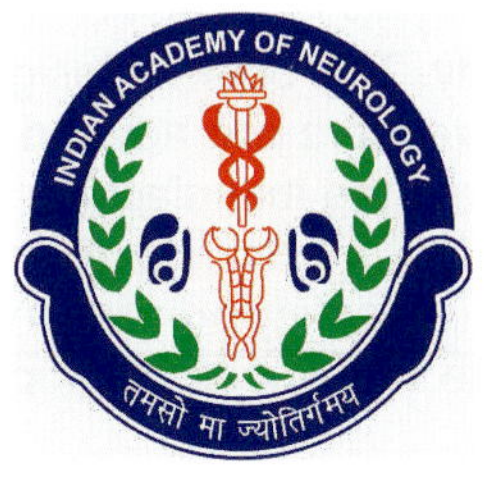

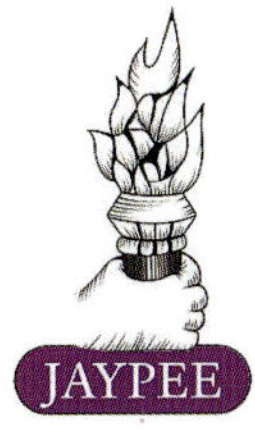

JAYPEE BROTHERS MEDICAL PUBLISHERS
The Health Sciences Publisher
New Delhi | London

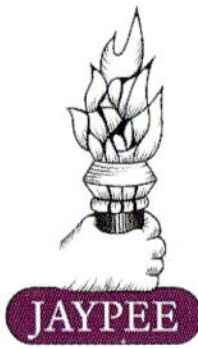

Jaypee Brothers Medical Publishers (P) Ltd

Headquarters
EMCA House
23/23-B, Ansari Road, Daryaganj
New Delhi 110 002, India
Landline: +91-11-23272143, +91-11-23272703
+91-11-23282021, +91-11-23245672
E-mail: jaypee@jaypeebrothers.com

Corporate Office
Jaypee Brothers Medical Publishers (P) Ltd.
4838/24, Ansari Road, Daryaganj
New Delhi 110 002, India
Phone: +91-11-43574357
Fax: +91-11-43574314
E-mail: jaypee@jaypeebrothers.com

Overseas Office
JP Medical Ltd.
83, Victoria Street, London
SW1H 0HW (UK)
Phone: +44-20 3170 8910
Fax: +44(0)20 3008 6180
E-mail: info@jpmedpub.com

Website: www.jaypeebrothers.com
Website: www.jaypeedigital.com

IAN Reviews in Neurology 2024: Dementia / ***Sita Jayalakshmi, Sangeeta Ravat***

First Edition: **2025**

ISBN: 978-93-5696-887-5

Printed at: Samrat Offset Pvt. Ltd.

Contributors

Abhishek Chowdhury MD DM
Consultant Neurologist
Apollo Multispeciality Hospital
Kolkata, West Bengal, India

Amitabha Ghosh MD MRCP(UK) CCST FRCP(London, Edinburgh)
Director and Head
Department of Neurology
Apollo Multispeciality Hospital
Kolkata, West Bengal, India

Anu Gupta DM(Neurology)
Associate Professor
Department of Neurology
Neurosciences Centre
All India Institute of Medical Sciences
New Delhi, India

Aparna Venugopal MSc(Speech Language Pathology)
PhD Scholar (Speech Pathology and Audiology)
Department of Speech Pathology and Audiology
National Institute of Mental Health and Neurosciences, Bengaluru
Speech Therapist (Karnataka Brain Health Initiative)
Department of Neurology
National Institute of Mental Health and Neurosciences (NIMHANS)
Bengaluru, Karnataka, India

Apoorva Pauranik MD DM
Director
Pauranik Academy of Medical Education
Ex-Professor
Department of Medicine/Neurology
MGM Medical College and MY Hospital
Indore, Madhya Pradesh, India

Arpita Roychoudhury MSc MPhil
Consultant Clinical Psychologist
Apollo Multispeciality Hospital
Kolkata, West Bengal, India

Ashwani Bhat MD(Internal Medicine) DM(Neurology)
Associate Professor
Department of Neurology
Himalayan Institute of Medical Sciences
Swami Rama Himalayan University
Dehradun, Uttarakhand, India

Asish Vijayaraghavan MD DM PDF
Assistant Professor
Department of Neurology
Sree Chitra Tirunal Institute for Medical Sciences and Technology (SCTIMST)
Thiruvananthapuram, Kerala, India

Atanu Biswas MD DM
Professor
Department of Neuromedicine
Bangur Institute of Neurosciences
IPGMER and SSKM Hospital
Kolkata, West Bengal, India

Avanthi Paplikar PhD Postdoctoral Fellowship (N-SERB, NIMHANS)
Founder and Speech Language Pathologist
SpeakUp Centre for Speech Therapy and Neuro Rehabilitation
Associate Professor and Research Coordinator
Department of Speech and Language Studies
Dr SR Chandrasekhar Institute of Speech and Hearing
Bengaluru, Karnataka, India

Christian Dansereau PhD
Neuroscientist and Computer Scientist
Perceiv Research Inc. (Perceiv AI)
Montreal, Quebec, Canada

Debjyoti Dhar DM
Consultant Neurologist
Max Super Speciality Hospital
Lucknow, Uttar Pradesh, India

Deenadayal Boopalan BNYS MD(Naturopathy)
Research Associate
ICMR-National Institute of Epidemiology
Chennai, Tamil Nadu, India

Durjoy Lahiri MD DM
Assistant Professor
Department of Neurology
Queen's University
Kingston, Ontario, Canada

Faheem Arshad MD DM(Neurology)
Assistant Professor
Department of Neurology
National Institute of Mental Health and Neurosciences (NIMHANS)
Bengaluru, Karnataka, India

Ganaraja VH DM DrNB(Neurology)
Assistant Professor
Department of Neurology
National Institute of Mental Health and Neurosciences (NIMHANS)
Bengaluru, Karnataka, India

Gautam Das DPM MD DM
Specialist Neurologist
Department of Neuromedicine
Bangur Institute of Neurosciences
IPGMER and SSKM Hospital
Kolkata, West Bengal, India

Howard J Rosen MD
Professor
Department of Neurology
UCSF Memory and Aging Center
San Francisco, California, USA

Ishwarya Thiruvuru MD(General Medicine)
Neurology Resident
Sri Ramachandra Institute of Higher Education and Research
Chennai, Tamil Nadu, India

Kuntal Biswas MD
Senior Resident
Department of Neuromedicine
Bangur Institute of Neurosciences
IPGMER and SSKM Hospital
Kolkata, West Bengal, India

Mani Tolety MBBS
Vice President
Alzheimer's and Related Disorders
Society of India (ARDSI) Hyderabad
Deccan Chapter
Hyderabad, Telangana, India

Manjari Tripathi DM(Neurology)
FNASc FRCP(Edinburgh)
Professor and Unit Head
Department of Neurology
NIH Fellow (UCLA)
Neurosciences Centre
All India Institute of Medical Sciences
New Delhi, India

MM Samim DM(Neurology)
Senior Resident
Department of Neurology
National Institute of Mental Health and
Neurosciences (NIMHANS)
Bengaluru, Karnataka, India

Mohammed Faruq MBBS PhD
Senior Principal Scientist
Genomics and Molecular Medicine
CSIR - Institute of Genomics and
Integrative Biology
Civil Lines, New Delhi, India

Najamus Saquib MBBS DPM
Consultant Psychiatrist
Asha Geriatric Psychiatric Unit
Asha Hospital
Hyderabad, Telangana, India

Nirmal Surya MD DNB(Neurology) FIAN
MNAMS FAAN
Chairman
Surya Neuro Centre
Assistant Professor
Bombay Hospital Institute of Medical
Sciences
Mumbai, Maharashtra, India

Pinki Singh PhD MASLP
Assistant Professor (SLP)
NSCB Medical College
Jabalpur, Madhya Pradesh, India

Porrselvi AP PhD
Founder and Cognitive
Neuropsychologist
Unified Brain Health Care
Chennai, Tamil Nadu, India

Priya Treesa Thomas PhD(Psychiatric
Social Work)
Additional Professor
Department of PSW
National Institute of Mental Health and
Neurosciences (NIMHANS)
Bengaluru, Karnataka, India

PT Alexander MD DM
Postdoctoral Fellow in Cognitive
Neurosciences
Department of Neurology
National Institute of Mental Health and
Neurosciences (NIMHANS)
Bengaluru, Karnataka, India

Ramshekhar N Menon MD DM PDF
Commonwealth Fellow
Professor
Department of Neurology
Sree Chitra Tirunal Institute for Medical
Sciences and Technology (SCTIMST)
Thiruvananthapuram, Kerala, India

**Ranganathan Lakshmi
Narasimhan** MD DNB DM DNB FEBN
FRCP(London, Glasgow) FAAN FACP FIAN
PhD
Head and Professor
Department of Neurology
Sri Ramachandra Institute of Higher
Education and Research
Chennai, Tamil Nadu, India

Ratnavalli Ellajosyula MD DM
Consultant Neurologist and Specialist
in Cognitive Neurology and Adjunct
Professor
Manipal Hospital
Annasawmy Mudaliar Hospital
Neurocare Clinic
Manipal Academy of Higher Education
(MAHE)
Bengaluru, Karnataka, India

Ravi Prakash Singh MD DM
Senior Resident
Department of Neurology
National Institute of Mental Health and
Neurosciences (NIMHANS)
Bengaluru, Karnataka, India

Ravi Yadav MD DM
Professor
Department of Neurology
National Institute of Mental Health and
Neurosciences (NIMHANS)
Bengaluru, Karnataka, India

Rithvik Ramesh MD DM(Neurology)
Associate Professor
Sri Ramachandra Institute of Higher
Education and Research
Chennai, Tamil Nadu, India

Saadiya Hurzuk MSc(Dementia
Studies)
Psychologist
Alzheimer's and Related Disorders
Society of India (ARDSI) Hyderabad
Deccan Chapter
Hyderabad, Telangana, India

Saranya B Gomathy MD DM
Assistant Professor
Department of Neurology
Jawaharlal Institute of Postgraduate
Medical Education and Research
(JIPMER)
Puducherry, India

Himanshi Kapoor PhD
Senior Research Associate
Genomics and Molecular Medicine
Division
CSIR - Institute of Genomics and
Integrative Biology
Civil Lines, New Delhi, India

Sinjan Ghosh MD(Internal Medicine)
DM(Neurology)
Postdoctoral Fellowship in Cognitive
and Behavioral Neurology
University of Toronto, Canada
Consultant Neurologist
Fortis Healthcare
Kolkata, West Bengal, India

Sneha Rozelena Anthony MSc
(Speech Language Pathology)
Speech, Language Pathologist
Department of Neuro Rehabilitation
Institute of Neurosciences
Kolkata, West Bengal, India

Sonali Bhattad MD DM
Consultant Neurologist
Manipal Hospital
Bengaluru, Karnataka, India

Souvik Dubey MD DM
Assistant Professor
Department of Neuromedicine
Bangur Institute of Neurosciences
IPGMER and SSKM Hospital
Kolkata, West Bengal, India

S Sandeep Kumar MD DM
Consultant Neurologist
Yashoda Hospitals
Hyderabad, Telangana, India

Subasree Ramakrishnan
DM(Neurology)
Additional Professor
Department of Neurology
National Institute of Mental Health and Neurosciences (NIMHANS)
Bengaluru, Karnataka, India

Subhash Kaul MD DM
Consultant Neurologist
Department of Neurology
Krishna Institute of Medical Sciences (KIMS)
Secunderabad, Telangana, India

Suman Kushwaha DM(Neurology)
Professor and Head
Department of Neurology
Institute of Human Behaviour and Allied Sciences (IHBAS)
Dilshad Garden, New Delhi, India

Suvarna Alladi DM
Professor and Head
Department of Neurology
National Institute of Mental Health and Neurosciences (NIMHANS)
Bengaluru, Karnataka, India

Urvashi Shah PhD
Consultant Neuropsychologist
Department of Neurology
King Edward Memorial Hospital (KEMH)
Mumbai, Maharashtra, India

Vaibhav Seth DM DRNB MRCP
SCE(Neurology)
Associate Consultant
Apollo Multispeciality Hospital
Kolkata, West Bengal, India

Preface

Dementia is currently the seventh leading cause of death and one of the major causes of disability and dependency among older people globally. According to the World Health Organization (WHO), currently more than 55 million people around the world are suffering from dementia. In India, an estimated prevalence of dementia in people aged more than 60 years is 7.4%. The WHO recognizes dementia as a public health priority. In May 2017, *the World Health Assembly endorsed the global action plan on the public health response to dementia 2017–2025*. The plan provides a comprehensive blueprint for action—for policymakers, international, regional, and national partners, and WHO in the following areas: Addressing dementia as a public health priority; increasing awareness of dementia and creating a dementia-inclusive society; reducing the risk of dementia; diagnosis, treatment, and care; information systems for dementia; support for dementia carers; and research and innovation (https://www.who.int/news-room/fact-sheets/detail/dementia).

While there is no cure for degenerative dementias, recent emergence of disease-modifying drugs represents a paradigm shift and breakthrough in the management of Alzheimer's disease. However, in recent years, the recognition of rapidly progressive dementias has gained increased attention as physicians encounter cases where cognitive decline progresses at an accelerated pace, over a matter of weeks or months. Providing care and support for a person living with dementia is challenging with high caregiver burden. Recognition of these cases and early intervention will help in slowing of the progression of disease and improve the outcomes.

Though there is no cure for dementia, a lot can be done for persons with dementia and their caregivers. The present book, *"IAN Reviews in Neurology: Dementia"*, collates state-of-the-art diagnostic and therapeutic developments in the management of dementia that may hold hope for countless persons with dementia and their caregivers. We are confident that this compilation will be of immense value to neurologists, psychologists, and physicians dealing with dementia patients.

Sita Jayalakshmi
Sangeeta Ravat

Acknowledgments

As the Editors of the book "*IAN Reviews in Neurology: Dementia*," we feel immensely happy that we had the opportunity to contribute for the academic activities of Indian Academy of Neurology. This was a gratifying experience.

First of all, we are extremely grateful to all the eminent authors for submitting the chapters in a restricted time and meticulously preparing the manuscripts. We convey our special thanks to Dr Alladi Suvarna, Professor and Head from NIMHANS, Bengaluru, for being with us all the way, right from the start, providing immense guidance as we undertook this project. We express our sincere gratitude to Dr Sudhindra Vooturi who helped us with editing and technical compilation.

We sincerely thank Dr Debashish Chowdhury, the President, Dr Meenakshi Sundaram, the Secretary, and all the executive committee members of Indian Academy of Neurology for their constant support during the preparation of this book.

We thank the publication team at M/s Jaypee Brothers Medical Publishers(P) Ltd, Ms Chetna Malhotra (Senior Director—Professional Publishing, Marketing and Business Development) and Ms Nedup Bhutia Pillai (Assistant Manager—Print Publishing), for their professional approach and support in bringing out this compilation.

Sita Jayalakshmi
Sangeeta Ravat

Contents

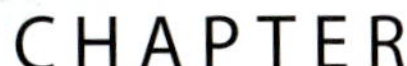

CHAPTER

1

Human Cognition: Structure–Function Relationships

Ashwani Bhat, Gautam Das

ABSTRACT

Cognitive neurology is to neurology what quantum physics is to physics: Apparently precise and localized yet like a vast expanse of merely 3 pounds inside the cranial vault. Although humans have been fascinated by this aspect of the brain for many centuries, the many mysteries and some of the finer nuances have only been solved in the past century or so. The concept of different brain areas responsible for different brain functions was introduced by Brodmann in the early 20th century and later consolidated by works like those of Broca, Wernicke, Gerstman, and others.

Since then, we have come a long way from the concept of structural localization to functional localization and the introduction of networks and circuits. The complex cognitive functions in humans have their origin not only in the various anatomical areas but arise from a complex interplay between the various brain areas and the connections thereof. A more holistic approach that has gained attention in the last couple of decades is the network theory, which focuses on three large scale networks of the human brain, namely the default mode network, the central executive, and the salience network.

The objective of this chapter is to explain the role of the individual brain areas and their connections in the genesis of human cognition and behavior. Although it is an endless topic, we will try to introspect over how the various structures synchronously orchestrate to achieve the complex cognitive states that no other known species or machine can achieve.

Keywords: Human cognition, Behavior, Neuroanatomy, Neural connections, Networks.

INTRODUCTION

"The human brain has 100 billion neurons each neuron connected to 10,000 other neurons. Sitting on your shoulders is the most complicated object in the known-universe."

—Michigan Kaku, American Physicist

There are four things to keep in mind while dealing with any biological system, as Tinbergen so astutely explained in 1951.[1]

These include phylogeny, selection, ontogeny, and mechanism.

- *Phylogeny and selection*: From insectivores, who primarily used their brains for sensation and movement, primates evolved a more complex brain with well-developed anterior and posterior association areas. Thus humans differed from other animals due to their larger brains, increased cortical grey matter, and cerebral cortical folds and a well-developed prefrontal cortex, which evolved from a granular one in early mammals.[2]
- *Development (Embryology)*: Although this aspect is beyond the scope of this chapter, what is astonishing is that the hundred billion neurons that we have and their connections develop from the tip of a 3-mm neural tube.
- *Mechanism*: The idea of brain areas responsible for different cognitive functions was introduced several hundred years ago by Broadman and later on consolidated by the work of Broca, Wernicke, and other important landmarks like the case of Phineas Gage and HM (Henry Gustav Molaison). The development of computed tomography (CT), magnetic resonance imaging (MRI), functional MRI,

and PET encouraged neuroscientists to identify the cognitive domains connected with each location. This chapter addresses this aspect of brain from four perspectives: Structural/topological (area-specific), structural/hodological (pathway-specific), functional, and the network perspective, respectively.

"THE HUMAN BRAIN FROM THE TOPOLOGICAL PERSPECTIVE"

The functional regions of the brain can be divided into the limbic region, the paralimbic zone or the mesocortex, the isocortical regions, and the most advanced idiotypic cortex, comprises the corticoid and allocortical regions.[3] However, this perspective ignores the contribution that individual areas have in the genesis of cognition. So, let us try to virtually dissect the various brain areas responsible for the same.

Frontal Lobes

The larger frontal lobes in humans and their unique density and organization of synapses enable regions of comparable dimensions to analyze more sophisticated data than the primitive brain **(Fig. 1)**.[4] The cognitive and motor functions of the frontal lobe are categorized into five reciprocally coupled subcortical circuits, as originally suggested by Alexander De Long and Strick.[5] Here, we will focus on the anatomical substrates for the cognitive functions **(Flowchart 1)**.

Dorsolateral Prefrontal Cortex and Circuit

Dorsolateral prefrontal cortex (DLPFC) originates from Broadman areas 9 and 46. The medial prefrontal cortex is considered to be important in monitoring, planning, and manipulation of information. The posterior part of DLPFC and its connections to subcortical structures are responsible for the attentional processes via inputs from medial and lateral parieto-occipital areas as well as from superior temporal lobe via the superior longitudinal fasciculus.[5] Although left and right DLPFC have different functions, this circuit is primarily concerned with executive function, generating hypothesis and impairment of flexibility for maintaining or set shifting as well as planning strategy, generation and activation of remote memories.[5,6] Dysfunction primarily leads to dysexecutive syndrome.

The Orbitofrontal Cortex and Circuit

The orbitofrontal cortex (OFC) comprises Broadman regions 10 and 11. This circuit has multiple interconnections and reciprocal connections with basal ganglia, thalamus limbic, and different heteromodal and unimodal and limbic cortices for polysensory and emotional inputs. The medial OFC plays a crucial role in personality, decision-making, social norms, and serves as a significant neural substrate for social cognition and theory of mind.[7] Dysfunction primarily leads to social inappropriateness, disinhibition.

The Anterior Cingulate Circuit[5]

The anterior cingulate circuit starts from Broadman area 24. The primary role of the circuit is to regulate motivated behavior, reversal, learning, reward processes, and appraisal. The circuit's lesions manifest as akinetic mutism, abulia, hypokinesia, or apathy.

The Frontopolar Cortex/Rostral Prefrontal Cortex[8]

The frontopolar cortex has a role in multitasking, "Theory of Mind" and prospective memory.[8] The frontopolar

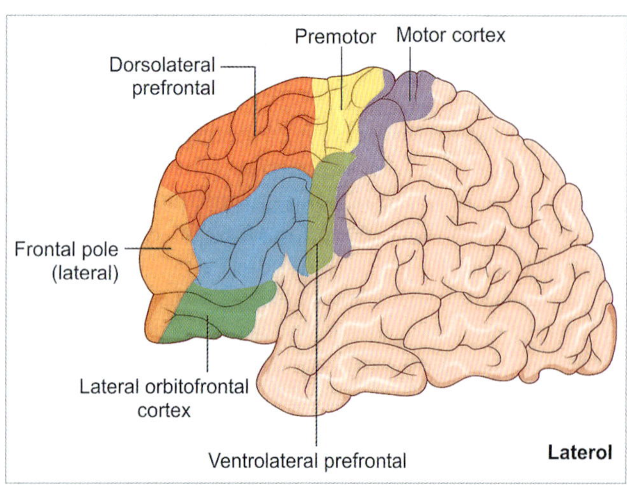

FIG. 1: The frontal lobes.

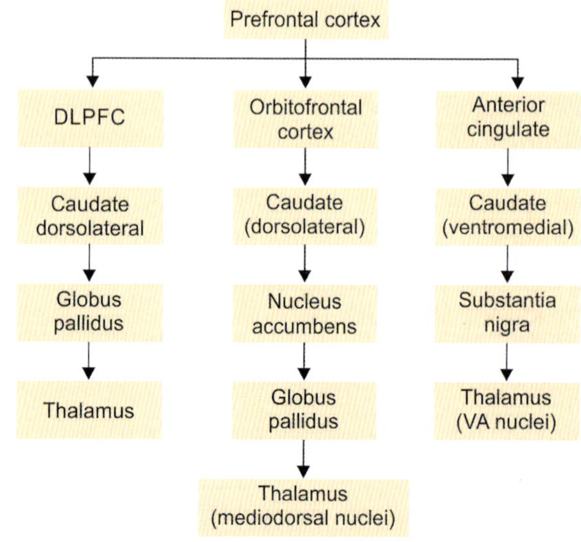

FLOWCHART 1: The frontal lobe circuits for cognition.

cortex also plays a crucial role in metacognition, which refers to the capacity to strategically plan, monitor, and evaluate one's cognitive functions.[9]

The Temporal Lobes

The temporal lobes are positioned below the sylvian fissure. The temporal lobes can be anatomically and functionally divided into medial, middle, and lateral regions, as well as the temporal poles.[9] The functions of the temporal lobes and corresponding association areas are concerned with vision, audition, semantics, episodic memory, and language **(Fig. 2)**.

- *Vision and visuoperceptual function*: "The ventral visual pathway": Visual recognition is done via the ventral visual stream, also known as the "What" pathway. The hierarchical system processes basic visual inputs into more complex representations. Simple inputs are processed posteriorly, while the anterior parts process more complicated and specific visual information.[10] An important feature of these association areas is invariant object recognition. The ability to distinguish intricate and different entities remains "invariant" as we move toward the anterior and inferior parts of the cortex, notably inferior temporal cortex area V5. It is unaffected by stimulus size, direction, contrast, color, or movement. Lesions in these regions cause visual agnosia. Faces and nonfacial things are processed by the fusiform face area, while the para hippocampal place area processes images of locations, landmarks, buildings, and settings.
- *Auditory functions*: The auditory representation system is arranged from posteriorly extending from the superior temporal gyrus (STG) to the anterior parts into planum-temporale, posterior superior temporal gyrus, and the temporal junction. The ventral auditory stream focuses on auditory processing information, while the dorsal auditory stream is responsible for processing sound, position, and movement.[11]
- *The medial temporal lobes (MTLs)*: The functions have been described in detail in the section on "Memory."
- *The temporal poles*: The temporal pole is linked to various advanced cognitive functions such as visual processing for complex objects and face recognition, autobiographical memory, naming and word-object labeling, semantic processing in all forms, and socioemotional processing.[7]

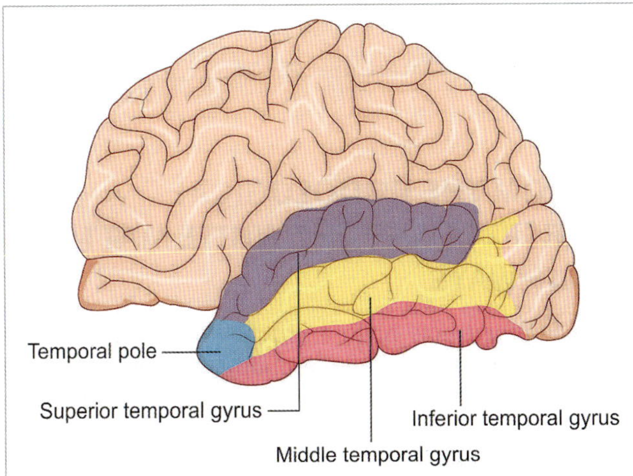

FIG. 2: The temporal lobes.

The Parietal lobe

The human parietal lobe consists of an anterior and a posterior part.[12] All sensory modalities are processed in the anterior parietal lobe, while cognitive tasks involve the posterior parietal lobe.[12] The intraparietal sulcus is critical for communication between the superior, inferior parietal lobules, and premotor cortex.[13] It encodes sensory-motor attention and short-term memory. The dorsal visual pathway from the occipital regions mostly connects to the superior parietal lobule, intraparietal sulcus, and precuneus. In the left hemisphere, the inferior parietal lobule and temporoparietal junction are critical to language and number processing, while in the right, they are involved in visuospatial attention and social cognitive functions.[12,13] Parietal-hippocampal connections are involved in formation of episodic memory **(Fig. 3)**.

Occipital Lobes

The primary visual cortex is located in the calcarine sulcus in the occipital lobe.

The V1 area has a comprehensive representation of the visual field, with the lower meridian represented superiorly, while the upper meridian is represented inferiorly. The diversity in this area is mostly associated with the cross-sectional area of the optic tract and the volumes of the magnocellular and parvocellular pathway, which accounts for variations in visual acuity among individuals.[14] V2 represents the contralateral visual field, divided into dorsal and ventral halves, while V3 is similarly divided into dorsal and ventral portions.[15] The cortical regions responsible for visual motion perception and color perception are typically found in the extrastriate cortex, such as area V5 or the medial temporal area for motion perception, and region V4 on the ventral surface of the occipital lobe for color patterns.[15] The V4 regions have a retinotopic organization. Damage to its anterior and lateral regions causes visual object agnosia, whereas damage to the posterior regions causes

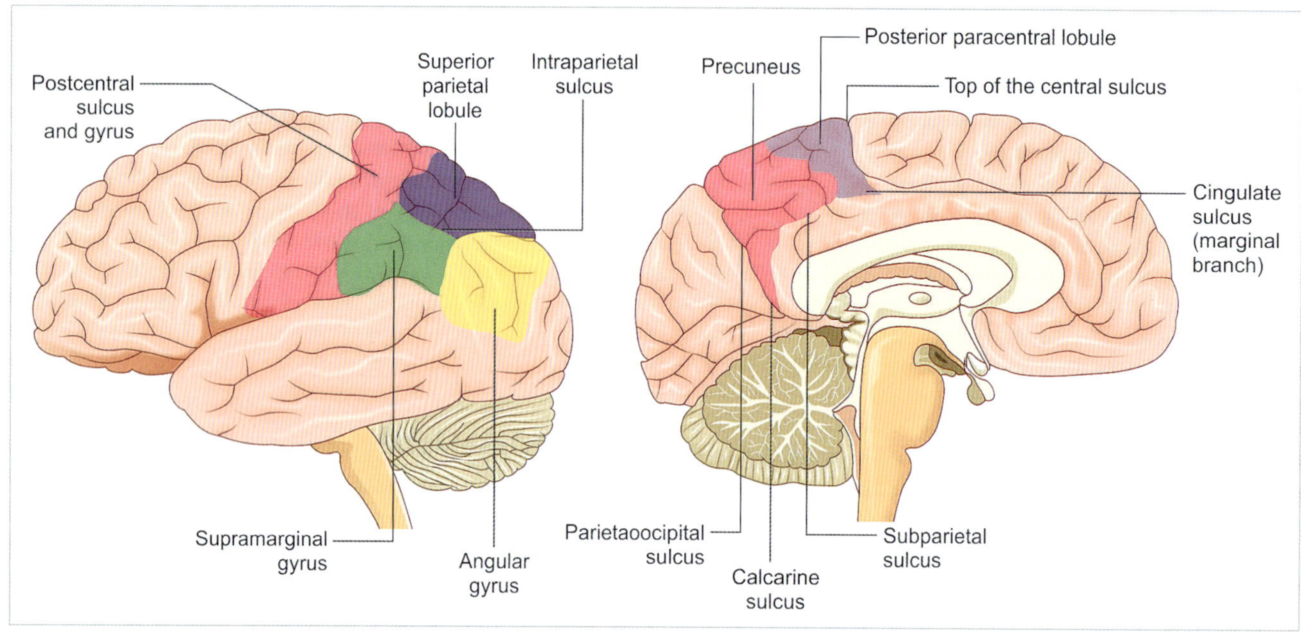

FIG. 3: The parietal lobe.

prosopagnosia, a disorder of facial recognition. A portion of the information originates not just from the occipital cortices but also from the subcortical pathways.[16] The coordinated and goal-directed actions involve the combined effort and processing of both the dorsal and the ventral streams. The dorsal stream is associated with vision for action, while the ventral stream is linked to vision for perception. The visual processing does not occur in a linear manner, but rather follows a temporal hierarchy in signal processing across the visual map and visual cortices, in addition to the spatial hierarchy that is known.[16] Thus the visuospatial function is a combined result of the complex processing in the temporal and occipital lobes **(Fig. 4)**.

The Basal Ganglia

The basal ganglia are intricately connected with the cortex and the thalamus via the cortico-striato-thalamocortical loop.[9] It has been suggested that the pathways described earlier (in **Flowchart 1**) have very soft boundaries and partial and frequent, asymmetric overlaps, which is responsible for the integration of cognitive motor sensory and effective information.[17]

The cerebellum: Recently, there has been an interest in the role of cerebellum in cognition. Cerebellar lesions are proposed to lead to the "cerebellar cognitive affective syndrome" or "Schmahmann's syndrome," which comprises of executive dysfunction, language, and visuospatial dysfunction along with behavioral dysfunction.

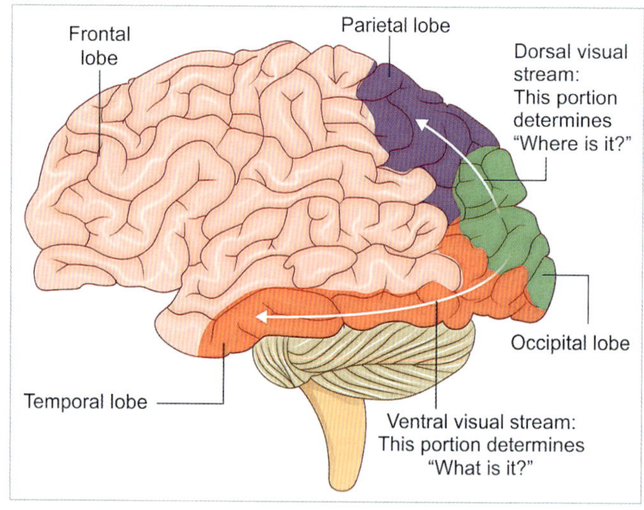

FIG. 4: The occipital lobe and visual pathways.

"FROM THE HODOLOGICAL PERSPECTIVE": THE WHITE MATTER PATHWAYS

White matter tracts have a crucial role in regulating, enhancing, screening, and distributing signals to various cortical and subcortical regions to facilitate both serial and parallel processing within the brain. Diffusion tensor imaging has allowed for the detailed mapping of these pathways into association fibers, commissural fibers, and projection fibers.[18]

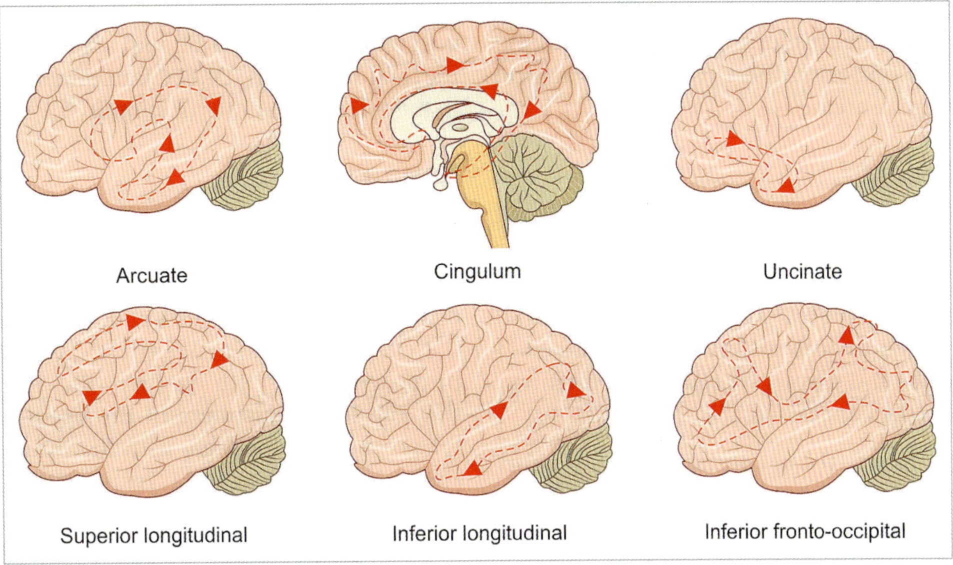

FIG. 5: White matter association tracts.

White Matter Tracts Connecting Different Regions of the Brain

Association fibers link the brain to cortical and sub-cortical areas. The fibers are predominantly long association fibers, such as the arcuate fasciculus, superior longitudinal fasciculus, inferior longitudinal fasciculus, uncinate fasciculus, cingulate fibers, and several occipital tracts **(Fig. 5)**.[18]

The arcuate fasciculus is traditionally known as a pathway between the anterior and posterior language regions. However, new imaging and functional approaches have led to the development of several models.[19] For example, the Catani model describes the arcuate fasciculus as a medial direct tract connecting the superior temporal lobe region with Broca's region in the inferior frontal lobe.[19] Additionally, there is a lateral indirect pathway that consists of an anterior and a posterior branch. The anterior portion of the indirect pathway links the Broca's region to the Geschwind's region in the inferior parietal lobe, while the posterior segment of this pathway connects the Geschwind's region to the Wernicke's region. The direct segment focuses on integrating auditory and motor functions, verbal memory, and forming semantic concepts.[20,21] The lateral segment, also known as the indirect pathway, is involved in naming, auditory phoneme-semantic coordination, and syntax.[19,22]

The superior longitudinal fasciculus (SLF) consists of three branches. The first branch links the superior parietal lobule with the superior frontal gyrus. This is responsible for the visuospatial coordination of the upper body and trunk.[23] The SLF-2 on the right side is associated with visual spatial coordination, attention, and visuospatial working memory and visuospatial function. The SLF-2 on the left side acts similarly to SLF-1.[23] SLF-3 is considered equivalent to the indirect branch of arcuate fasciculus.

The cingulate fasciculus extends from the amygdala and parahippocampal gyrus to the orbitofrontal lobe. Short fibers from the cingulate connect to several regions along its whole length, including the cingulate cortex, superior and medial frontal gyrus, paracentral lobule, precuneus, cuneus, lingular, and fusiform gyrus. The dorsal part of the cingulate cortex is responsible for the default mode network, whereas the ventral part connects the amygdala and parahippocampal cortex to the retrosplenial areas, forming the network for spatial orientation. The uncinate fasciculus connects the anterior part of the temporal lobe with the orbital and orbito-frontal cortices. It is crucial for lexical retrieval, semantic association, naming, and social cognition.[24]

The inferior longitudinal fasciculus links the occipital areas to the temporal lobe. It is involved in transmitting visual information crucial for tasks such as recognizing objects and faces, reading, and representing items visually.[25] The inferior fronto-occipital fasciculus is involved in tasks related to reading, writing, and other semantic and syntactic components of language.[26]

The Commissural Fibers

Commissural fibers facilitate the transfer of information between the two hemispheres of the brain, contributing significantly to the coordination of motor, perceptual, and cognitive functions. The corpus callosum is the greatest bundle of nerve fibers, connecting the two hemispheres of the brain and lies above the lateral ventricles.[27] The anterior commissure is a tiny bundle of fibers that is split into an anterior and posterior branch. The anterior fibers link the amygdala, fusiform gyrus, and temporal poles, whereas the posterior fibers connect the ventral temporal and occipital areas.[20]

Projection Fibers

The fibers are categorized as ascending and descending fibers. The ascending fibers link subcortical structures to cortical structures through the thalamus. The three primary descending routes are the corticospinal, corticobulbar, and corticorubral. The fornix is classified as a projection fiber and plays a crucial role in memory, particularly within the Papez circuit.[21]

Short association fibers: These consist of several short U-shaped fibers and interlobar association tracts.[21] Key neural pathways consist of the frontal aslant tract, the frontal operculum pathway, and the ventral occipital bundle of Wernicke.[28] The frontal aslant tract links the posterior part of Broca's region with the presupplementary motor area, the medial prefrontal cortex, and the anterior cingulate cortex.[28] This tract plays a significant role in language processing and is predominantly located on the left side in the majority of righthanded individuals. Lesions can cause changes in fluency or reduced speech initiation (mutism).[28]

"FROM THE FUNCTIONAL PERSPECTIVE"

The structure or the pathway-based approaches explain the neuroanatomical substrates in a detailed manner but fail to explain the individual cognitive domains comprehensively. The first and foremost of the domains is attention as all other domains are dependent on it.

Attention

Attention is the selective capacity to focus on one thing and not another. It is classified into Sustained attention, Divided attention, and Selective attention.[29] Top-down voluntary attention is used to plan and carry out goal-directed selection for stimuli and reactions, while automatic attention is the bottom-up detection of stimuli that are important to behavior, especially when they are novel and stand out. In the real world, attention is a culmination of both the above processes for which multiple models have been described.[30] The ascending reticular activating system (ARAS) in the brainstem is crucial for attention by activating cortical regions. Neural networks originating from the reticular formation travel through the reticular nuclei in the thalamus and then project to various regions of the cerebral cortex. The cortical regions mutually affect the ARAS in a reciprocally connected manner. Finally, all the above processes are governed by our motivational state (limbic system) and the long-term goals (DLPFC), culminating in the attention to the selected stimulus or stimuli.[30]

Language

Another one of most fascinating of the cognitive domains is the language which not only allows us to communicate among us but also as a medium of internal dialogue.[31] The earliest model of language also known as the classical model or Wernicke-Lichtheim model was proposed in the 19th century. The accepted view was that the left hemisphere of the brain was responsible for processing language, with the inferior frontal gyrus (IFG) housing the area responsible for producing speech (Broca's area) and the superior temporal lobe housing the area responsible for processing and comprehending speech (Wernicke's area). Recent models have categorized the linguistic anatomical foundations into a dorsal and a ventral pathway. The Hickok and Poeppel model states that the auditory and phonological processing systems are arranged bilaterally in the left and right dorsal STG and mid-posterior superior temporal sulcus (STS), respectively.[32] The paths divide into a ventral and a dorsal stream on both sides. The streams are predominantly located on the left side. The ventral stream processes auditory information into semantic meaning. The posterior middle temporal gyrus (MTG) and posterior inferior temporal sulcus (pITS) are responsible for deciphering the syntax and semantics of speech. The anterior middle temporal gyrus (aMTG) serves as a combinatorial network.[32] The left dorsal stream comprises the Sylvian-parietotemporal area (Spt) along the parietal–temporal boundary, together with the anterior insula, premotor cortex, and the posterior inferior frontal gyrus (pIFG). This section of the dorsal stream transforms auditory stimuli into motor action. The ventral and dorsal streams have extensive links with the widely distributed conceptual network in the brain. These connections decode spoken speech and plan spoken articulation by retrieving meaning and concepts from a semantic conceptual framework.[32]

Memory

A memory is an enduring neural representation that manifests in ideas, experiences, or behaviors. Although there are many classification systems, we will broadly describe memory into short- and long-term memory.

- *Short-term memory*: It is described as information that is temporarily available and has a restricted storage duration. Baddley and Hitch suggested that working memory is a complicated system with multiple components that alter information storage to enhance

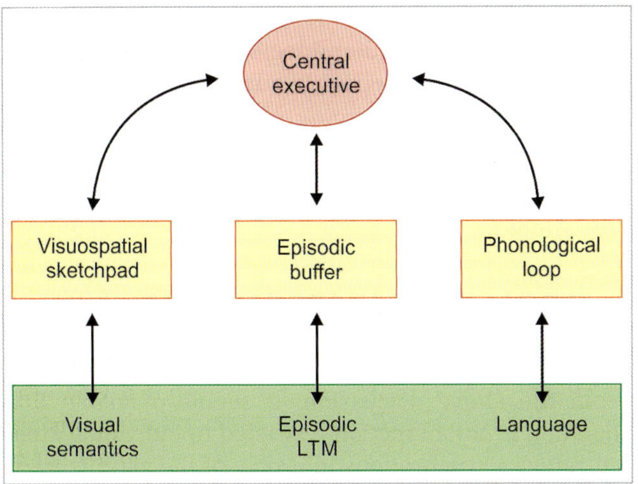

FIG. 6: Model for working memory Baddeley and Hitch.

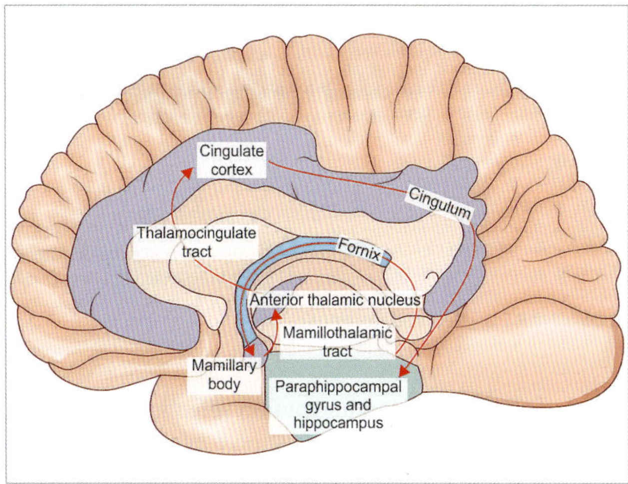

FIG. 7: Papez circuit.

cognitive function.[33] The three subcomponents are the phonological loop (verbal working memory), visuospatial sketchpad (visual-spatial working memory), and the central executive (DLPFC), which includes the attentional control system. The "episodic buffer" is a component introduced later that modulates and integrates various sensory input[33] **(Fig. 6)**.

- *Long-term memory*: Schacter and Tulving first proposed the classification of long-term memory. It categorizes the memory into declarative and nondeclarative forms. Episodic memory is personal and self-referential. It pertains to recollections of deliberate occurrences in our lives that have a distinct origin in time, space, and circumstances. Semantic memory encompasses information about the world, ourselves, and other individuals. Episodic learning can occur either consciously through intentional efforts or inadvertently without conscious attempts to memorize information. For instance, we might recall a scenario from a memory seminar where the memory circuit diagram was being drawn on the board, assuming we were attentive. We may be able to identify the identical diagram upon each subsequent viewing.[34] The MTL is necessary for encoding and transferring episodic memories, but the memory traces themselves are thought to be stored in the cortex.[34,35] Visual information is processed in the occipital lobes while spatial information is communicated through the dorsal visual pathway to the parahippocampal cortex, and then to the medial entorhinal cortex, while other qualities such as shape, size, color, and texture are transmitted along the ventral visual pathway to perirhinal cortex, and subsequently to the lateral entorhinal cortex.[35] Concurrently, there is a parallel connection between the mentioned characteristics and semantic and lexical information. The medial and lateral entorhinal cortices are components of the Papez circuit, which includes the hippocampus, fornix, mammillary bodies, and mammillothalamic tract, anterior thalamic nucleus, cingulate gyrus, entorhinal cortex, and hippocampus. Within the Papez circuit, information from the hippocampal formation is sent to the dentate gyrus and CA3 for associative processing and facilitating subsequent retrieval. The CAl region is intended to offer a "timestamp" for this information, establishing a temporal sequence for events.[36] The connection between the human OFC, vmPFC, and anterior cingulate cortex allows reward and emotional value to be integrated into episodic memory, facilitating the remembering of where a reward was encountered. During retrieval, the visual cortex decodes the memory circuit from the neocortex and reconstructs the episode stored in the MTL **(Fig. 7)**.

Praxis

Praxis neuroanatomy consists of two subsystems: The praxis conceptual system and the praxis production system.[37] The conceptual system comprises the concepts necessary for generating movements. These concepts are retained as "praxicons" in the left inferior parietal lobule. The praxicons store information about objects, actions, and the sequence of activities. The production system includes the superior parietal lobule, supplementary motor area (SMA), and premotor cortex. It is responsible for generating motions by transmitting signals to the primary motor cortex. Some studies propose that object use requires information from the ventral and dorsal streams, which is combined by the inferior parietal lobe.[37,38] The affordance competition hypothesis proposes

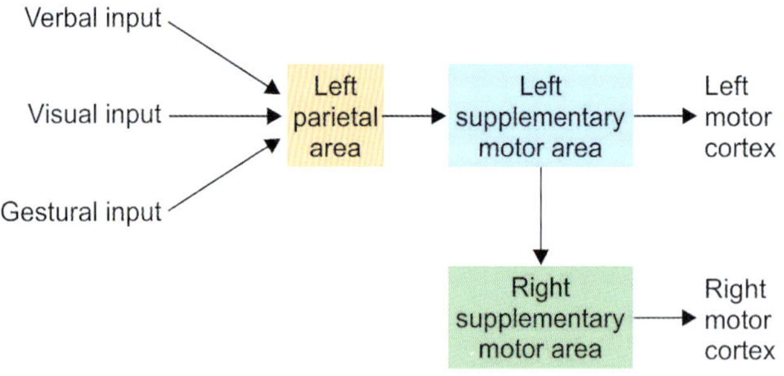

FLOWCHART 2: Neuroanatomy of praxis.

that action specification and action selection are carried out by the same neural circuits spread across many brain areas.[38] Information on object and action knowledge is stored in the inferior parietal lobule. The superior parietal lobule stores engrams related to executing sequential actions and visuospatial and kinesthetic elements. When we need to take action, conceptual engrams are triggered in the inferior parietal lobule, followed by the activation of kinesthetic engrams in the superior parietal lobule. The impulses are then transmitted to the supplementary motor cortex on both sides, which is in-charge of motor movement planning. The SMA stimulates the premotor cortex bilaterally, which then activates the corresponding primary motor cortex to commence movement **(Flowchart 2)**.[39]

Visuospatial and Visuoperceptual Domains

These domains have been described in the sections on the "what" and "where" pathways, respectively. To simplify, the visuospatial function is primarily ascribed to the parietal lobe. The right parietal lobe is responsible for attending to both the hemispaces, while the left parietal lobe is responsible for attending to the right hemispace. So, a right parietal lesion causes left hemineglect/hemi-inattention, but a left parietal lesion does not cause right hemineglect, because the right hemispace also has representation in the undamaged right parietal lobe.

Executive function and other frontal lobe-related domains: These have been described in detail in the section on frontal lobes.

"FROM THE PERSPECTIVE OF THE NETWORKS"

From the above discussion, it seems plausible that cognition is not a function restricted to individual areas but rather a synchronous interplay of the various areas and the connections thereof. This is where the "network theory" comes into play.[39,40] These are classified as the executive network, the salience network, and the default-mode network.

The default-mode network decreases its activity during tasks that demand high level of attention and tasks that are non-self-referential. It is activated when the brain is in a resting state.[41] However, recent studies have pointed out that this network is involved in complex cognitive tasks like abstract thought and memory. The activity of this network increases when we think about ourselves, imagine the future or the past, create mental imagery, or are involved in social cognition such as empathy, moral judgment, and reward-based decision making.[41]

The central executive also known as the frontoparietal network (FPN) consists of the DLPFC and the lateral posterior parietal cortex. The role of this network is primarily related to cognitive effort, task selection, and executive function, using input from other brain networks to actively process information, and supporting higher-order cognitive functions, such as attentional control and working memory **(Fig. 8)**. The FPN is also essential for

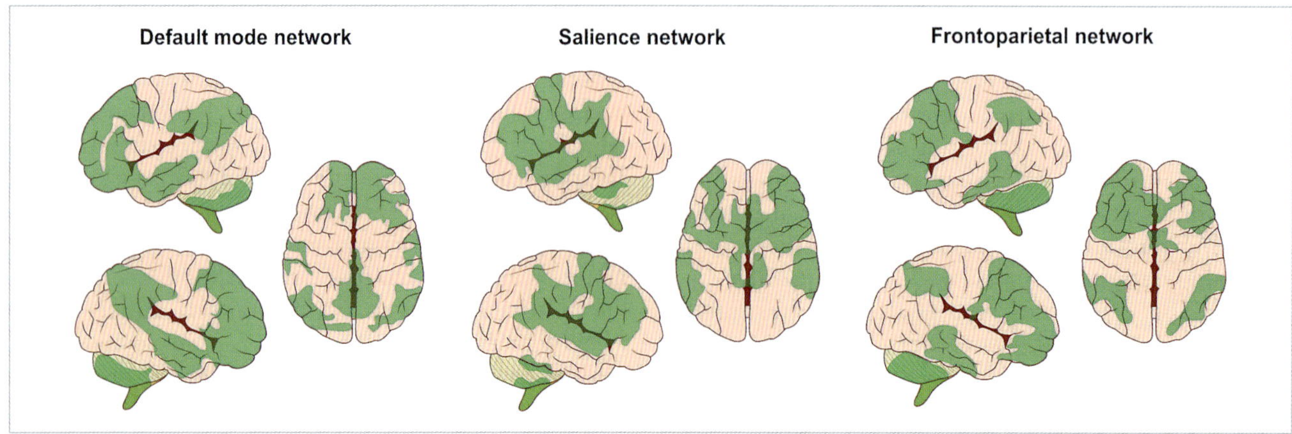

FIG. 8: The major brain networks.

decision-making in the context of goal-directed behavior in rule-based problem-solving.[42]

The salience network consists of the anterior insula and the dorsolateral anterior cingulate cortex.[43] The primary role of this network is to act as a switch between the self-referential DMN and the externally directed FPN.[44] It is responsible for the allocation of salience stimuli and their selection between the top-down and bottom-up mechanisms of attention control.[44] Other important functions include processing reward, emotion, motivation, and pain. Disorders within this structure are correlated with many cognitive affective dysfunctions, including those associated with both psychiatric disorders and neurodegenerative diseases. Overactivity is mainly associated with affective disorders and neuroticism.[44]

CONCLUSION

There have been many new developments in the field of neuroscience in the last couple of decades, especially in terms of connections and networks. This has all been possible due to the advancements in imaging, especially the functional imaging. However, the role of individual areas in the genesis of cognition and behavior cannot be underestimated. It is in certain ways analogous to the Schrodinger's cat. We do not know what is happening inside the box until we open it.

"Symptoms must be viewed as expressions of disturbances in a system, not as direct expressions of focal loss of neuronal tissue."

—AL Benton, 1981

REFERENCES

1. Nesse RM. Tinbergen's four questions: Two proximate, two evolutionary. Evol Med Public Health. 2018;2019(1):2.
2. Glasser MF, Goyal MS, Preuss TM, Raichle ME, Van Essen DC. Trends and properties of human cerebral cortex: Correlations with cortical myelin content. NeuroImage. 2014;93:165-75.
3. Mesulam M. Neurocognitive networks and selectively distributed processing. Revue Neurologique. 1994;150(8-9):564-9.
4. Semendeferi K, Damasio H, Frank R, Van Hoesen GW. The evolution of the frontal lobes: a volumetric analysis based on three-dimensional reconstructions of magnetic resonance scans of human and ape brains. J Hum Evol. 1997;32(4):375-88.
5. Alexander GE, DeLong MR, Strick PL. Parallel Organization of Functionally Segregated Circuits Linking Basal Ganglia and Cortex. Annu Rev Neurosci. 1986;9(1):357-81.
6. Ngetich R, Zhou J, Zhang J, Jin Z, Li L. Assessing the Effects of Continuous Theta Burst Stimulation Over the Dorsolateral Prefrontal Cortex on Human Cognition: A Systematic Review. Front Integr Neurosci. 2020;14:35.
7. Herlin B, Navarro V, Dupont S. The temporal pole: From anatomy to function—A literature appraisal. J Chem Neuroanatomy. 2021;113:101925.
8. Volle E, Gonen-Yaacovi G, de Lacy Costello A, Gilbert SJ, Burgess PW. The role of rostral prefrontal cortex in prospective memory: A voxel-based lesion study. Neuropsychologia. 2011;49(8):2185-98.
9. Kiernan JA. Anatomy of the Temporal Lobe. Epilepsy Res Treat. 2012;2012:1-12.
10. Goodale MA. Transforming vision into action. Vision Res. 2011;51(13):1567-87.
11. Read H. Functional architecture of auditory cortex. Curr Opin Neurobiol. 2002;12(4):433-40.
12. Bzdok D, Hartwigsen G, Reid A, Laird AR, Fox PT, Eickhoff SB. Left inferior parietal lobe engagement in social cognition and language. Neurosci Biobehav Rev. 2016;68:319-34.
13. Derbie AY, Dejenie MA. Intra Parietal Sulcus Area 1–2 and Angular Gyrus Differentiates Visual Short-Term Memory and Sustained Attention Activities. Ann Neurosci. 2022;29(2-3):166-9.
14. Stensaas SS, Eddington DK, Dobelle WH. The topography and variability of the primary visual cortex in man. J Neurosurg. 1974;40(6):747-55.
15. Galletti C, Fattori P. The dorsal visual stream revisited: Stable circuits or dynamic pathways? Cortex. 2018;98:203-17.
16. Bridge H, Thomas OM, Minini L, Cavina-Pratesi C, Milner AD, Parker AJ. Structural and Functional Changes across the Visual Cortex of a Patient with Visual Form Agnosia. J Neurosci. 2013;33(31):12779-91.
17. Sousa G, Aurelio M, de A, Mary K, Ferraz R, Alice I, et al. Basal ganglia for beginners: the basic concepts you need to know and their role in movement control. Front Syst Neurosci. 2023;17:1242929.
18. Forkel SJ, Friedrich P, Thiebaut de Schotten M, Howells H. White matter variability, cognition, and disorders: a systematic review. Brain Struct Funct. 2021;227(2):529-44.
19. Catani M, Jones DK, ffytche DH. Perisylvian language networks of the human brain. Ann Neurol. 2004;57(1):8-16.
20. Ku J, Morrison EH. Neuroanatomy, Anterior White Commissure. In: StatPearls [Internet]. Treasure Island (FL): StatPearls Publishing; 2024.
21. Guevara M, Guevara P, Roman C, Mangin JF. Superficial white matter: A review on the dMRI analysis methods and applications. Neuroimage. 2020;212:116673.
22. Ivanova MV, Zhong A, Turken A, Baldo JV, Dronkers NF. Functional Contributions of the Arcuate Fasciculus to Language Processing. Front Hum Neurosci. 2021;15:672665.
23. Porto de Oliveira JVM, Raquelo-Menegassio AF, Maldonado IL. What's your name again? A review of the superior longitudinal and arcuate fasciculus evolving nomenclature. Clin Anat. 2021;34(7):1101-10.
24. Bubb EJ, Metzler-Baddeley C, Aggleton JP. The cingulum bundle: Anatomy, function, and dysfunction. Neurosci Biobehav Rev. 2018;92:104-27.
25. Zemmoura I, Burkhardt E, Herbet G. The inferior longitudinal fasciculus: anatomy, function and surgical considerations. J Neurosurg Sci. 2022;65(6):590-604.

26. Andelman-Gur MM, Gazit T, Strauss I, Fried I, Fahoum F. Stimulating the inferior fronto-occipital fasciculus elicits complex visual hallucinations. Brain Stimulation. 2020;13(6): 1577-9.
27. Goldstein A, Covington BP, Mahabadi N, Mesfin FB. Neuroanatomy, Corpus Callosum. In: StatPearls [Internet]. Treasure Island (FL): StatPearls Publishing; 2024.
28. Catani M, Mesulam MM, Jakobsen E, Malik F, Martersteck A, Wieneke C, et al. A novel frontal pathway underlies verbal fluency in primary progressive aphasia. Brain. 2013;136 (Pt 8):2619-28.
29. McDowd JM. An Overview of Attention: Behavior and Brain. J Neurol Phys Ther. 2007;31(3):98-103.
30. Sarter M, Givens B, Bruno JP. The cognitive neuroscience of sustained attention: where top-down meets bottom-up. Brain Res Rev. 2001;35(2):146-60.
31. Alderson-Day B, Fernyhough C. Inner speech: Development, cognitive functions, phenomenology, and neurobiology. Psychol Bull. 2015;141(5):931-65.
32. Hickok G. The cortical organization of speech processing: Feedback control and predictive coding the context of a dual-stream model. J Commun Disord. 2012;45(6):393-402.
33. Baddeley A. Working memory. Curr Biol. 2010;20(4):R136-40.
34. Danieli K, Guyon A, Bethus I. Episodic Memory formation: A review of complex Hippocampus input pathways. Prog Neuropsychopharmacol Biol Psychiatry. 2023;126:110757.
35. Greene P, Howard M, Bhattacharyya R, Fellous JM. Hippocampal Anatomy Supports the Use of Context in Object Recognition: A Computational Model. Comput Intell Neurosci. 2013;2013:294878.
36. Sugar J, Moser M. Episodic memory: Neuronal codes for what, where, and when. Hippocampus. 2019;29(12):1190-205.
37. Gross RG, Grossman M. Update on apraxia. Curr Neurol Neurosci Rep. 2008;8(6):490-6.
38. Rounis E, Humphreys G. Limb apraxia and the "affordance competition hypothesis." Front Hum Neurosci. 2015;9:429.
39. Ptak R, Doganci N, Bourgeois A. From Action to Cognition: Neural Reuse, Network Theory, and the Emergence of Higher Cognitive Functions. Brain Sci. 2021;11(12):1652.
40. Bressler SL, Menon V. Large-scale brain networks in cognition: emerging methods and principles. Trends Cogn Sci. 2010;14(6):277-90.
41. Smallwood J, Bernhardt BC, Leech R, Bzdok D, Jefferies E, Margulies DS. The default mode network in cognition: a topographical perspective. Nat Rev Neurosci. 2021;22(8):503-13.
42. Valera-Bermejo JM, De Marco M, Mitolo M, Cerami C, Dodich A, Venneri A. Large-Scale Functional Networks, Cognition and Brain Structures Supporting Social Cognition and Theory of Mind Performance in Prodromal to Mild Alzheimer's Disease. Front Aging Neurosci. 2021;13:766703.
43. Seeley WW. The Salience Network: A Neural System for Perceiving and Responding to Homeostatic Demands. J Neurosci. 2019;39(50):9878-82.
44. Schimmelpfennig J, Topczewski J, Zajkowski W, Jankowiak-Siuda K. The role of the salience network in cognitive and affective deficits. Front Hum Neurosci. 2023;17:1133367.

CHAPTER

2 Global and Local Burden of Dementia

Gautam Das, Souvik Dubey, Atanu Biswas

ABSTRACT

Dementia is a chronic illness. A number of patients with dementia have been increased over past few decades due to both population growth and population ageing. It is expected to rise further. There are strong evidences supporting the importance of modifiable risk factors. Globally, there is heterogeneity among the countries regarding the prevalence, mortality, risk factors, cost generated, and also the trends of these. Dementia is a leading cause of mortality, both globally and locally. The epidemiology of dementia is closely related with sociodemographic index (SDI). Risk factors, mortality, and prevalence of dementia vary in male and female. Dementia has an immense impact on societal costs, and its direct and indirect components. Nationally, the dementia burden has been distributed unevenly across states and subpopulations. 61% of people with dementia live in low- and middle-income countries (LMICs), whereas 74% of the costs occur in high-income countries (HICs). Life expectancy in India has steadily increased from 42.9 years in 1960 to 70.4 years in 2020. This rising longevity is associated with increased prevalence of dementia. The diversity of the country has been reflected in heterogeneity in dementia prevalence. The need for public health planning efforts and policy to address the halting of dementia progression.

Keywords: Burden, Cost, Dementia, Global, Mortality, Prevalence.

WHY IT IS NECESSARY TO MEASURE THE BURDEN OF DEMENTIA?

"Burden" according to Britannica dictionary means "to make (someone) hold or carry something heavy or accept or deal with something difficult: to put a heavy burden on (someone)." In that sense, dementia adds burden to our life. Burden estimation is important to establish health priorities and to plan perfectly in a resource-constrained context. In many middle-income countries, the profile of burden has shifted from communicable to noncommunicable diseases. Burden estimation help us to understand the reason behind the alteration in the course, dementia prevalence, or risk factors.

THE NECESSITY TO MEASURE THE BURDEN OF DEMENTIA

Population growth and population ageing are increasing, as well as the number of people with dementia. Modifiable risk factors for dementia plays an important role. A decreasing trend in dementia incidence potentially due to increase in educational attainment and improvements in the management of cardiovascular disease and its risk factors has been observed in developed countries.[1-3] In Japan and China, there are increases in age-specific prevalence, which is a function of disease incidence and duration.[4,5]

Globally, the number of people affected by dementia was estimated to have increased by 117% between 1990 and 2016, largely due to population ageing.[6] Demographic analyses suggest that these patients are driven by decreases in fertility coupled with increases in life expectancy, which together lead to large changes in the age structure of the population.[7,8]

The 2020 update to the *Lancet* Commission on dementia prevention, intervention, and care highlighted the evidence for 12 modifiable risk factors for dementia: Low education, hypertension, hearing impairment, smoking, midlife obesity, depression, physical inactivity, diabetes, social isolation, excessive alcohol consumption, head injury, and air pollution.[9] Curbing the effects of these factors through public health interventions remains the key for reduction of dementia prevalence. Studies have shown that education and the prevalence and treatment of cardiovascular diseases might be key in explaining previous and future trends in dementia prevalence.[10,11] So, risk factors and its changes are important in predicting dementia prevalence, in forming policy decisions, health system planning, and allocation of resources.

Global prevalence of dementia in 2019 and forecasted prevalence in 2050 was estimated in Global Burden of Disease (GBD) study. Dementia prevalence was found to be higher in women than men and increased with age, doubling about every 5 years until 85 years of age in both 2019 and 2050. In 2050, the prevalence of dementia in men globally was forecasted to be 0.5% among those aged 40–69 years, 6.5% among those aged 70–84 years, and 23.5% among those aged 85 years and older. In women, global forecast was projected to be 0.6% among those aged 40–69 years, 8.5% among those aged 70–84 years, and 30.5% among those aged 85 years and older **(Figs. 1A and B)**.[12]

They estimated a much larger percentage change in all age dementia prevalence between 2019 and 2050 due to population ageing, and an even larger percentage change in the all-age number of prevalent cases, due to a combination of population ageing and population growth. In 2019, they estimated 57.4 million individuals living with dementia globally. The number would increase to 83.2 million in 2030, 116.0 million in 2040, and 152.8 million in 2050, and there will be more women than men with dementia globally in 2019 (female to male ratio 1.69 in 2019) and 1.67 in 2050. The study revealed that the percentage change between 2019 and 2050 in total number of dementia cases was highest for the low sociodemographic index (SDI) (a composite indicator of total fertility rate, mean years of education in individuals older than 15 years, and lag-distributed income per capita.[8]) quintile (330%) and lowest for the high-middle SDI quintile (113%) and high SDI quintile (140%).

The percentage change in age standardized rates between 2019 and 2050 was also highest for the low SDI quintile (8.2%) and lowest for the low-middle SDI quintile (1.3%). They exhibited evidence of large variability in the projected increases. It has been revealed in that study, the decomposition of percentage change in projected dementia cases indicated a fairly small overall effect of changing prevalence, which included an increase in prevalence due to GBD risk factors for all regions, except high income Asia Pacific,

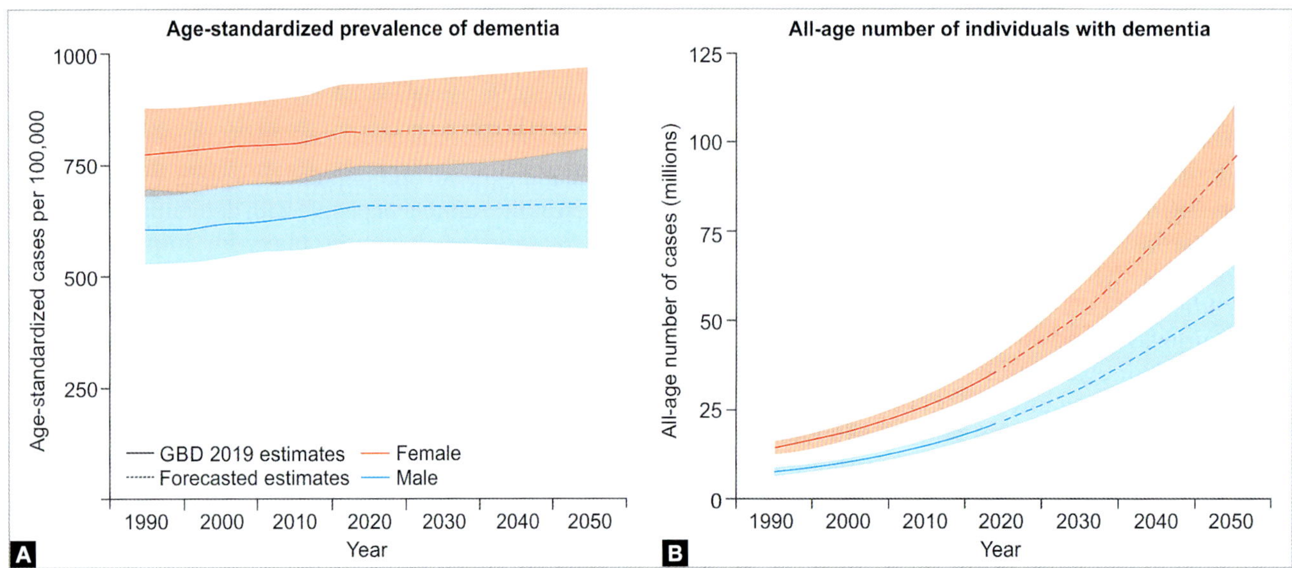

FIGS. 1A AND B: Estimated trends in the global (A) age-standardized dementia prevalence and (B) all-age number of cases, with 95% uncertainty intervals, 2019–2050.

Source: Estimation of the global prevalence of dementia in 2019 and forecasted prevalence in 2050: An analysis for the Global Burden of Disease Study 2019.[12]

and a decrease in prevalence due to the added effect of trends in education in this analysis.

Although there were increases for every country, the smallest increases were projected in high-income Asia Pacific (53%) and western Europe (74%), whereas the largest estimated increases were in north Africa and the Middle East (367%) and eastern sub-Saharan Africa (357%).

Population growth is responsible for most of the increases in dementia prevalence in sub-Saharan Africa but contributes little in East Asia and west Europe. In central Europe, eastern Europe, and high-income Asia Pacific anticipated declines in populations serve to partly counteract the effect of population ageing. Population ageing is expected to lead to increases in projected dementia cases in every region; the largest projected increases due to population ageing are observed in east Asia, and north Africa and the middle East.

GLOBAL MORTALITY FROM DEMENTIA

The GBD Study 2019 revealed the mortality burden from dementia.[6,12] They code for—decubitus ulcer, malnutrition, sepsis, pneumonia, urinary tract infections, falling from bed, senility, dehydration, hip fracture, and bedridden status as indicators of severe disease. The attributable risk of pneumonia was the highest (attributable risk 0.31). The next were dehydration (0.15), urinary tract infections (0.12), and decubitus ulcer (0.06). The proportion of individuals who died with dementia and had any end-stage disease marker in the year before death was 0.59, and who died without dementia this became 0.35.

Overall, the study estimated 1.62 million deaths due to dementia globally in 2019. Far more deaths occurred in women (1.06 million) than men (0.56 million) giving a female to male ratio of 1.94. The female to male ratio for age standardize rates was 1.19, suggesting that a portion of the sex difference was independent of the higher life expectancy in women. Between 1990 and 2019, the increase in age standardized mortality rates (ASMRs) among males (5.1%) was higher than females (3.0%). Among males, the largest increase was observed for low SDI countries (9.6%).

As revealed by the GBD Study, the total number of deaths from dementia increased with SDI quintile, from 62.1 thousand deaths in the low SDI quintile to 563.2 thousand deaths in the high SDI quintile. However, the age standardized rates were not significantly different between SDI quintiles, indicating that differences in the numbers stem from differences in population size and population age structure **(Figs. 2 and 3)**.[12,13]

The countries with the highest ASMR due to dementia were Afghanistan (30.79 deaths per 100,000 person-years), Mozambique (29.74), and Vietnam (29.71). The countries with the lowest ASMR due to dementia were Bangladesh (18.23), India (19.12) and Nepal (19.51). The study revealed that in 1990 dementia was the 20th leading cause death globally comparing all-age mortality rates and the 6th leading cause of death among individuals 70 years and older. However, by 2019, deaths due to dementia were estimated to rank 7th globally across all ages and 4th among individuals 70 years and older **(Fig. 4)**.[14]

Dementia subtypes also influence the degree of caregiver burden. Lewy body disease (LBD) patients have a higher caregiver burden than those of Alzheimer's disease (AD) patients, may be due to the increased rate of neuropsychiatric symptoms in LBD patients. Mood disorders and motor features also compound the burden. Similarly patients with frontotemporal degeneration (FTD) have higher burden than AD patients due to higher rate of behavioral and psychiatric symptoms. Vascular dementia patients have more burden than AD patients due to initial part of the disease but as disease progresses, the load decreases with vascular one. On average vascular and mixed dementia have more burden than AD patients **(Figs. 5 to 7)**.[14,15]

DOES DEMENTIA COST?

As some studies revealed that the ways of estimation of dementia cost are varied, some of the cost concepts are as:[16-18]

- *Direct medical costs*: Refer to formal medical care system, such as costs of hospital care, drugs, diagnostic tests, and visit to the clinic.
- *Direct social costs*: (sometimes called "direct nonmedical costs") refer to formal services provided outside of the medical care system, includes care in residential or nursing homes or other long-term care facilities, and community services such as home care, food supply, and transport.
- Indirect costs refer to informal care provided by family members, friends, and others and production losses by people with dementia. This informal care can be described in three domains: Personal or basic activities of daily living (ADLs, such as eating, hygiene, toilet visits, and dressing), support in instrumental ADLs (IADLs, more complex activities such as shopping, preparing food, and financial transactions), and supervision (to prevent dangerous events).

There is a close relationship between dementia severity and resource use and costs. Currency and inflation also count in estimating the cost of dementia care.

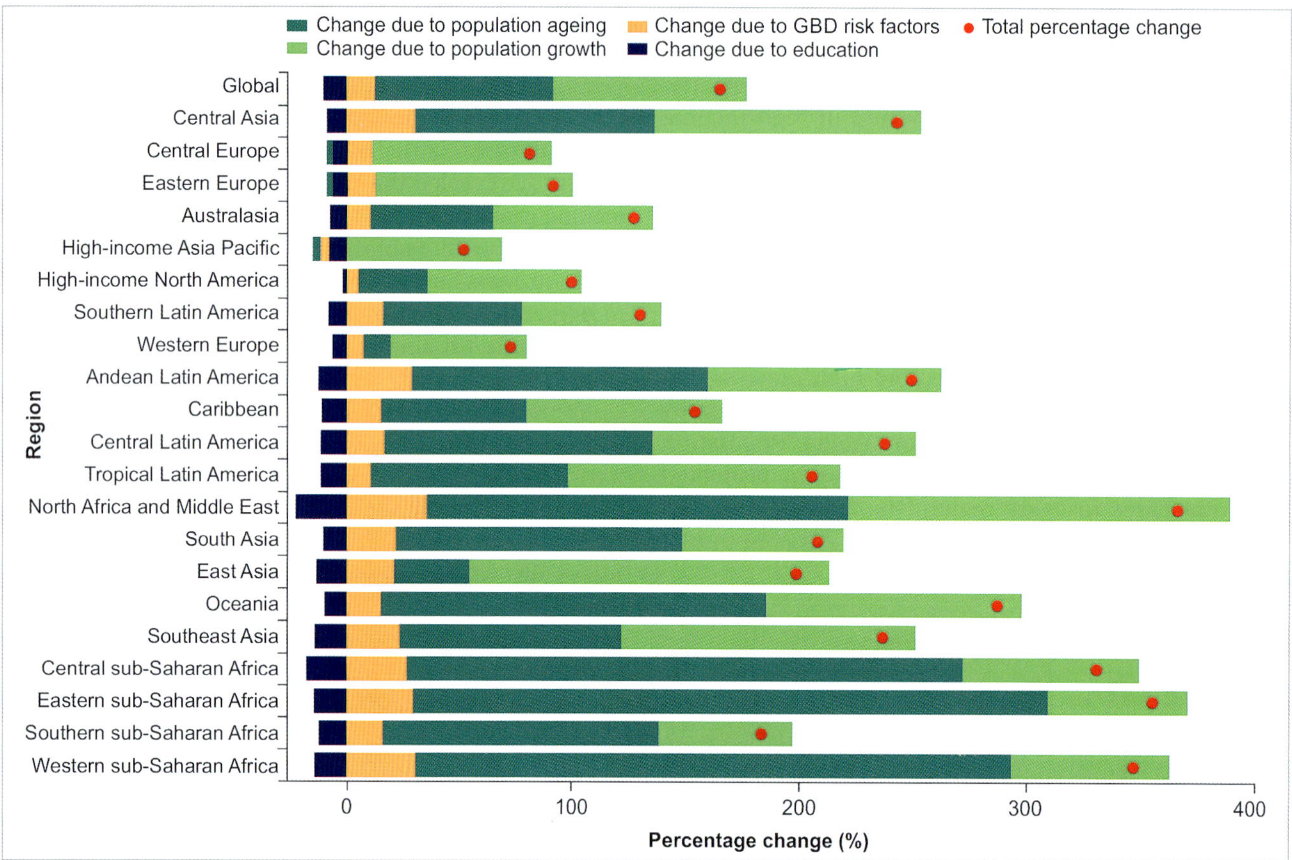

FIG. 2: Decomposition of percentage change in the number of individuals with dementia between 2019 and 2050 globally and by world region.

(GBD: Global Burden of Disease, Injuries, and Risk Factors Study)

Source: Estimation of the global prevalence of dementia in 2019 and forecasted prevalence in 2050: an analysis for the Global Burden of Disease Study 2019.[12]

GLOBAL COST ESTIMATES[19]

High-income countries (HICs) accounted for 74% of the costs even though 61% of people with dementia live in low- and middle-income countries (LMIC). Direct costs of dementia, as a proportion of global GDP (gross domestic product), have increased from 0.59% in 2010 to 0.76% in 2019. Between 2010 and 2019, the global costs of dementia increased by 62%.[12] There was also a shift in the distribution of costs from HIC to LMIC, partially reflected by an increase in the numbers of people with dementia in LMIC, mainly linked to more rapid population aging, but also on higher estimates for informal care. Also, the World Bank (WB) classification had changed by 2019, and many countries had been "promoted" upward in the classification due to economic growth, resulting in more people with dementia particularly in upper-middle-income countries.

As was found in the 2010 and 2015 estimates, the impact of informal care is greater than direct costs in LMIC but not as much as in the 2019 estimates. Although total costs did not differ greatly between severity levels, per-person costs were very different; globally, annual cost per person with mild dementia was US $15.899, for moderate dementia it was US $26,859, and for severe dementia $36,180. The weighted average annual cost per person with dementia was US $23,764.

The main reasons for the increased cost are: Increase in numbers of people with dementia and a higher estimate of informal care costs. National policy on health and social care and local systems of treatment and support are increasingly becoming more important for meeting the needs of people with dementia and their caregivers.

About half of the costs were related in informal care with a gradient in relation to country income level: 44% in HIC and 85% in low-income countries.[20] Given the expected future increase in numbers of people with dementia—combined with changes in family structure, migration, urbanization, demography, and female labor force participation rates—particularly in LMIC, it is unrealistic to expect that unpaid care can be a sustainable care option at the same level as today.[18] This will be the most unfortunate part of the story.

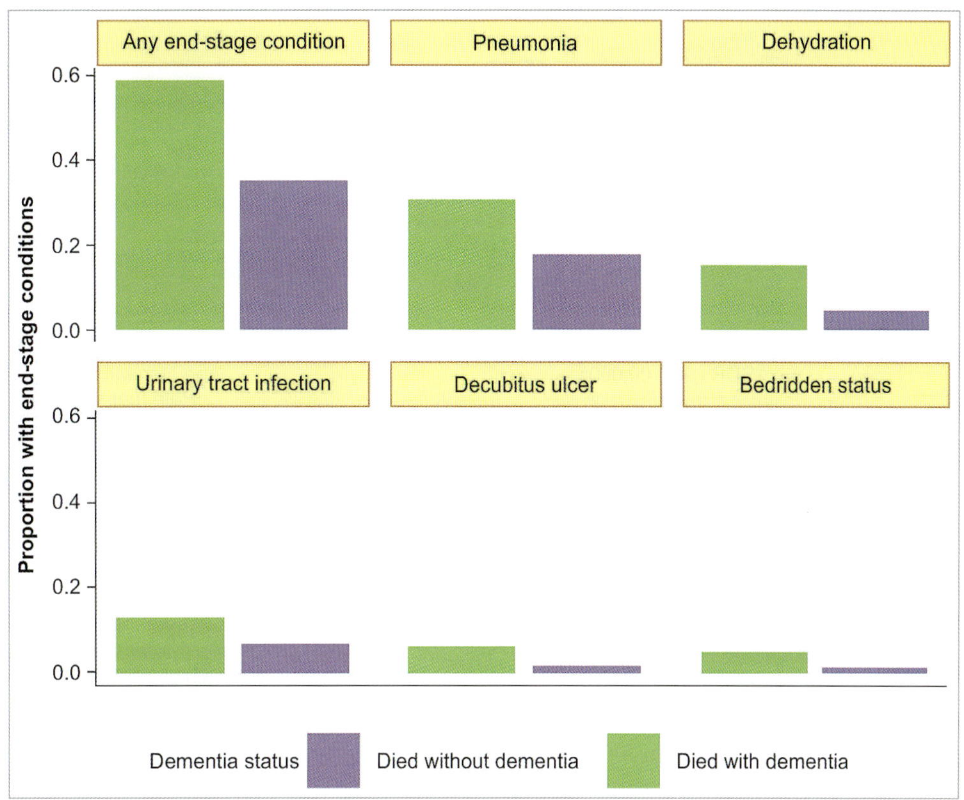

FIG. 3: Proportion of individuals who died with end-stage conditions in the last year before death for all conditions combined and the conditions with the top five excess proportions, shown separately for individuals who died with and without dementia. These estimates are derived from linked clinical and death records from 2003 to 2017 in the Emilia Romagna region of Italy. They are assumed to apply globally and over the time period considered in this study.

Source: Global mortality from dementia: Application of a new method and results from the Global Burden of Disease Study 2019.[13]

The annual household cost of caring for a person with dementia in India, depending on the severity of the disease, ranged between INR 45,600 to INR 202,450 in urban areas and INR 20,300 and INR 66,025 in rural areas, and the costs increased with increasing severity of the disease process. Extrapolating these costs, nationally, it was estimated that households would be spending INR 23,330 crores. The total money spent is similar in urban and rural areas.[21]

The geriatric health services in India have perceptibly changed in the recent past; however, this is not commensurate with the felt-needs. The health of the elderly in India is constrained by, not just availability and accessibility, but also, affordability of services. The national health accounts indicate that nearly 90% of the health expenditure in India is Out-of-Pocket (OOP) expenditure.[22] With burgeoning elderly population, managing the costs for care, even at the household level through OOP expenses, is not a perceivable viability. Public health needs to step in for developing systems of management and care.

TRENDS OF CHANGING BURDEN IN PEOPLE WITH DEMENTIA

Incidence Trends from 1990 to 2019

Globally, the incidence of dementia increased by 147.95% from 1990 to 2019, with 2.92 million cases in 1990 and 7,24 million cases in 2019. Regarding sex, the age-standardized incidence rate (ASIR, per 100,000 population) of dementia increased in both men and women over this period. From 1990 to 2019, the incidence rate in the 70–74 age group was the fastest growing over time.[14] The ASIRs (age-standardized incidence rates) of dementia were positively related to SDI levels (SDI is an indicator to evaluate the level of social development in a country or region considering the education rate, economic situation, and total fertility rate). The ASIRs (per 100,000 population) for dementia increased most in the high-middle SDI regions, while in areas with a low-SDI and low-middle SDI decreasing trends were observed.

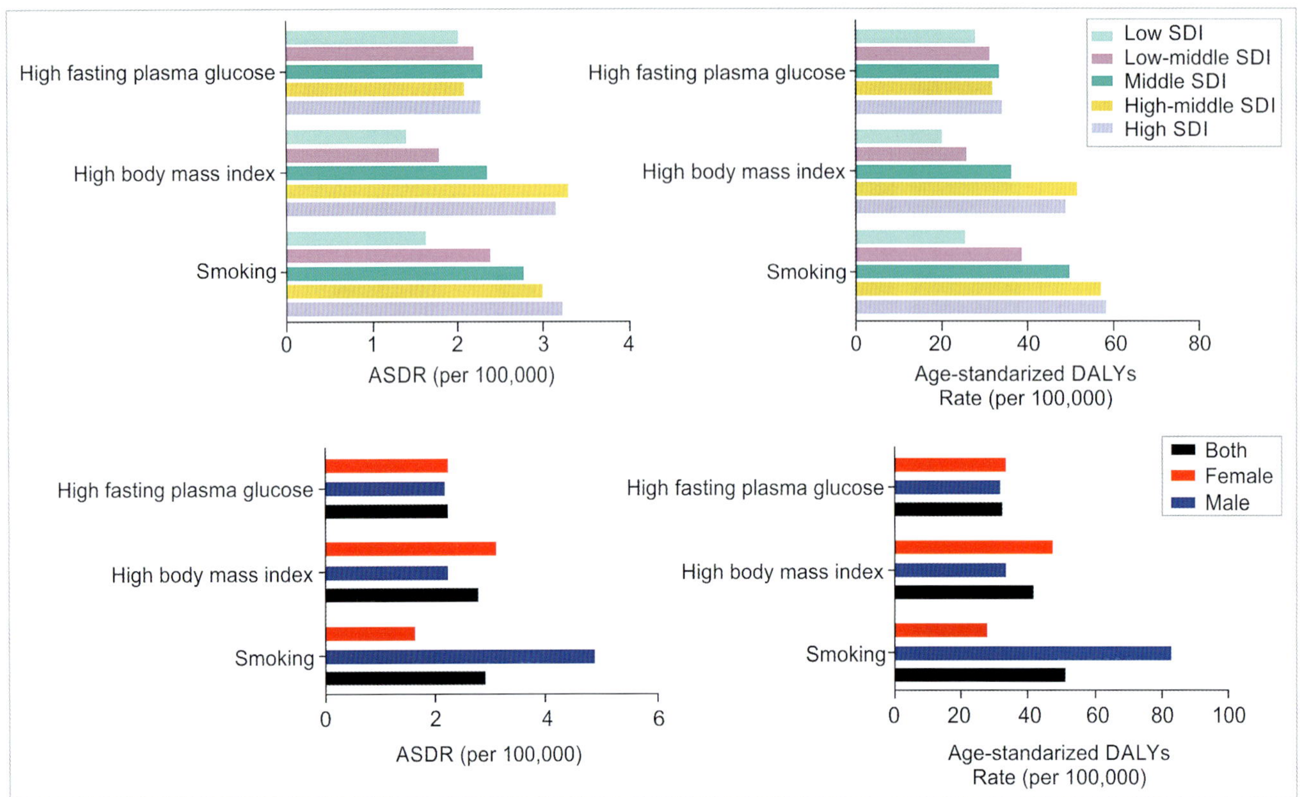

FIG. 4: Impact of risk factors on the disease burden of Alzheimer's disease by SDI region and gender, 2019. (A) Contribution of three risk factors for death and DALYs in different SDI regions; (B) Contribution of three risk factors to death and DALYs in both sexes.

(ASDR: age-standardized death rate; DALYs: disability-adjusted life-years; SDI: sociodemographic index)

Source: Global, regional, and national burden of Alzheimer's disease and other dementias, 1990–2019.[14]

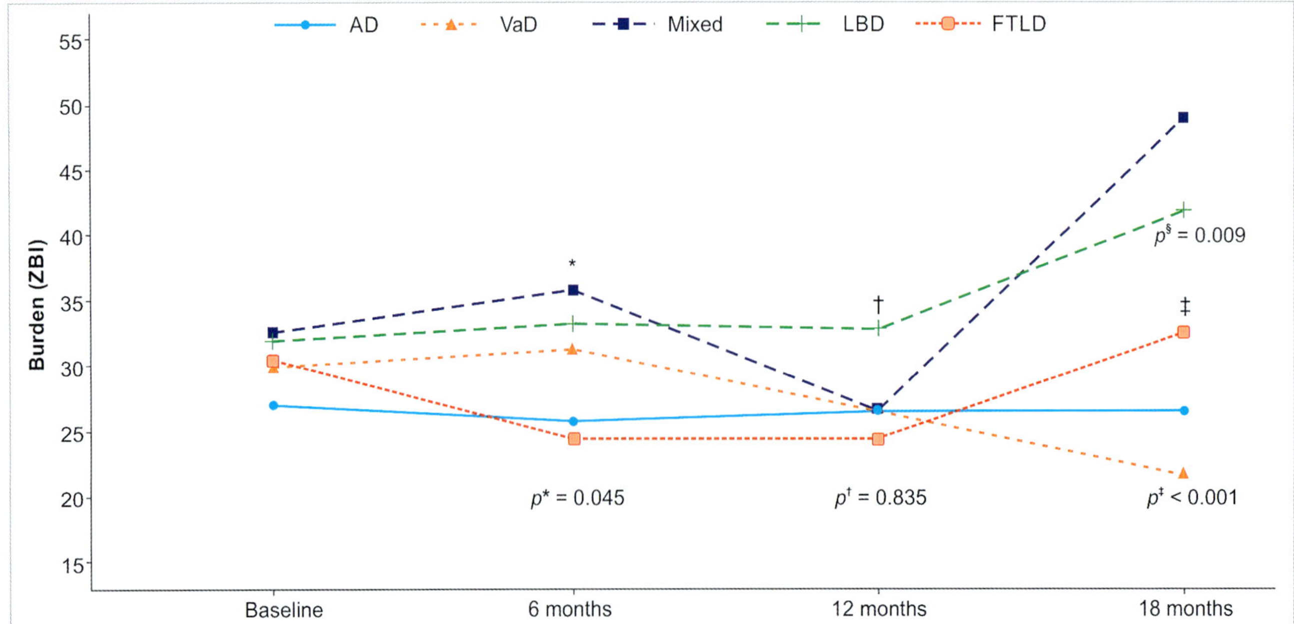

FIG. 5: The trajectory of Zarit Burden Interview scores in different dementia subtypes.

Source: Wen-Chien Huaang, et al.[15]

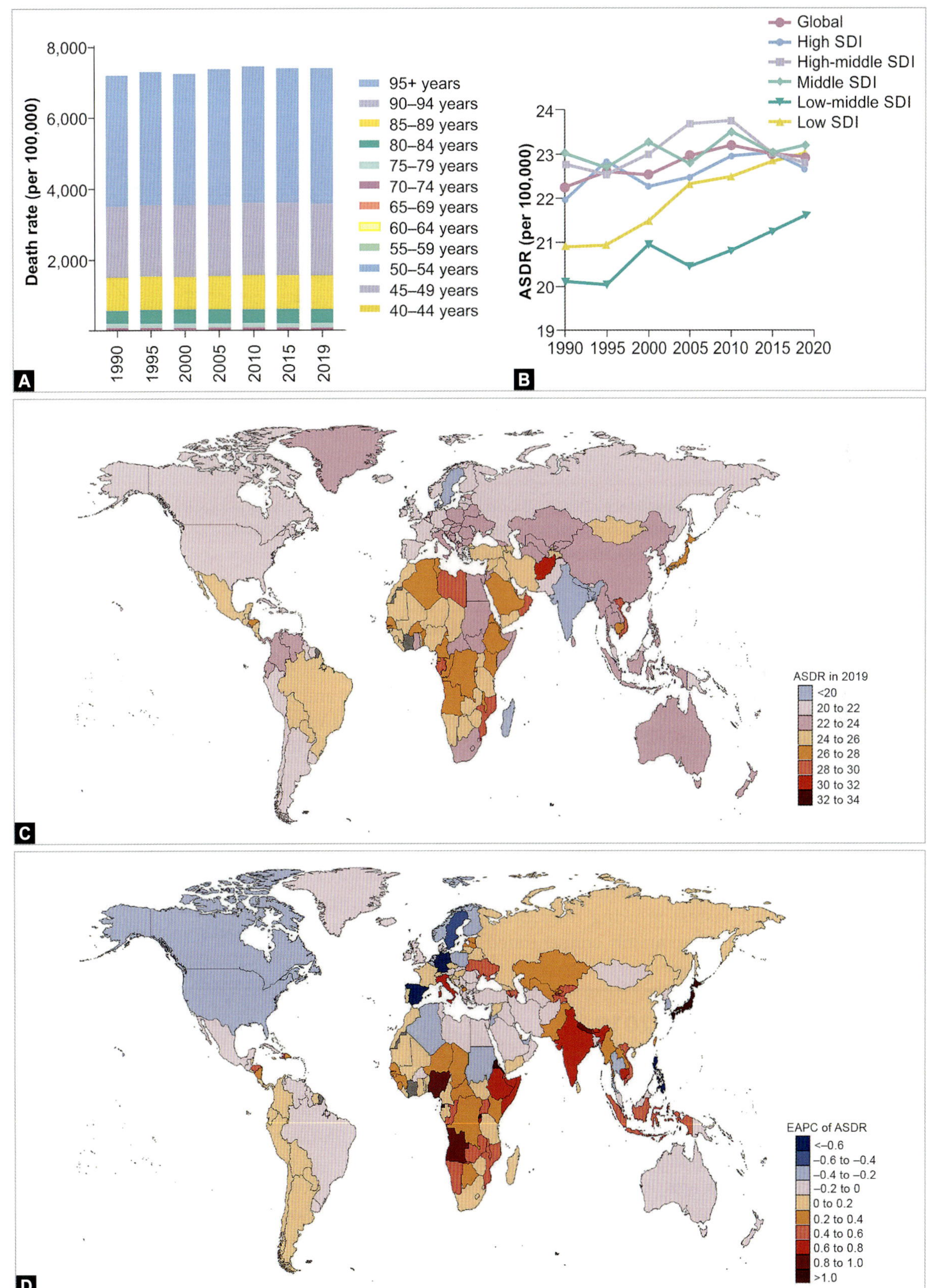

FIGS. 6A TO D: Distribution of the incidence of Alzheimer's disease and other dementias in 204 countries and territories from 1990 to 2019 by age group and sociodemographic index (SDI) region. (A) Incidence rate in each age group; (B) Correlations between the age-standardized incidence rates (ASIRs) of Alzheimer's disease and other dementias.

(ASDR: age-standardized death rate from publication; EAPC: estimated annual percentage change)

Source: Global, regional, and national burden of Alzheimer's disease and other dementias, 1990–2019.[14]

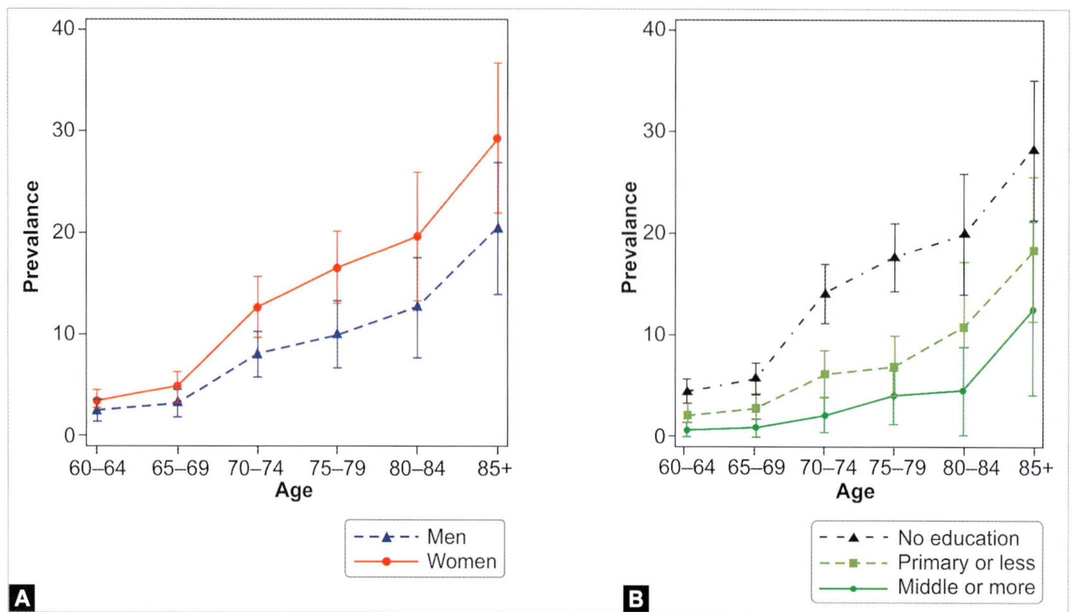

FIGS. 7A AND B: Age-specific dementia prevalence rates by sex, urbanity, and education. (A) Mean age-specific dementia prevalence rate by sex [95% confidence interval (CI)]; (B) Mean age-specific dementia prevalence rate by education (95% CI).

Source: Prevalence of dementia in India: National and state estimates from a nationwide study.[26]

Prevalence Trends from 1990 to 2019

Globally, in 2019, the number of dementia patients was 160.84% higher than that observed in 1990, which was 51.62 million. The ASPR (age-standardized prevalence rate, per 100,000 population) in all the SDI regions showed an upward trend, with the highest in the high-middle SDI region, while ASPRs in the middle SDI region showed the fastest increase. Compared with men, women had a higher ASPR. However, there was a larger upward trend in the male ASPR. The prevalence rate increased with age. From 1990 to 2019, the prevalence rate in the 80–84 age group was the fastest growing over time. Notably, the younger patients were mainly concentrated in lower SDI regions.

Death Trends from 1990 to 2019

Global deaths due to dementia increased from 0.56 million in 1990 to 1.62 million in 2019. The age-standardized death rate (ASDR) also increased. From 1990 to 2019, the overall ASDR proportions in women were higher than those in men though increased in both. The death rate increased with age. From 1990 to 2019 death cases in >95 age group showed the fastest growth over time. In 2019, the ASDRs were highest in the middle SDI and low SDI regions. The low SDI regions had the largest increase in the ASDR. The lower the SDI, the higher the proportion of the younger people who died due to dementia.[14]

Disability-adjusted Life Years Trend from 1990 to 2019

Between 1990 and 2019, the number of disability-adjusted life years (DALYs) due to dementia worldwide increased from 9.66 million to 25.28 million. In 2019, the burden of dementia was consistently higher in women than in men. From 1990 to 2019, the number of DALYs in the 80–84 age group showed the fastest growth over time.

Risk Factors

Based on GBD 2019, high fasting blood glucose, high body mass index (BMI), and smoking were the major risk factors for dementia. In the high-middle SDI group, risk factors had the highest impact on the dementia burden. Risk factors had the least impact on the disease burden in the low-SDI regions. Smoking contributed the most to the disease burden in areas with the high-SDI group. Men were more affected by risk factors than women. Women are more susceptible to metabolic risk factors, such as high BMI; men are to behavioral risk factors, such as smoking.

The rapid development in the social economy has intensified the social competition and life pressure experienced by the people; this stress is often accompanied by harmful living habits (smoking, excessive alcohol consumption, and lack of physical activity). The regions with higher SDIs were more affected by these risk factors.

DEMENTIA BURDEN AT NATIONAL LEVEL

Dementia prevalence among individuals aged 60 and older in India is 7.4%, and ASPR of dementia is 8.0%. The sex gap in prevalence increases with age. Individuals without formal education have much higher prevalence than their educated counterparts.[14] This difference is especially apparent in the 70–74 and 75–79 age groups.

Cross-state variation in dementia prevalence is considerable. It is lowest in Delhi at 4.5% and highest in Jammu and Kashmir at 11.0%. The ASPR is 6.3% in men and 9.6% in women. The large sex difference in prevalence is likely attributable to females being older and less educated **(Fig. 7)**. Prevalence rate is higher in rural than in urban areas. If prevalence remains the same, the number of people with dementia is projected to reach 16.9 million in 2036 due to the growth in the older Indian population.[23] The rapid rise in risk factors for cardiovascular disease in India may increase dementia risk.[23] Different levels of educational attainment across states could contribute to cross-state differences in various dementia risk factors, such as undernutrition, uncontrolled cardiovascular disease, and exposure to indoor air pollution **(Fig. 7 and Table 1)**.[24]

CONCLUSION

Global economic costs of dementia were estimated to reach US $1313.4 in 2019. 61% of people with dementia live in LMICs, whereas 74% of the costs occur in HICs. There is a great need for more cost studies, and long-term care infrastructure particularly in LMICs. Discussions of a framework for global cost comparisons are needed. The different cross-national studies have postulated that low prevalence in the developing countries could be due to various factors including shorter life expectancy and differential mortality. There may be different risk

TABLE 1: Sample characteristics and dementia prevalence among adults 60 years and older in India.

	LASI ages 60+		Dementia prevalence[c]			
	N[a]	%[b]	Population-representative	95% CI	Age-standardized	95% CI
ALL	31,477	100.0	7.43	(6.35–8.51)	8.01	(6.83–9.18)
Age						
60–64	10,134	32.4	294	(2.08–3.80)	NA	NA
65–69	8,845	29.4	4.01	(2.93–5.09)	NA	NA
70–74	5,746	17.6	10.30	(8.14–12.47)	NA	NA
75–79	3,362	10.3	13.34	(10.93–15.75)	NA	NA
80–84	1,942	5.8	16.25	(11.31–21.19)	NA	NA
85+	1,448	4.6	25.41	(19.31–31.51)	NA	NA
Sex						
Male	15,106	49.2	5.77	(4.40–7.14)	6.30	(4.81–7.79)
Female	16,371	50.8	9.03	(7.50–10.57)	9.63	(8.01–11.26)
Urbanicity						
Urban	10,756	30.7	5.34	(4.32–6.37)	5.98	(4.80–7.16)
Rural	20,721	69.4	8.35	(7.08–9.61)	8.91	(7.58–10.24)
Education						
None	16,894	60.3	10.29	(8.62–11.97)	10.48	(8.79–12.17)
Primary school or less (up to standard 7)	7,562	20.3	4.52	(3.28–5.77)	5.05	(3.65–6.45)
Middle school or more (standard 8 and higher)	7,021	19.4	1.54	(0.64–2.44)	2.35	(1.13–3.57)

[a]Refers to unweighted sample.
[b]Values are weighted using survey weights to represent the population.
[c]Survey weights are also applied to estimate the prevalence rate for the population.
(CI: confidence interval; LASI: Longitudinal Aging Study in India; NA: not applicable)
Source: Prevalence of dementia in India: National and state estimates from a nationwide study. (LASI-DAD: Diagnostic Assessment of Dementia for the Longitudinal Aging Study in India).[26]

and protective factors operating among them than in developed countries with higher incidence rates. Despite relative consistency in overall prevalence across studies, the proportion of prevalent dementia caused by AD varies, likely in part to reflect longer survival of AD cases relative to stroke-related dementia or other dementias. Incident cases, particularly the onset of dementia, are challenging to determine with precision. This problem increases with changing life-styles and breakdown of traditional social security systems.[25] One reason is temporal sequence; by observing the disease and the risk factor at the same time, we cannot be certain that the risk factor was present before the onset of disease. A subtler reason is that associations found with prevalent cases might be in fact factors associated with survival with disease, rather than with risk of developing disease in the first place. Or, at least, the strength of association observed with a particular risk factor based on prevalent cases may be misleading, because it largely represents an association with survival. With all these challenges we should face and move forward to win the battle against dementia.

ACKNOWLEDGMENTS

- Major portions of the data are shared from "Global Burden of Disease Study 2019". We are grateful to Emma Nichols, Jainnie D Steinmetz, Stein Emil Vollset et al., for their article "Estimation of the global prevalence of dementia in 2019 and forecasted prevalence in 2050: an analysis for the Global Burden of Disease Study 2019"; published in *Lancet Public Health,* 2012. We again thank Emma Nichols for the article "Global mortality from dementia: Application of a new method and results from the Global Burden of Disease Study 2019".
- We thank Xue Li, Xiaojin Feng, Xiadong Sun, et al., for the article "Global, regional, national burden of Alzheimer's disease and other dementias, 1990-2019" published in *Frontiers Iin Aging Neuroscience,* 10/10/2022. We shared from this article.
- We are thankful to Anders Wimo, Katrin Seeher, Rodrigo Cataldi, et al., as they allow us to share from their article "The worldwide costs of dementia in 2019", published in *Alzheimer's & Dementia,* 2022.
- We are thankful to Jinkook Lee, Erik Meijer, Kenneth M Langa, et al., as we shared from their article "Prevalence of dementia in India: National and state estimates from a nationwide study", published in *Alzheimer's & Dementia,* 2022.
- We are grateful to Wen-Chein Huaang, Ming-Che Chang, Wen-Fu Wang, and Kai-Ming Jhang for allowing us to share from their article "A comparison of Caregiver Burden for Different Types of Dementia: An 18-Month Retrospective Cohort Study". *Frontiers in Psychology.* 17th January, 2022.
- Many thanks to Girish N Rao and Srikala Bharath as they permitted me to share from their article "Cost of Dementia Care in India: Delusion or Reality?" published in *Indian Journal of Public Health,* Volume 57, Issue 2, April–June, 2013.
- Special thanks to our colleagues Madhusree Chakrabarty, Deep Subhra Ghosh, and Bidisha Bhattacharya for their heartiest effort and support.

REFERENCES

1. Wolters Fj, Chibnik LB, Waziry R, Anderson R, Berr C, Beiser A, et al. Twenty-seven-year time trends in dementia incidence in Europe and the United States: the Alzheimer Cohorts Consortium. Neurology. 2020;95(5):e519-31.
2. Matthews FE, Stephen BCM, Robinson L, Jagger C, Barnes LE, Arthur A, et al. A two-decade dementia incidence comparison from the Cognitive Function and Ageing Studies I and II. Nat Common. 2016;7:11398.
3. Satizabal CL, Beiser AS, Chouraki V, Chėne G, Dufouil C, Seshadri S. Incidence of dementia over three decades in the Framingham Heart Study. N Engl J Med. 2016;374:523-32.
4. Dodge HH, Buracchio TJ, Fisher GG, Kiyohara Y, Meguro K, Tanizaki Y, et al. Trends in the prevalence of dementia in Japan. Int J Alzheimer's Dis. 2012;2012:956354.
5. Wu Y-T, Ali G-C, Guerchet M, Prina AM, Chan KY, Prince M, et al. Prevalence of dementia in mainland China, Hong Kong and Taiwan: an updated systematic review and meta-analysis. Int J Epidemiol. 2018;47:709-19.
6. Nichols E, Szoeke CEI, Vollset SE, Abbasi N, Abd-Allah F, Abdela J, et al. Global, regional, and national burden of Alzheimer's disease and other dementias, 1990-2016. Lancet Neurol. 2019; 18(1):88-106.
7. Lutz W, Sanderson W, Scherbov S. The coming acceleration of global population ageing. Nature. 2008;451:716-19.
8. Wang H, Abbas KM, Abbasifard M, Abbasi-Kangevari M, Abbastabar H, Abd-Allah F, et al. Global age-sex-specific fertility, mortality, healthy life expectancy (HALE), and population estimates in 204 countries and territories, 1950-2019: a comprehensive demographic analysis for the Global Burden of Disease Study 2019. Lancet. 2020;396:1160-203.
9. Livingston G, Huntley J, Sommerlad A, Ames D, Ballard C, Banerjee S, et al. Dementia prevention, intervention, and care: 2020 report of the Lancet Commission. Lancet. 2020;396(10248):413-46.
10. Langa KM, Larson EB, Crimmins EM, Faul JD, Levine DA, Kabeto MU, et al. A comparison of the prevalence of dementia in the United States in 2000 and 2012. JAMA Int Med. 2017;177(1):51-8.

11. Skoog I, Bőrjesson-Hanson A, Kern S, Johansson L, Falk H, Sigström R, et al. Decreasing prevalence of dementia in 85-year olds examined 22 years apart: the influence of education and stroke. Sci Rep. 2017;7(1):6136.
12. Nichols E, Steinmetz JD, Vollset SE, Fukutaki G, Chalek J, Abd-Allah F, et al. Estimation of the global prevalence of dementia in 2019 and forecasted prevalence in 2050: an analysis for the Global Burden of Disease Study 2019. Lancet Public Health. 2022;7:e105-25.
13. Emma Nichols, Abd-Allah F, Abdoli A, Abosetugn AE, Abrha WA, Abualhasan A, et al. Global mortality from dementia: Application of a new method and results from the Global Burden of Disease Study 2019. Azheimer's Dement. 2021;7:e 12200.
14. Li X, Feng X, Sun X, Hou N, Han F, Liu Y. Global, regional, and national burden of Alzheimer's disease and other dementias, 1990-2019. Front Aging Neurosci. 2022;14:937486.
15. Huang WC, Chang MC, Wang WF, Jhang KM. A Comparison of Caregiver Burden for Different Types of Dementia: An 18-Month Retrospective Cohort Study. Front Psychol. 2022;12:798315.
16. James SL, Abate D, Abate KH, Abay SM, Abbafati C, Abbasi N, et al. Global, regional, and national incidence, prevalence, and years lived with disability for 354 diseases and injuries for 195 countries and territories, 1990-2017: a systematic analysis for the Global Burden of Disease Study 2017. Lancet. 2018;392(10159):1789-858.
17. Wimo A, Jőnsson L, Winblad B. An estimate of the total worldwide societal costs of dementia in 2005. Alzheimers Dement. 2017;3(2):81-91.
18. Winblad B, Wimo A, Jőnsson L (Eds). The Worldwide Direct Costs and Costs of Informal Care of Dementia. ICAD; 2006.
19. OECD, Eurostat, WHO. (2017). A System of Health Accounts 2011: Revised Edition. [online] Available from https://www.oecd.org/en/publications/a-system-of-health-accounts-2011_9789264270985-en.html [Last accessed July, 2024].
20. Wimo A, Winblad B, Jőnsson L. The worldwide societal costs of dementia: estimates for 2009. Alzheimers Dement. 2010;6(2):98-103.
21. Rao GN, Bharath S. Cost of Dementia Care in India: Delusion or Reality? Indian J Public Health. 2013;57(2):71-7.
22. MOHFW. National Health Health Accounts India 2004-05 with provisional estimates from 2005-06 to 2008-09. National Health Accounts Cell, Ministry of Health and Family Welfare, Government of India, New Delhi, 2009.
23. Vas CJ, Pinto C, Panikker D, Noronha S, Deshpande N, Kulkarni L, et al. Prevalence of dementia in an urban Indian population. Int Psychogeriatr. 2001;13(4):439-50.
24. Rajkumar S, Kumar S, Thara R. Prevalence of dementia in a rural setting: a report from India. Int J Geriatr Psychiatry. 1997;12:702-7.
25. Lee J, Meijer E, Langa KM, Ganguli M, Varghese M, Banerjee J, et al. Prevalence of dementia in India: National and state estimates from a nationwide study. Alzheimers Dement. 2023;19(7):2898-912.

CHAPTER

3

Clinical Approach to Dementia Diagnosis

Abhishek Chowdhury, Arpita Roychoudhury, Amitabha Ghosh

ABSTRACT

The approach to diagnosis of degenerative dementias such as Alzheimer's disease (AD) has undergone a sea change in recent years. Availability of increasingly sophisticated imaging, such as amyloid- and tau-positron emission tomography (PET) scans and biofluid biomarkers has revolutionized the diagnoses of these diseases. Nevertheless, for now, a robust clinical approach still remains the core around which the presence or absence of these biomarkers has to be interpreted. This chapter is an overview of such a clinical approach.

Keywords: Dementia, Alzheimer's disease, Diagnosis, Biomarkers.

INTRODUCTION

Dementia is an umbrella term for diseases that can cause significant cognitive decline to the extent that it affects functions of daily living. According to the World Health Organization, currently, more than 55 million people around the world are suffering from dementia. In India, the estimated prevalence of dementia in people aged more than 60 years is 7.4%.[1] Of all degenerative dementias, Alzheimer's disease (AD) is the most prevalent worldwide.

In 2011, the National Institute on Aging and the Alzheimer's Association Workgroups in the United States (US) proposed revised clinical diagnostic guidelines for AD.[2] Dementia is diagnosed when a person has cognitive or behavioral impairment that involves at least two of the following domains: Memory, executive function, visuospatial abilities, language function, personality, and behavior. Assessment of these patients should include both history taking from the patient and a knowledgeable informant, and an objective cognitive assessment. Moreover, there should be a definite decline from previous levels of functioning and symptoms must be severe enough to interfere with daily routine activities. It is also important that these symptoms should not be explained by delirium or a major psychiatric disorder.

Around this time there was an increased recognition of AD as a clinicopathological continuum beginning years, or decades, before the onset of clinical symptoms.[3,4] A preclinical stage, an early symptomatic stage, and the stage of established dementia were recognized. This realization that AD could be diagnosed well before the occurrence of dementia led to the more recent biomarker-based diagnosis of AD. Similar approaches have been taken for other non-AD dementias such as frontotemporal dementia (FTD).[5]

Mild cognitive impairment (MCI) is included in the early symptomatic stage of dementia. It is diagnosed when the decline in cognitive abilities affects one or more of the cognitive domains but does not interfere with the activities of daily living.[3] It can be classified as amnestic and nonamnestic types based on whether memory is affected. Amnestic MCI could be a prodromal stage of AD.

ETIOLOGY OF DEMENTIA

Dementia may result from any pathology that damages brain tissue. Neurodegenerative dementias are caused by excessive accumulation of abnormal and misfolded protein aggregates in neurons and glia. These abnormal protein deposits can alter normal neuronal function, ultimately leading to cell death. These proteins can be classified into six major groups: Amyloid-beta (Aβ), microtubule-associated protein tau, TAR DNA-binding protein 43 (TDP-43), fused in sarcoma (FUS), alpha-synuclein, and prion protein. Dementia can therefore be classified into pathological subtypes depending upon the abnormal protein deposits, and into clinical syndromes based on the clinical features. Different pathologies can cause similar clinical syndromes.

Currently, no treatment can cure or reverse disease progression in degenerative dementias. Hence, all efforts should be made to rule out reversible causes. Based on this discussion, dementia can be classified into the following:

- Degenerative dementia
- Reversible dementia

The major types of degenerative dementia are:

- *AD and its variants*:[6] [*Pathological proteins*: Aβ and hyperphosphorylated tau (p-tau)]
    - Typical AD
    - Atypical or variant AD
        - Logopenic variant
        - Posterior variant
        - Frontal variant
- *FTD*:[7] (*Pathological proteins*: Tau, TDP-43, and FUS):
    - Behavioral variant frontotemporal dementia (bvFTD)
    - Language variant FTD:
        - Semantic variant primary progressive aphasia (svPPA) [also called semantic dementia (SD)]
        - Nonfluent variant primary progressive aphasia (nfvPPA) [also called progressive nonfluent aphasia (PNFA)]
    - Motor frontotemporal degeneration syndromes:
        - Corticobasal syndrome
        - Progressive supranuclear palsy
        - FTD with motor neuron disease (FTD-MND)
- *Lewy body dementia*[8]: (*Pathological protein*: α-synuclein)
    - Dementia with Lewy bodies (DLB)
    - Parkinson's disease dementia (PDD)
- *Vascular dementia*:[9]Although degenerative, it is not caused by the accumulation of abnormal proteins.
- *Prion disease*: Creutzfeldt–Jakob disease (*Pathological protein*: Prion proteins)

Causes of Reversible Dementia

As discussed, a low threshold should be kept to identify any potentially treatable cause of cognitive impairment. Encountering certain atypical features during the evaluation of dementia should raise the suspicion of potentially reversible dementia **(Table 1)**. These red flag signs[10] are:

- Acute or subacute onset of symptoms
- Rapid cognitive decline
- Younger age of onset
- Prominent fluctuations
- Exposures to various drugs and toxins
- History of high-risk behaviors
- Unexplained findings on neurological examination

HISTORY AND EXAMINATION

Dementia is mainly a clinical diagnosis. A comprehensive history should be taken from the patient as well as a reliable informant, preferably the one who stays the most with the patient. Patients presenting with cognitive symptoms may have memory problems, language-related problems, visuospatial difficulties, or attention- and decision-making-related problems. Clinicians will do well

TABLE 1: Reversible causes of dementia.

Etiology	Causes
Vascular	Subdural hematoma, cerebral venous thrombosis, central nervous system (CNS) vasculitis, and posterior reversible encephalopathy syndrome (PRES)
Infectious	Bacterial, viral, fungal, or parasitic encephalitis/meningitis
Nutritional	Alcoholism, vitamin B12, and niacin deficiency
Toxic–metabolic	Dyselectrolytemia, hepatic encephalopathy, renal failure, thyroid/parathyroid dysfunction; heavy metal, toluene, lithium toxicity; chronic benzodiazepine usage, and carbon monoxide poisoning
Autoimmune/ Inflammatory	Autoimmune encephalitis, multiple sclerosis, anti-myelin oligodendrocyte glycoprotein (anti-MOG) antibody syndrome, acute disseminated encephalomyelitis (ADEM), systemic inflammatory diseases, and sarcoidosis
Neoplastic	CNS tumors, lymphoma, and paraneoplastic encephalitis
Iatrogenic	Medication overuse, radiation-induced, and substance abuse
Others	Normal pressure hydrocephalus, nonconvulsive status epilepticus, and hypoxia

to remember that a complaint of "forgetfulness" does not necessarily point to amnesia and other cognitive domains should be equally explored. Patients with problems with attention may be unable to concentrate or maintain a train of thoughts. Episodic memory impairment may present as difficulty remembering recent events, misplacing objects, or making repetitive statements, whereas patients with language impairments may have difficulty in naming and understanding conversations, saying grammatically incorrect sentences, or mispronouncing words. Patients getting lost in familiar places or having difficulty finding objects may have visuospatial problems. A detailed history is necessary to find out the cognitive domain that is initially affected, pattern of cognitive decline, and the temporal course of the disease. It is important to ask about any decline in daily living activities from premorbid levels.

It is also important to know about the onset and progression of symptoms. An acute or subacute onset or rapidly progressive symptoms may point toward nondegenerative causes of dementia. Presence of associated motor symptoms like slowness, tremors, myoclonus, gait unsteadiness, limb weakness, or fasciculations should be ascertained. Psychiatric symptoms, such as depression, delusions, hallucinations, change in personality, or socially inappropriate behavior, if present, should be noted.

History of vascular risk factors like diabetes, hypertension, smoking, or previous stroke should be taken as these may be risk factors for vascular dementia and may also contribute to other dementias. History of any malignancy or autoimmune disease may suggest autoimmune or paraneoplastic etiology. Efforts should also be made to look for the presence of sleep-related disorders such as rapid eye movement (REM) sleep behavior disorder (RBD), sleep apnea, or excessive daytime sleepiness. RBD in a patient with cognitive symptoms could suggest the presence of degenerative dementia with α-synuclein pathology such as DLB or PDD.

In the elderly, polypharmacy is common and various medications especially anticholinergics and sedatives may significantly affect cognition. A comprehensive check of the patient's medications should be done and any possible offending agent needs to be identified. Also, history of any potential high-risk behaviors or exposure to any toxins including excessive alcohol intake should be taken.

A detailed family history, especially among first-degree relatives, is also very important in the evaluation of dementia. Younger age of onset with a family history of dementia, parkinsonism, psychiatric illness, or amyotrophic lateral sclerosis may suggest a genetic etiology. Although genetic testing is not routinely recommended for dementia evaluation, patients with strong family histories could benefit from genetic testing by having a confirmed molecular diagnosis.

Clinical Examination

A thorough neurological examination along with testing for visual or hearing impairment should be carried out in all patients with dementia. Neurological examination may be normal in patients with dementia such as AD. There may be evidence of Parkinsonism in certain dementias such as dementia with Lewy body (DLB), PDD, corticobasal syndrome, or progressive supranuclear palsy. Dementia patients with prominent gait disturbance may have normal pressure hydrocephalus or associated Parkinsonism. Patients of vascular dementia may have focal neurological deficits resulting from vascular insults in the past. Fasciculations and atrophy may suggest the presence of motor neuron disease, especially if seen in association with bvFTD.

NEUROPSYCHOLOGICAL TESTING

An objective cognitive assessment with neuropsychological testing is an important part of dementia evaluation. Neuropsychological testing helps differentiate normal aging from pathological cognitive impairment, and evaluate severity of cognitive impairment, different subtypes of dementia, and functional status due to cognitive or behavioral decline, among other things. Cognitive evaluation includes global dementia screening tests such as the mini-mental state examination (MMSE),[11] Montreal cognitive assessment (MoCA),[12] Addenbrooke's cognitive examination-III (ACE-III),[13] among others. More detailed tests could be used to evaluate individual cognitive domains such as attention, executive function, episodic memory, semantic memory, language, praxis, visuospatial and visuoperceptual functions, behavior, social cognition and affect. A comprehensive neurocognitive toolbox (ICMR-NCTB) in multiple languages has been developed by the Indian Council of Medical Research for use in Indian literate subjects.[14] Tests such as the ACE-III have also been validated for Indian low-literate and illiterate subjects.[15] It is, however, important to guard against interpreting test scores and impaired domain functions in isolation. Cognition is a dynamic interplay within the brain's structural and functional networks, and an astute neuropsychologist recognizes that impairment in one domain could very well be due to damage somewhere else in the network.

After a thorough history-taking, neurological examination, and objective cognitive assessment, a reasonable clinical diagnosis of dementia subtypes can often be made. The clinical features of common dementia subtypes are as follows:

- *AD and its variants*:[6]
    - *Typical AD*: Early and progressive episodic memory impairment with or without involvement of other cognitive domains; objective evidence of hippocampal amnestic syndrome
    - Atypical or variant AD:
        - *Logopenic variant*: Word-finding difficulties, impaired repetition, circumlocution, phonemic paraphasias; spared semantic, syntactic, and motor speech abilities
        - *Posterior variant*: Biparietal dorsal variant presenting with Bálint syndrome, Gerstmann syndrome, limb apraxia, neglect; occipito-temporal ventral variant presenting with apperceptive agnosia, prosopagnosia
        - *Frontal variant*: Predominant features include early apathy, disinhibition, impairment of executive functions like planning and organizational skills.
- *FTD*:
    - *bvFTD*:[7] Early behavior and personality changes include disinhibition, apathy, lack of sympathy or empathy, and perseverative behavior, as well as hyperorality and prominent executive dysfunction.
    - *svPPA*:[16] An early, predominant, and progressive aphasia characterized by impaired single-word comprehension, and impaired confrontational naming. Other features include impaired object knowledge, surface dyslexia or dysgraphia, and preserved speech production and repetition.
    - *nfvPPA*:[16] An early, predominant, and progressive aphasia characterized by agrammatism or apraxia of speech. There may be impaired comprehension of syntactically complex sentences. Single-word comprehension and object knowledge are generally spared.
- *DLB*:[8] Progressive cognitive impairment (prominent impairment of attention, executive function, and visuospatial abilities) with associated Parkinsonism, early visual hallucinations, fluctuation of attention and alertness, and RBD
- *Vascular dementia*:[9] Patterns of cognitive impairment may vary depending upon the site of vascular insult.

LABORATORY INVESTIGATIONS

All patients with suspected cognitive impairment should have structural brain imaging [magnetic resonance imaging (MRI) or computed tomography (CT)], complete blood count, liver and renal function tests, estimation of glycemic control, serum thyroid-stimulating hormone (TSH), and vitamin B12 levels. Other laboratory tests such as electroencephalography (EEG), cerebrospinal fluid (CSF) analysis, antibody testing for autoimmune encephalitis, venereal disease research laboratory test (VDRL) testing, etc., may be done whenever there is a clinical suspicion.

For degenerative dementias, early and accurate diagnosis is becoming increasingly important with clinical drug trials beginning to show some success in early symptomatic AD. A prolonged preclinical and prodromal period can precede clinical symptoms in AD. It has been found that molecular biomarkers may be positive in this period, much before clinical deterioration or structural changes appear in neuroimaging.

The most commonly used neuroimaging techniques to study dementia include structural MRI and positron emission tomography (PET). PET imaging may have glucose metabolism [F-Fluorodeoxyglucose (FDG)-PET] or abnormal protein accumulation (amyloid and tau) as their targets.

Structural Imaging in Dementia

Magnetic resonance imaging (MRI) is preferred over CT scan. Primarily, it helps rule out nondegenerative or treatable causes of dementia. It also helps in differentiating degenerative dementias based on their characteristic pattern of atrophy. Recommended MRI protocol for dementia patients[17] include:

- *T2-weighted and fluid-attenuated inversion recovery (FLAIR) magnetic resonance (MR) sequences*: To identify signal abnormalities
- *T1-weighted MR sequences*: To assess the pattern and extent of atrophy [global atrophy score, medial temporal lobe atrophy (MTA) score, and Koedam—posterior/parietal atrophy score]
- *Diffusion-weighted MR images (DWI)*: May show areas of diffusion restriction (acute ischemia, for example) or signal alterations suggestive of Creutzfeldt–Jakob disease
- *Susceptibility-weighted MR images (SWI)*: To identify microbleeds and superficial siderosis

Typical MRI changes in various dementia subtypes:

- *AD*: The most common imaging finding is cortical atrophy predominantly involving temporoparietal regions symmetrically.
    - *Typical AD*: Mesial temporal atrophy (hippocampus, entorhinal cortex, and perirhinal cortex); precuneus and posterior cingulate atrophy (especially in early-onset AD)

  - *Posterior variant*: Parietotemporal or occipitotemporal cortical atrophy; may be asymmetric
  - *Logopenic variant*: Atrophy involves the left temporoparietal junction including the left inferior parietal lobule, lateral posterior temporal lobe, and perisylvian cortical region.
  - *Frontal variant*: Frontal lobe atrophy with relative mesial temporal lobe sparing
- *Frontotemporal spectrum disorders*: The most common imaging finding is frontotemporal atrophy with relative preservation of posterior cortices.
  - *bvFTD*: Atrophy of orbitofrontal cortex, prefrontal cortex, anterior cingulate along with atrophy of the adjacent insular cortex and anterior temporal lobes
  - *svPPA*: Asymmetric (more commonly left than right) involvement of the anterior and inferior temporal lobes
  - *nfvPPA*: Atrophy of left inferior frontal lobe posteriorly and insula with a widening of the left perisylvian fissure
- *Dementia with Lewy bodies and Parkinson's disease dementia*: Diffuse mild cortical atrophy with no distinct regional pattern
- *Vascular dementia*:
  - *Small vessel disease and Binswanger's disease*: White matter hyperintensities, enlarged Virchow-Robin spaces, and lacunar infarcts
  - *Cerebral amyloid angiopathy*: Cerebral microbleeds located peripherally at the cortical gray-white matter interface and progressively diffuse white matter hyperintensities
  - *Hereditary vasculopathies—cerebral autosomal dominant arteriopathy with subcortical infarcts and leukoencephalopathy* (CADASIL): Extensive white matter damage with prominent involvement of anterior temporal lobes and external capsule.
- *Creutzfeldt-Jakob disease*: DWI restriction mainly involving the superior frontal gyrus, insula, cingulate gyrus, and striatum and the presence of "cortical ribboning sign", "hockey stick sign", and "pulvinar sign"
- *Idiopathic normal pressure hydrocephalus*: Ventriculomegaly, Evans index >0.3, acute callosal angle, disproportionately enlarged subarachnoid space hydrocephalus (DESH), and prominent aqueductal flow voids

Functional Imaging in Dementia

In patients with dementia, metabolic changes in the brain can be detected much before anatomical changes are seen on structural imaging. These metabolic changes are detected by functional brain imaging such as PET and single-photon emission computed tomography (SPECT). PET imaging commonly uses radioactive glucose analogue ^{18}F-FDG and in dementia shows areas of hypometabolism in specific areas of brain, whereas SPECT imaging shows alterations in regional blood flow.

Moreover, SPECT with ^{123}I-ioflupane could be used for dopamine-transporter imaging and could be of importance in patients with Parkinson's disease and DLB. PET imaging is more commonly used than SPECT for dementia diagnosis.

^{18}F-FDG PET imaging can help in differentiating various degenerative dementias, especially in early disease when structural imaging is not explanatory.[18] In AD, it shows early hypometabolism in the posterior cingulate cortex and precuneus followed by hypometabolism in bilateral temporoparietal lobes. Frontal hypometabolism occurs late in the disease. In behavioral variant of frontotemporal dementia, there may be hypometabolism in bilateral frontal lobes, whereas in semantic dementia there is predominant hypometabolism in the anterior temporal lobes. In progressive nonfluent aphasia, there is predominant hypometabolism in the left inferior or middle frontal and precentral gyrus. In dementia with Lewy bodies, there is global cortical hypometabolism, especially in the visual association cortex of the occipital lobe with preserved metabolism of the posterior cingulate gyrus (cingulate island sign) and primary visual cortex (occipital tunnel sign). However, there is no specific pattern of hypometabolism in vascular dementia, which may be seen to patchily affect different areas of the brain.

Amyloid- and tau-based PET imaging: Using specific tracers, abnormal accumulation of amyloid and tau in the brain can be identified in vivo using PET imaging. Carbon 11-labeled Pittsburgh Compound B, which binds to amyloid β protein, was the first radiotracer to be used for amyloid PET imaging. However, because of its short half-life, it was replaced later by other radiotracers with longer half-life such as ^{18}F-florbetapir, ^{18}F-flutemetamol, and ^{18}F-florbetaben. These compounds bind nonspecifically to white matter and areas of amyloid deposition with little or no uptake in normal gray matter. Whereas a normal amyloid PET scan will show only a white matter pattern, a positive amyloid scan will show a loss of gray-white differentiation.[18] Tau-specific ligands for PET imaging such as ^{18}F flortaucipir have also been developed to study abnormal tau deposition in the brain in various neurodegenerative diseases.[19]

In AD, there is a widespread amyloid deposition in the cortex. However, amyloid scans may also be positive in normal elderly population and other dementias. If an amyloid PET scan is negative, the likelihood of the patient having AD is very minimal. Vascular dementia and FTD usually have negative amyloid scans. Patients with cerebral amyloid angiopathy may show amyloid deposition. Patients with DLB may or may not show amyloid deposition.

Other Neuroimaging Techniques

Special MRI techniques may also be used to assess brain structure and function in patients with dementia. These are diffusion tensor imaging (DTI), functional MRI (fMRI) with blood oxygenation level-dependent (BOLD) imaging, quantitative susceptibility mapping, and arterial spin labeling.

Cerebrospinal Fluid Biomarkers

The AD biomarker assays currently used for clinical diagnosis include CSF levels of Aβ42, Aβ40, total tau (t-tau), and phosphorylated tau at position 181 (p-tau181). CSF levels of Aβ42 decrease and CSF t-tau and p-tau181 levels start to increase after the formation of amyloid plaques and neurofibrillary tangles in the brain.

So in AD:
- CSF Aβ42 and Aβ42/Aβ40 ratio decreases
- CSF t-tau and t-tau/Aβ42 ratio gets elevated
- CSF p-tau181 and p-tau181/Aβ42 ratio get elevated

Blood Based Biomarkers

Currently, biomarkers such as plasma levels of Aβ42/Aβ40 ratio, p-tau, neurofilament light chain (NfL), and glial fibrillary acidic protein (GFAP) are under research and can provide rapid, cost-effective, and noninvasive diagnostic tools in the evaluation of AD and other dementias.

Genetic Testing

Genetic testing is not routinely recommended in the evaluation of dementia as mostly these dementias are sporadic in nature and have a polygenic mode of inheritance. However, in some cases, genetic testing could be beneficial. Young-onset dementia patients usually have atypical features and getting a precise diagnosis could help avoid unnecessary testing. It could also help in better prognostication of the disease, help family members ascertain their individual risk, and help them in family planning. Further, if patients have an accurate diagnosis they could partake in appropriate clinical trials and could benefit from targeted presymptomatic therapies whenever some of these become available.

The modified Goldman score[20] is a scoring system that helps to categorize the risk of having a causal mutation by assessment of the family history.
- *Score 1*: Autosomal dominant, where three individuals are affected over two generations with one person being a first-degree relative of the others.
- *Score 2*: Familial aggregations, where three members of a family are affected but not meeting the criteria of score 1.
- *Score 3*: Where there is one other affected relative (Score 3.5—if the age of the onset of dementia in the affected relative is above 65 years).
- *Score 4*: No or unknown family history

The most common mutations for autosomal dominant AD are in presenilin 1 *(PSEN1)*, presenilin 2 *(PSEN2)*, and amyloid precursor protein *(APP)* genes.[21] However, these are seen in <1% of all AD patients. In sporadic AD, APOEe4 increases the risk whereas APOEe2 protects against AD. In FTD, mutations in the microtubule-associated protein tau *(MAPT)*, progranulin *(GRN)*, and chromosome 9 open reading frame 72 (*C9orf72)* together account for the majority of the disease in autosomal dominant families.[22]

CONCLUSION

The approach to diagnosis of degenerative dementias such as AD and FTD has undergone remarkable change in recent years. Availability of increasingly sophisticated imaging, such as amyloid- and tau-PET scans, biofluid biomarkers, and freely accessible genetic tests have revolutionized the diagnoses of these diseases. For example, the demonstration of amyloid positivity in the brain is now essential to diagnose AD pathology. Nevertheless, a robust clinical approach still remains the core around which the presence or absence of these biomarkers has to be interpreted, even as more and more revised criteria for the diagnosis of AD and other diseases evolve.

REFERENCES

1. Lee J, Meijer E, Langa KM, Ganguli M, Varghese M, Banerjee J, et al. Prevalence of dementia in India: National and state estimates from a nationwide study. Alzheimers Dement. 2023;19(7):2898-912.
2. McKhann GM, Knopman DS, Chertkow H, Hyman BT, Jack CR Jr, Kawas CH, et al. The diagnosis of dementia due to Alzheimer's disease: Recommendations from the National Institute on Aging-Alzheimer's Association workgroups on diagnostic guidelines for Alzheimer's disease. Alzheimers Dement. 2011;7(3):263-9.
3. Jack CR Jr, Knopman DS, Jagust WJ, Petersen RC, Weiner MW, Aisen PS, et al. Tracking pathophysiological processes in Alzheimer's disease: An updated hypothetical model of dynamic biomarkers. Lancet Neurol. 2013;12(2):207-16.
4. Jack CR Jr, Bennett DA, Blennow K, et al. NIA-AA Research Framework: Toward a biological definition of Alzheimer's disease. Alzheimer's Dement. 2018;14:535-62.
5. Benussi A, Alberici A, Samra K, Russell LL, Greaves CV, Bocchetta M, et al. Conceptual framework for the definition

of preclinical and prodromal frontotemporal dementia. Alzheimers Dement. 2022;18(7):1408-23.

6. Dubois B, Feldman HH, Jacova C, Hampel H, Molinuevo JL, Blennow K, et al. Advancing research diagnostic criteria for Alzheimer's disease: The IWG-2 criteria. Lancet Neurol. 2014;13(6):614-29.
7. Rascovsky K, Hodges JR, Knopman D, Mendez MF, Kramer JH, Neuhaus J, et al. Sensitivity of revised diagnostic criteria for the behavioural variant of frontotemporal dementia. Brain. 2011;134(Pt 9):2456-77.
8. McKeith IG, Boeve BF, Dickson DW, Halliday G, Taylor JP, Weintraub D, et al. Diagnosis and management of dementia with Lewy bodies: Fourth consensus report of the DLB Consortium. Neurology. 2017;89(1):88-100.
9. Sachdev P, Kalaria R, O'Brien J, Skoog I, Alladi S, Black SE, et al. Diagnostic criteria for vascular cognitive disorders: A VASCOG statement. Alzheimer Dis Assoc Disord. 2014;28(3):206-18.
10. Day GS. Reversible dementias. Continuum (Minneap Minn). 2019;25(1):234-53.
11. Folstein MF, Folstein SE, McHugh PR. "Mini-mental state". A practical method for grading the cognitive state of patients for the clinician. J Psychiatr Res. 1975;12:189-98.
12. Nasreddine ZS, Phillips NA, Bédirian V, Charbonneau S, Whitehead V, Collin I, et al. The Montreal Cognitive Assessment, MoCA: A Brief Screening Tool For Mild Cognitive Impairment. J Am Geriatr Soc. 2005;53(4):695-9.
13. Hsieh S, Schubert S, Hoon C, Mioshi E, Hodges JR. Validation of the Addenbrooke's Cognitive Examination III in frontotemporal dementia and Alzheimer's disease. Dement Geriatr Cogn Disord. 2013;36(3-4):242-50.
14. Iyer GK, Paplikar A, Alladi S, Dutt A, Sharma M, Mekala S, et al. Standardising Dementia Diagnosis Across Linguistic and Educational Diversity: Study Design of the Indian Council of Medical Research-Neurocognitive Tool Box (ICMR-NCTB). J Int Neuropsychol Soc. 2020;26(2):172-86.
15. Paplikar A, Varghese F, Battacharyya B, Shukla V, Tripathi M, Biswas, et al. Dementia diagnosis using Addenbrooke's Cognitive Examination in low literates and illiterates in three Indian languages. Alzheimers Dement. 2023;19:e077702.
16. Gorno-Tempini ML, Hillis AE, Weintraub S, Kertesz A, Mendez M, Cappa SF, et al. Classification of primary progressive aphasia and its variants. Neurology. 2011;76(11):1006-14.
17. Furtner J, Prayer D. Neuroimaging in dementia. Wien Med Wochenschr. 2021;171:274-81.
18. Zukotynski K, Kuo PH, Mikulis D, Rosa-Neto P, Strafella AP, Subramaniam RM, et al. PET/CT of dementia. AJR Am J Roentgenol. 2018;211(2):246-59.
19. Tian M, Civelek AC, Carrio I, Watanabe Y, Kang KW, Murakami K, et al. International consensus on the use of tau PET imaging agent 18F-flortaucipir in Alzheimer's disease. Eur J Nucl Med Mol Imaging. 2022;49(3):895-904.
20. Rohrer JD, Guerreiro R, Vandrovcova J, Uphill J, Reiman D, Beck J, et al. The heritability and genetics of frontotemporal lobar degeneration. Neurology. 2009;73(18):1451-6.
21. Bertram L, Tanzi RE. Thirty years of Alzheimer's disease genetics: The implications of systematic meta-analyses. Nat Rev Neurosci. 2008;9(10):768-78.
22. Pottier C, Ravenscroft TA, Sanchez-Contreras M, Rademakers R. Genetics of FTLD: Overview and what else we can expect from genetic studies. J Neurochem. 2016;138:32-53.

CHAPTER 4

Neuropsychology Testing for Assessment of Dementia in a Diverse Multilingual Context

Urvashi Shah, Porrselvi AP

ABSTRACT

This chapter delves into the complexities of diagnosing and understanding dementia in culturally and linguistically diverse populations. It explores the challenges of applying neuropsychological tests in a multilingual world, highlighting potential biases in test norms and interpretation. It recommends specific strategies and best practices for conducting culturally sensitive assessments, equipping clinicians with the necessary tools to navigate the crucial aspect of dementia diagnosis. A comprehensive list of assessment options available in India, categorized as screening tools and comprehensive batteries are tabled. Screening tools offer a quick evaluation of cognitive function, while comprehensive batteries offer a more in-depth analysis of the various cognitive domains. The chapter highlights the need for comprehensive and sensitive assessments for a more nuanced understanding of dementia in diverse cultures.

Keywords: Dementia, Diagnosis, Neuropsychological tests, Multilingualism, India.

INTRODUCTION

Globally, demographic transitions, improved healthcare systems, and increased longevity have created a daunting reality of an exponential increase in elderly populations who are at risk for dementia. In low- and middle-income countries (LMICs) where the majority population of dementia is expected to reside,[1] there is a looming public healthcare crisis and an unmet need to diagnose and intervene early, to recommend disease-specific treatments, maintain quality of life, and reduce the burden of dementia.

Dementia is a multifaceted neurodegenerative disorder that transcends the realm of age-related cognitive decline. Characterized by a progressive deterioration in cognitive function that significantly impairs an individual's ability to perform activities of daily living (ADLs), it poses a significant diagnostic challenge due to its complex and multifaceted clinical presentation.

The onset of dementia is a gradual insidious process that goes largely unrecognized in the early years due to mistaken, normal aging cognitive loss. Clinical dementia diagnosis is based on symptom presentation and there is a significant diagnostic delay due to numerous factors. Initially, caregivers do not report due to cultural belief systems regarding normal aging and the stigma associated with the diagnosis,[2] but there is also reluctance on the part of clinicians to provide a label until the symptoms are more pronounced and clinically evident. To arrive at the diagnosis, the clinicians must establish cognitive and functional impairment and rule out other causes. The establishment of true impairment, beyond normal aging, requires detailed neuropsychological evaluation with robust standardized tools.

COMPREHENSIVE NEUROPSYCHOLOGICAL EVALUATION

Dementia is not a monolithic entity. It encompasses a heterogeneous spectrum of etiologies, each with distinct neuropathological signatures and corresponding cognitive profiles. Neuropsychological assessment has emerged as a vital tool in navigating this complex clinical landscape. A comprehensive evaluation includes use of standardized cognitive tests to sample abilities in different cognitive domains and integrates information from clinical interviews (presenting symptoms, premorbid function, medical comorbidities, mood, and family history), behavioral observations, clinical record reviews, and collateral information. Established diagnostic criteria, such as those outlined in the Diagnostic and Statistical Manual of Mental Disorders, Fifth Edition (DSM-5) and the International Classification of Diseases, 10th Revision (ICD-10), provide a standardized framework for dementia diagnosis[3,4] and both acknowledge the value of a comprehensive neuropsychological assessment as a tool in the overall evaluation and diagnostic process.

UTILITY OF A NEUROPSYCHOLOGICAL EVALUATION

For the clinician, neuropsychology evaluations in dementia are useful for establishing the clinical diagnosis, for prognosis, and for tracking treatment outcomes.

- *Differential diagnosis*: Cognitive impairment profiles help differentiate normal aging from mild cognitive impairment (MCI), neurodegenerative dementia from reversible dementia due to depression, and different types of dementia such as Alzheimer's disease (AD) versus frontotemporal dementia (FTD).
- *Tracking progression*: Tracking changes in performance over time, neuropsychological assessment allows clinicians to monitor disease progression and inform treatment decisions.
- *Competency evaluation*: Test performance helps estimate capacity for managing finances, inheritance-related legal matters, driving, independent travel, and decisions-making. The competency assessment guides clinicians and families about the care required for the person with dementia (PwD).
- *Rehabilitation*: The cognitive profile of relative strengths and weaknesses guides rehabilitation planning and ensures that a PwD remains independent and productive as long as possible.

TEST CHARACTERISTICS

Multidomain Testing

Testing should include assessment of major cognitive domains with standardized tests that have undergone rigorous cultural adaptations and adequately stratified normative data. It is critical that testing assesses the key cognitive domains (attention, processing speed, memory, language executive function, and visual spatial function) as there are signature clinical profiles for the distinct types of dementia. It is also important to recognize that the extent and severity of the condition changes with progression and profiles may shift depending on the level of the disease advancement. For instance, AD, the most prevalent form of dementia, is characterized primarily by progressive memory decline, but with advancing disease, there are impairments in executive function, while vascular dementia often manifests with difficulties in attention, processing speed, and executive functioning. Hence, a multidomain assessment is an important part of cognitive evaluation in dementia.

Test Standardization and Normative Data

In several LMICs with diverse sociodemographic and multilingual populations, selecting a suitable, culturally adapted, standardized instrument with appropriate sensitivity and specificity is crucial for accurate diagnosis. However, this can be challenging. The application of neuropsychological tests, traditionally developed in the west and normed on different language and cultural groups, poses a significant challenge in assessing dementia in populations with educational and language diversity. Cognitive processes develop in culturally distinctive ways and the cultural backgrounds can influence test performance. For instance, tasks that rely on language skills or literacy may disadvantage individuals from cultures with different communication styles or educational backgrounds. Stimuli for the verbal, language-based tests need significant adaptations in countries such as India with diverse populations (e.g., Indian adaptations of Addenbrooke Cognitive Examination III[5]). Even for the "culture-free" visual tests such as the Visual Object and Space Perception (VOSP) Battery, stimuli appear to be processed differently by various cultures and require population-specific normative data.[6] The lack of resources and low priority for development of population-specific norms and standardization of instruments result in potential biases arising from both test norms and score interpretation.

Normative comparison is the cornerstone of neuropsychological testing and comparing a patient's performance to a reference group of the same age, education, ethnicity, and gender cannot be ignored. Test norms, which represent the average performance of a specific demographic group, may not be generalizable to individuals from diverse cultural or linguistic backgrounds. The clinician must be extremely cautious in pronouncing a diagnosis if tests lack appropriate age and education-stratified norms. Without the education norms, for example, person 1 with an impoverished, rural background and primary level of education may fail several tests (floor effect) and be misclassified as having dementia, while person 2 of the same age from a sophisticated, urban background with a postgraduate degree may pass the same tests (ceiling effect) and be misclassified as normal. With regards to age norms, in the normal elderly, there is a natural, progressive decline with age and there is a marked difference between the performance of a "young-old" (65–79 years) and "old-old" (≥80 years) age categories.[7] Normative data that treats age as a homogenous construct and does not have age-stratified scores may falsely label a person in the old-old age category as impaired.

IMPACT OF DIVERSITY

The effectiveness of a neuropsychological assessment hinges on a nuanced understanding of the individual undergoing evaluation. Administering these tests within a multilingual context presents several complexities and influences of factors such as socioeconomic, education, and language background.

Socioeconomic Background

Socioeconomic status (SES) can exert an influence on test performance. Individuals from lower SES backgrounds may have had less access to educational opportunities, potentially leading to lower baseline scores on cognitive measures. Conversely, higher SES may not equate to superior cognitive performance but rather reflect advantages in test-taking strategies or familiarity with the testing format.[8]

Educational Background

A test bias against low levels of education may be present in the dementia screening tests and a low level of education may itself be a risk factor for dementia. In LMICs with large numbers of illiterates from low socioeconomic backgrounds, to avoid false-positive diagnosis, it is critical to modify tests and collect specific norms for this group.[9]

Cognitive Reserve

There are intraindividual differences in the extent of cognitive reserve. Educational attainment and occupational complexity are significant contributors to cognitive reserve, the brain's capacity to withstand neurodegenerative processes. Higher levels of education are associated with a greater ability to compensate for neuropathology, potentially delaying the onset of dementia symptoms or masking them on cognitive testing.[10] This underscores the importance of interpreting test results within the context of an individual's educational background.

Language: A Multifaceted Challenge

Language presents a unique set of challenges in dementia assessment for multilingual populations.

Impact of Language Proficiency

Performance on language-based tasks within neuropsychological tests can be significantly influenced by an individual's proficiency in the test language. Individuals with limited proficiency may be disadvantaged, leading to an underestimation of their cognitive abilities. While testing bilinguals or multilinguals, the language of test administration and patient responses is extremely important to ensure that the test instructions have been understood and the patient has an opportunity to respond optimally. Ideally, patients should be tested in their most proficient language and the examiner needs to evaluate for language proficiency either through self-reports or objective measures.[11] The proficiency of the examiner in the testing language is equally important and when the examiner is not fluent, trained interpreters should be available to facilitate the administration.

Linguistically Validated Test Versions

Clinicians must be cautious of potential biases introduced by translated versions without proper validation. However, the availability of culturally and linguistically validated versions of neuropsychological tests remains limited, particularly for less commonly spoken languages.

Primary Language and Bilingualism

Identifying the individual's primary language is crucial. Dementia can disproportionately affect an individual's dominant or nondominant language, depending on the specific pathology. Bilingualism, on the other hand, has been associated with a cognitive protective effect,[12] potentially delaying the onset of dementia.[13] However, the complex interplay between language and cognitive decline in bilingual individuals necessitates careful consideration during assessment.

Test Administration and Multilingualism

In countries such as India, the phenomenon of translanguaging is common, wherein bilinguals and multilinguals access different languages to maximize communication. There is fluid language usage and it is common for people to shift across languages in daily conversation. Hence, instructions across languages and scoring to allow for "borrowed words" from other languages need to be considered while assessing bilinguals and multilinguals in India. In certain tests such as the confrontation naming and verbal fluency (phonemic and semantic fluency), the current expert recommendation for India is to allow patients to respond in more than one language and score for all responses in the native or other language. It has been suggested that this method of administration is more ecologically valid for bilingual India.[11]

Test Norms

There has been evidence that bilinguals may have advantages over monolinguals in executive tasks and disadvantages in language-based tasks,[14] indicating that there should be separate norms for monolinguals versus bilinguals. However, recent findings from the study in India, wherein tests were simultaneously standardized in multiple languages, suggested that separate normative data might not be required for bilinguals and multilinguals.[11]

BARRIERS IN NEUROPSYCHOLOGICAL TESTING

Interpretation of the test data requires a careful understanding of factors that may affect test performance. Cognitive testing is impacted by multiple factors such as patient cooperation and motivation, status of hearing and vision, and test wiseness and bilingualism/multilingualism, underscoring the need for a trained neuropsychologist to conduct a dementia evaluation.

Patient Motivation

Patients may lack insight, be defensive, anxious about a testing situation, and depressed, and may deny any problems, often stating that they have agreed to the testing on the behest of a family member. They may also devalue a "paper pencil" test as being unimportant to help reach a diagnosis. In all these situations, the level of cooperation may fluctuate, requiring the skills of a trained neuropsychologist to elicit the optimal performance.

Hearing and Vision

Cognitive evaluation requires comprehension of the test instructions and processing of visual stimulus. The aging process impacts vision and hearing and it is not uncommon for the elderly to forget to carry/or not want to use a hearing aid or not bring their reading spectacles. Cognitive testing needs to be sensitive to any sensory barriers that will undermine the performance of the elderly during the session.

Test Wiseness

Test-taking sophistication or "test wiseness" is the knowledge of how to respond optimally to psychological tests, which is gained through experience of having undergone previous similar testing. The exposure to these experiences is limited in nonwestern cultures and varies in a country based on whether the patient dwells in rural or urban settings. The lack of "test wiseness" impacts performance on timed tests and comprehension of complex test instructions, sometimes needing modifications in instructions and administration procedures.[15]

DEMENTIA ASSESSMENT TOOLS

Tests for dementia can be divided into two broad categories of instruments:

Screening Tests

Dementia screening tests serve as the initial line of assessment in identifying potential cognitive decline. These brief, easy-to-administer tests are designed to quickly assess an individual's cognitive functions and are useful for early identification of individuals at risk and who may warrant further evaluation. Administration of screening tests requires training but may be administered by healthcare professionals.

- *Advantages*: Screening tests prioritize brevity and ease of administration, often relying on simple tasks such as immediate and delayed memory recall, clock drawing, or basic orientation questions.
- *Disadvantages*: A screening test is not capable of assessing individual cognitive domains thoroughly and may lack adequate assessment of a particular domain [e.g., executive function in Mini-Mental Status Examination (MMSE)]. Screening tests are often low in sensitivity and classification accuracy and use of these tests alone may miss individuals with true cognitive impairment.
- *Considerations in a multilingual context*: While translated versions of screening tests may be available, language-based tasks in the screening tool may disadvantage individuals with limited proficiency in the translated language and ensuring cultural appropriateness is crucial (e.g., items in the naming tests). Clinicians must consider the availability of culturally adapted versions of screening tests or to use tests with minimal language dependence.

Comprehensive Assessment Battery Approach

Comprehensive neuropsychological test batteries offer an in-depth evaluation of an individual's cognitive functioning across multiple domains. These batteries typically involve a series of standardized tests that provide a detailed cognitive profile. Administration of test batteries requires expert, trained neuropsychologists.

- *Advantages*: Unlike screening tests, comprehensive batteries delve deeper, employing a wider range of tasks to assess various cognitive domains, such as memory, attention, executive function, language, visuospatial skills, and processing speed. This detailed profile allows for a more nuanced understanding of an individual's cognitive strengths and weaknesses, leading to a more accurate diagnosis.
- *Disadvantages*: Increased testing time, need for trained, skilled professionals for administration and interpretation
- *Considerations for diverse populations*: When selecting a test battery for culturally diverse populations, the availability of culturally adapted versions or culturally neutral tests becomes paramount. Culturally adapted versions involve modifications to the test stimuli, administration procedures, or scoring criteria to minimize the influence of cultural background on performance. Culturally neutral tests, on the other hand, rely on selected tasks with minimal language or cultural dependence, such as visuospatial puzzles or abstract reasoning tasks.

By strategically employing both screening tests and comprehensive assessment batteries, clinicians can navigate the complexities of dementia diagnosis in culturally diverse populations. In India, with the sociocultural, educational, and linguistic diversity, identifying a single test for the entire country is quite challenging. A number of screening tools and test batteries have been standardized with appropriate adaptations, multiple language translations, and normative data **(Table 1)**. The choice of instrument will depend on the specific purpose of the assessment, available resources

TABLE 1: Neuropsychology tests for dementia evaluation in India.

Test name	Age range	Languages	Domains
Screening tools			
Hindi Mental State Examination (HMSE)[16]	55+ years	Hindi	Orientation, memory, and attention language
Montreal Cognitive Assessment[17,18]	55–85 years	Hindi, Tamil, Urdu, Bengali, Telugu, Kannada, Malayalam, Gujarati, Marathi, and Punjabi	Visuospatial/executive functions, naming, memory, attention, language, and abstraction
Addenbrooke's Cognitive Examination-III (ACE-III)—Indian adaptation[5,9,19,20]	50+ years	Hindi, Telugu, Kannada, Malayalam Urdu, Tamil, and Indian English, illiterate version	Orientation, attention, memory, language, fluency, and visuospatial skills
Kolkata Cognitive Battery (KCB)[21,22]	50–95 years (Bengali) 40+ years (Marathi)	Bengali and Marathi	Fluency, naming, mental state examination, calculation, visuoconstructional ability, and verbal memory
Hindi Cognitive Screening Test (HCST)[23,24]	60+ years	Hindi and Malayalam	Orientation, memory, attention language, praxis, and naming
Oxford Cognitive Screen Tamil (OCS-Tamil)[25]	Adults (Poststroke/vascular screening)	Tamil	Orientation, attention, language, visuospatial skills, memory, executive functioning, calculation, and praxis
Mini–Mental Status Examination (MMSE)[26]	Adults	Gujarati, Hindi, Indian English, Kannada, Malayalam, Marathi, Punjabi, Tamil, Telugu, Urdu, and Bengali	Orientation, attention, calculation, memory, and language
General Practitioner Assessment of Cognition (GPCOG)[27]	Elderly	Urdu and Hindi	Informant interview, orientation, visuospatial, and memory
Clinical Dementia Rating Scale (CDR)[28]	Older adults	Indian English, Hindi, Malayalam, Marathi, Tamil, Telugu, Urdu, Kannada, and Bengali	Memory, orientation, judgment and problem solving, community affairs, home and hobbies, and personal care
Dementia Assessment by Rapid Test (DART)[29]	55–84 years	Hindi	Language, memory, and visuospatial
Rowland Universal Dementia Assessment Scale (RUDAS)[30]	Older adults	Malayalam	Memory, praxis, language, and judgment, drawing and body orientation

Continued

Continued

Test name	Age range	Languages	Domains
Vellore Dementia Screening Questionnaire (VDSQ)[31]	Older adults	Tamil	Patient and informant questionnaire; memory, language, praxis, gnosis, executive function, and activities of daily living (ADLs)
Mini-Cog[32]	Older adults	Marathi, Hindi, and Urdu	Memory and visuospatial skills
Hindi Adaptation of Mattis Dementia Rating Scale (HMDRS)[33]	60–80 years	Hindi	Attention, memory, initiation and perseveration, construction, and conceptualization
Neuropsychological Evaluation Screening Tool (NEST)[34]	16–71 years	Hindi and English	Memory, executive function, attention, and visuospatial
Indian Adaptation of the Alzheimer's Disease Assessment Scale-Cognitive (ADAS-cog)[35]	60+ years	Hindi and Marathi	Word recall and recognition, commands, constructional praxis, ideational praxis naming, orientation, concentration, and executive function
Picture-based memory impairment screen for dementia (PMIS)[36]	55+ years	Malayalam	Memory
Comprehensive battery			
Indian Council of Medical Research-National Cognitive Toolbox (ICMR-NCTB)[37]	Adults	Indian English, Hindi, Bengali, Telugu, Kannada, and Malayalam	Attention and executive function, episodic memory, language, visuospatial ability, unilateral spatial neglect, and behavioral scales
PGI Battery of Brain Dysfunction[38]	20–59 years	Indian English	Attention, memory, visuospatial abilities, executive functions, and language
PGI Memory Scale[39]	20–45 years	Indian English	Memory
NIMHANS Neuropsychological Battery[40]	16–65 years	Indian English	Attention, memory, visuospatial abilities, executive functions, and language
NIMHANS Neuropsychological Battery for Elderly (NNB-E)[41]	55–80 years	Indian English	Attention, memory, visuospatial abilities, executive functions, language, and parietal focal signs
All India Institute of Medical Sciences Comprehensive Neuropsychological Battery[42]	15–80 years	Hindi	Sensorimotor, language, arithmetic, memory, intellectual abilities, and pathognomic scale
10/66 Dementia Research Group Cognitive Test Battery[43]	65+ years old	Indian English	Memory and fluency
Wechsler Adult Intelligence Scale Fourth Edition, India[44]	16 years to 84 years 11 months	Indian English	Working memory, processing speed, verbal comprehension, and perceptual reasoning as well as general cognitive ability [Full Scale Intelligence Quotient (IQ)]
Wechsler Memory Scale Third Edition, India[44]	16–89 years	Indian English	Memory
Wechsler Abbreviated Scale of Intelligence, Second Edition, India[44]	6–90+ years	Indian English	Verbal Comprehension Index (VCI) and Perceptual Reasoning Index (PRI) as well as general cognitive ability (Full Scale IQ)
Tamil Cognitive Assessment (TAM Battery)[45]	Older adults	Tamil	Orientation, attention, memory, language, executive function, processing speed, premorbid cognitive function, and performance validity

that include time and availability of trained professional, and the patient's background. It is crucial to prioritize culturally sensitive approaches throughout the assessment process, ensuring accurate and equitable diagnosis of dementia.

CONCLUSION

Neuropsychological assessment plays a pivotal role in diagnosing dementia across diverse populations. However, navigating the complexities associated with this process in a multilingual context requires a nuanced understanding of cultural, sociodemographic, and language background. Age, education, and SES, all exert an influence on test performance. There are efforts to develop universal, culture-fair tests, but language diversity presents a unique set of challenges and there are limited testing options for the illiterates and the very elderly. By acknowledging these complexities and adopting culturally sensitive practices, clinicians can ensure a more equitable and informative assessment process. This involves employing culturally adapted test versions when available, using alternative assessment techniques with minimal language dependence, and prioritizing a comprehensive understanding of the individual's background and communication preferences. The diagnosis of dementia can be a devastating and life-altering event. Selection of appropriate tools, sensitive test administration, and critical interpretation of test results will ensure that the PwD and the family are able to receive the correct diagnosis and make informed decisions regarding management, rehabilitation, and future planning.

REFERENCES

1. World Health Organization. World Health Statistics 2015. Geneva: World Health Organization. 2015.
2. Porrselvi AP, Shankar V. Status of Cognitive Testing of Adults in India. Ann Indian Acad Neurol. 2017;20(4):334-40.
3. World Health Organization. The ICD-10 Classification of Mental and Behavioural Disorders: Diagnostic Criteria for Research. Geneva: World Health Organization; 1994.
4. American Psychiatric Association. Diagnostic and Statistical Manual of Mental Disorders: DSM-5™, 5th edition. Washington, DC: American Psychiatric Publishing, Inc.; 2013.
5. Mekala S, Paplikar A, Mioshi E, Kaul S, Divyaraj G, Coughlan G, et al. Dementia diagnosis in seven languages: the Addenbrooke's Cognitive Examination-III in India. Arch Clin Neuropsychol. 2020;35(5):528-38.
6. Chatterjee S. Differences in object perception: a comparison of Indian and British participants on scene and silhouetted object perception tasks. PhD thesis. Glasgow: University of Glasgow; 2021.
7. Wong CG, Thomas KR, Edmonds EC, Weigand AJ, Bangen KJ, Eppig JS, et al. Neuropsychological Criteria for Mild Cognitive Impairment in the Framingham Heart Study's Old-Old. Dement Geriatr Cogn Disord. 2019;46(5-6):253-65.
8. Manly JJ, Jacobs DM, Sano M, Bell K, Merchant CA, Small SA, et al. The effect of literacy on neuropsychological test performance in Alzheimer's disease. Neurology. 2002;59(8):1231-9.
9. Bhattacharyya B, Paplikar A, Varghese F, Das G, Shukla V, Arshad F, et al. Illiterate Addenbrooke's Cognitive Examination-III in Three Indian Languages: An Adaptation and Validation Study. Arch Clin Neuropsychol. 2024:acad106.
10. Stern Y. Cognitive Reserve. Neuropsychologia. 2009;47(10): 2015-28.
11. Paplikar A, Alladi S, Varghese F, Mekala S, Arshad F, Sharma M, et al. Bilingualism and its implications for neuropsychological evaluation. Arch Clin Neuropsychol. 2021;36(8):1511-22.
12. Venugopal A, Paplikar A, Varghese FA, Thanissery N, Ballal D, Hoskeri RM, et al. Protective effect of bilingualism on aging, MCI, and dementia: A community-based study. Alzheimers Dement. 2024;20(4):2620-31.
13. Alladi S, Bak TH, Duggirala V, Surampudi B, Shailaja M, Shukla AK, et al. Bilingualism delays age at onset of dementia, independent of education and immigration status. Neurology. 2013;81(22):1938-44.
14. Celik S, Kokje E, Meyer P, Frölich L, Teichmann B. Does bilingualism influence neuropsychological test performance in older adults? A systematic review. Appl Neuropsychol Adult. 2022;29(4):855-73.
15. Fernandez AL. Modern neuropsychological tests for a diversity of cultural contexts. Clin Neuropsychol. 2019;33(8):1-8.
16. Ganguli M, Chandra V, Gilby JE, Ratcliff G, Sharma SD, Pandav R, et al. Cognitive test performance in a community-based nondemented elderly sample in rural India: The Indo-U.S. Cross-National Dementia Epidemiology Study. Int Psychogeriatr. 1996;8:507-24.
17. MoCA Cognition. Montreal Cognitive Assessment [online] Available from https://mocacognition.com/paper/ [Last accessed July, 2024].
18. Kaul S, Paplikar A, Varghese F, Alladi S, Sharma M, Dhaliwal RS, et al.; Consortium ICMRCTB. MoCA in five Indian languages: A brief screening tool to diagnose dementia and MCI in a linguistically diverse setting. Int J Geriatr Psychiatry. 2022;37(10).
19. Bajpai S, Upadhyay A, Sati H, Pandey RM, Chaterjee P, Dey AB. Hindi version of Addenbrooke's cognitive examination III: Distinguishing cognitive impairment among older Indians at the lower cut-offs. Clin Interv Aging. 2020;15:329-39.
20. Sharma D, Chaudhary P, Sheth M, Dalal D. Translation, Cultural Adaptation and Validation of ACE III for Assessment of Cognition for Gujarati Population. J Clin Diagn Res. 2018;12(6): 11-4.
21. Das SK, Banerjee TK, Mukherjee CS, Bose P, Biswas A, Hazra A, et al. An urban community-based study of cognitive function among non-demented elderly population in India. Neurol Asia. 2006;11:37-48.
22. Sundar U, Mukhopadhyay A, Shah N, Adsul B. Age-stratified normative cognitive scores in urban and rural populations: A community-based study. Ann Indian Acad Neurol. 2020;23: 403-5.

23. Tiwari SC, Tripathi RK. Development of an Education and Culture Fair Hindi Cognitive Screening Test (HCST) for the Elderly Population of India. Indian J Geriatr Mental Health. 2011;7(2):83-96.
24. Radhakrishnan PJ, Raghunath SP, Mohan D, Rajan R, Iype T. Normative scores for Malayalam cognitive screening test battery among older adults in Kerala, India. Ann Indian Acad Neurol. 2023;26:44-53.
25. Porrselvi AP, Venkateswaran P, Vijayanand S, Webb SS, Ramkumar S, Sneha CR, et al. The cultural and linguistic adaptation of the Oxford Cognitive Screen to Tamil. J Int Neuropsychol Soc. 2023;29(10):964-71.
26. Folstein MF, Folstein SE, McHugh PR. Mini-Mental State Examination. [online] Available from https://www.parinc.com/Products/Pkey/237 [Last accessed July, 2024].
27. Dhikav V, Jadeja B, Gupta P. Community Screening of Probable Dementia at Primary Care Center in Western India: A Pilot Project. J Neurosci Rural Pract. 2022;13(3):490-4.
28. Washington University School of Medicine in St. Louis. Knight Alzheimer Disease Research Center. CDR® Dementia Staging Instrument. [online] Available from https://knightadrc.wustl.edu/professionals-clinicians/cdr-dementia-staging-instrument/ [Last accessed July, 2024].
29. Swati B, Vishnubhatla S. Dementia Assessment by Rapid Test (DART): An Indian Screening Tool for Dementia. J Alzheimer Dis Parkinsonism. 2015;05(03).
30. Iype T, Ajitha BK, Antony P, Ajeeth NB, Job S, Shaji KS. Usefulness of the Rowland Universal Dementia Assessment scale in South India. J Neurol Neurosurg Psychiatry. 2006;77(4):513-4.
31. Stanley R, Kuruvilla A, Kumar S, Gayathri K, Mathews P, Abraham V, et al. The Vellore screening instruments and strategies for the diagnosis of dementia in the community. Int Psychogeriatr. 2009;21(3):539-47.
32. Mini-Cog©. Mini-Cog© Quick Screening for Early Dementia Detection. [online] Available from https://mini-cog.com/ [Last accessed July, 2024].
33. Gopaljee S, Dwivedi C, Pandey R. Psychometric evaluation of the Hindi adaptation of Mattis Dementia Rating Scale (HMDRS). Indian J Social Sci Res. 2011;8(1&2).
34. Chopra S, Kaur H, Pandey RM, Nehra A. Development of neuropsychological evaluation screening tool: An education-free cognitive screening instrument. Neurol India. 2018;66(2):391-9.
35. Panikker D, Bhatt A, Dikshit J, Vas CJ. The Indian adaptation of the Alzheimer's Disease Assessment Scale-Cognitive (ADAS-cog): Standardisation on a community-resident sample of older persons. Int J Geriatr Psychopharmacol. 2000;2(3):142-7.
36. Verghese J, Noone ML, Johnson B, Ambrose AF, Wang C, Buschke H, et al. Picture-based memory impairment screen for dementia. J Am Geriatr Soc. 2012;60(11):2116-20.
37. Iyer GK, Paplikar A, Alladi S, Dutt A, Sharma M, Mekala S, et al. Standardising Dementia Diagnosis Across Linguistic and Educational Diversity: Study Design of the Indian Council of Medical Research-Neurocognitive Tool Box (ICMR-NCTB). J Int Neuropsychol Soc. 2020;26(2):172-86.
38. Pershad D, Verma SK. Handbook of PGI Battery of Brain Dysfunction (PGIBBD). Agra: National Psychological Corporation; 1990.
39. Pershad D, Wig NN. Reliability and validity of a new battery of memory tests. Indian J Psychiatry. 1978;20:76-80.
40. Rao SL, Subbakrishna DK, Gopukumar K. NIMHANS Neuropsychological Battery Manual. Bangalore: NIMHANS Publications; 2004.
41. Tripathi R, Kumar JK, Bharath S, Marimuthu P, Varghese M. Clinical validity of NIMHANS neuropsychological battery for elderly: A preliminary report. Indian J Psychiatry. 2013;55:279-82.
42. Gupta S, Khandelwal SK, Tandon PN, Maheshwari MC, Mehta VS, Sundram KR, et al. The development and standardization of a comprehensive neuropsychological battery in Hindi-Adult form. J Pers Clin Stud. 2000;16:75-109.
43. Sosa AL, Albanese E, Prince M. Population normative data for the 10/66 Dementia Research Group cognitive test battery from Latin America, India, and China: A cross-sectional survey. BMC Neurol. 2009;9:48.
44. Pearson. Pearson Clinical India: Adapted and Standardized Assessments. [online] Available from https://pearsonclinical.in/resources/ [Last accessed July, 2024].
45. Porrselvi AP. TAM battery: Development and pilot testing of a Tamil computer-assisted cognitive test battery for older adults. Clin Neuropsychol. 2023;37(5):1005-24.

CHAPTER

5

Investigative Approach to Treatable Dementias

Vaibhav Seth, Suman Kushwaha

ABSTRACT

Most dementia cases are attributed to neurodegenerative causes. They have a uniform prognosis leading to progressive impairment in multiple cognitive domains. The course and progression may fluctuate but ultimately it leads to the death of the patient and a large-scale caregiver burden. The appropriate management of dementing illness is to be understood by treating clinicians. Not all dementias fall into the domain of Alzheimer's disease (AD) and there might be some component of reversible disease. This must be properly looked at with clinical examination and by appropriate imaging or diagnostic techniques. There are certain atypical features or red flags that should be appropriately sought while examining a patient with dementia in a cognition clinic.

Keywords: Reversible dementia, Cognition clinic, Red flags, Rapidly progressive dementia.

INTRODUCTION

A vast majority of dementia cases seen in clinical practice is attributed to neurodegenerative cases. They have a uniform prognosis leading to progressive impairment in multiple cognitive domains and ultimately death. The appropriate management of dementing illness is to be understood by treating clinicians. Not all dementing illnesses are Alzheimer's disease (AD) and there might be some component of reversible disease in them. This must be properly looked at with clinical examination and by appropriate imaging or diagnostic techniques.

There are certain atypical features or red flags that should be appropriately sought while examining a patient with dementia in a cognition clinic.[1]

These red flag symptoms are as follows:

- Rapidly progressive symptoms and cognition decline
- Symptoms at younger age
- Prominent fluctuations
- Acute or chronic high-risk exposures
- A history of high-risk behaviors (past or present)
- Unexplained or unanticipated findings on the neurologic examination
- Performance on neurocognitive testing that is incongruent with the clinical history

RAPIDLY PROGRESSIVE SYMPTOMS AND COGNITION DECLINE

The term "rapidly progressive dementia" (RPD) is used to describe a cognitive syndrome where there is an accelerated progression and decline leading to impairment in activities of daily living, as defined by the Diagnostic and Statistical Manual of Mental Disorders fourth edition. This progression and decline occurs within a relatively short time period, the cut-off for which varies but is commonly considered to be less than either 1 or 2 years.[2] The spectrum of RPD is highly variable and encompasses different groups of disorders like immune-mediated, infectious and metabolic encephalopathies, and prion diseases. There are other conditions also which include atypical rapid progression of other neurodegenerative diseases. The prion diseases have been considered prototypical RPDs. But the growing spectrum of immune-mediated neurodegeneration and toxic and metabolic plus infective encephalopathy is now considered in the differential diagnosis of prion disease. This needs thorough consideration and ruling out reversible causes. **Flowchart 1** illustrates different causes that can lead to RPD. All patients with RPDs should undergo proper testing to evaluate any reversible etiologies outlined as follows. This includes screening serum studies, neuroimaging [favoring magnetic resonance imaging (MRI)], and routine as well as at times advanced cerebrospinal fluid (CSF) analyses with electroencephalogram (EEG).[3]

Hematological Tests

Routine blood tests done on patients with RPD can provide important information and identify potentially reversible conditions. These conditions include systemic inflammation that can be checked by leukocyte counts and C-reactive protein levels. Electrolytes, markers of liver and kidney injury along with thyroid function can identify potentially reversible various metabolic disorders. Testing for specific infectious diseases such as human immunodeficiency virus (HIV) and syphilis and searching for systemic autoantibodies as well as certain vitamin deficiencies (e.g., vitamin B1, vitamin B12, and folic acid) can be helpful.

Neuroimaging

Computed tomography (CT) scan is important in the emergency setting to exclude intracerebral bleeding or acute hydrocephalus. These disorders can cause acute symptomatic deterioration in patients with chronic neurodegenerative changes. MRI brain is a better modality, and if done with gadolinium contrast administration, can identify tumors and inflammatory lesions, chronic vascular changes, microbleeds, edema, and others. Diffusion-weighted imaging (DWI) imaging can help to identify cortical ribboning, which can be seen in prion diseases. The magnetic resonance angiography is useful to identify vessel occlusion and also visualize stenosis in central nervous system (CNS) vasculitis.[3]

Magnetic resonance imaging abnormalities are reported to be mostly absent in the majority (70% or more) of patients with anti-N-methyl-D-aspartate receptor (anti-NMDAR) **(Fig. 1)** or antidipeptidyl-peptidase-like protein 6 (anti-DPPX) limbic encephalitis.[4] Sometimes individuals with other types of encephalitis

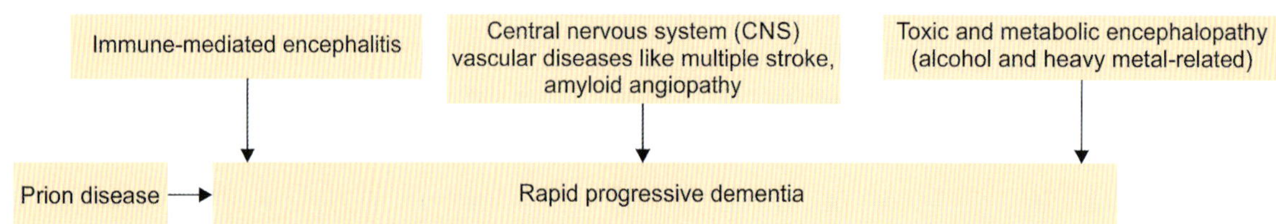

FLOWCHART 1: Different causes leading to rapid cognitive decline.

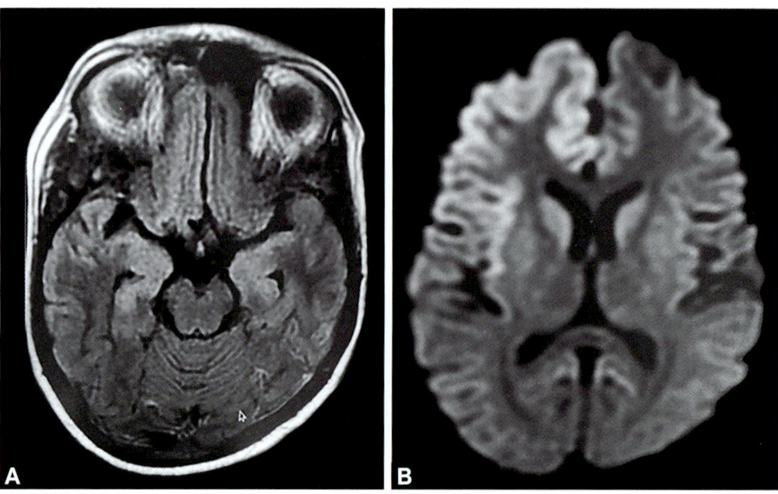

FIGS. 1A AND B: Magnetic resonance imaging (MRI) brain showing (A) T2 fluid-attenuated inversion recovery (FLAIR) hyperintensities in bilateral medial temporal lobes (right > left); and (B) diffusion-weighted imaging (DWI) images showing cortical ribboning in the right superior frontal gyrus and anterior cingulate region in a patient with anti-N-methyl-D-aspartate (anti-NMDA) receptor encephalitis.

Courtesy: Dr Annapurna Patwari, consultant radiologist, Kolkata, India.

are likely to show increased signal in the medial temporal lobes [anti-leucine-rich glioma-inactivated 1 (anti-LGI1), anticontactin-associated protein-like 2 (anti-CASPR2), anti-alpha-amino-3-hydroxy-5-methyl-4-isoxazolepropionic acid receptor (anti-AMPAR), and anti-gamma aminobutyric acid receptor (anti-GABAB receptor)], basal ganglia (antidopamine receptor 2), or multiple cortical and subcortical regions [anti-gamma aminobutyric acid-A (anti-$GABA_A$ receptor).[4]

Cerebrospinal Fluid Analysis

Lumbar puncture and CSF analyses are important diagnostic tools for identifying inflammatory CNS diseases and are essential for the evaluation of RPDs. In initial or emergency evaluation, elevated white blood cell (WBC) counts can rapidly identify encephalitis and meningitis. The CSF lacks a typical inflammatory response in people with prion diseases. In short, inflammatory CSF shall point toward nondegenerative cause of RPD and will need further evaluation. Some neoplastic conditions such as lymphoma and carcinomatous meningitis can have inflammatory CSF. Conversely, immune-mediated encephalitis can lack inflammatory signs in CSF. Strong suspicion is needed in such cases and needs evaluation with autoimmune and paraneoplastic encephalitis panel.

With respect to neurodegenerative dementia, highly sensitive and specific protein biomarker tests have been established for the early diagnosis of AD (p-tau, Aβ42, and the Aβ42/Aβ40 ratio) and Creutzfeldt–Jakob disease (CJD) [real-time quaking-induced conversion (RT-QuIC)]. CJD is also associated with extreme elevation of neuronal injury markers such as CSF total tau protein and neurofilament light chain.

Electroencephalogram Features

Electroencephalogram can detect epileptiform discharges or even nonconvulsive status epilepticus, which should be done urgently. Sometimes, periodic complexes are also to be seen in some patients of CJD. EEG abnormalities like extreme delta brush raise concern for N-methyl-D-aspartate (NMDA) encephalitis.

Nuclear Imaging

Cerebral ^{18}F-Fluorodeoxyglucose (^{18}F-FDG) positron emission tomography (PET) can reveal glucose hypometabolism in specific brain regions. This will be helpful in certain differential diagnoses for RPD like the presence of thalamic hypometabolism in fatal familial insomnia (FFI) or sporadic fatal insomnia or to delineate specific tumor entities. The ^{18}F-FDG PET scan can detect tissue hypometabolism in neurodegenerative diseases that precede MRI changes such as atrophy. Molecular tracers that bind to cerebral beta-amyloid (Aβ) (amyloid-PET) and tau (tau-PET) deposits can identify AD-related pathology at very early stage but are available in selected centers. Certain immune-mediated diseases can give rise to bilateral mesial temporal signal abnormalities on 18F-FDG PET scan. Another advantage offered by a whole-body PET scan is to rule out malignancy.[5]

SYMPTOMS AT YOUNG AGE

Although more likely in younger women (particularly women of childbearing age), autoimmune encephalitis is recognized in patients of all ages and both sexes. The high potential for reversibility justifies testing the CSF and blood for autoantibodies known to be associated with autoimmune encephalitis. Autoantibody testing should be considered in all patients meeting criteria for possible autoimmune encephalitis. They should have features such as subacute onset of memory deficits, altered mental status, or psychiatric symptoms. This should be coupled with at least one of the following: New focal CNS findings, unexplained seizures, CSF pleocytosis, or MRI features suggestive of encephalitis. Testing should likewise be considered in patients 60 years of age or older with characteristic CNS syndrome including unexplained faciobrachial dystonic seizures (FBDS); gait instability, brainstem dysfunction, and sleep disorder; or subacute confusion and memory loss.[6] When diagnostic uncertainty persists, additional disease-specific biomarkers may help to clarify the diagnosis (e.g., CJD-specific biomarkers like 14-3-3). In a similar fashion, empiric treatment of autoimmune encephalitis may be considered with close monitoring. Many causes of autoimmune encephalitis are treatment-responsive initially, but later on, may have a rapid decline and turn into CJD.[6]

PROMINENT FLUCTUATIONS

Prominent fluctuations are usually features of dementia with Lewy bodies. But they can also can also be a manifestation of reversible dementias.

There are various reversible dementia that can have fluctuations:

- *Sleep Apnea*: Sleep apnea patients have snoring and excessive daytime sleepiness as the predominant complaints but some patients may have systemic signs and symptoms like hypertension, depression, and cognitive decline. The mechanism postulated for cognitive decline is multifactorial. Some say due to small strokes that happen silently in such patients. The reason could be night time hypoxia with increased deposition of Abeta in brain coupled with decreased clearance. Sleep apnea also causes hippocampal atrophy.

- . Treatment of sleep apnea may improve cognition. Treatment with continuous positive pressure ventilation improves cognition impairment in the majority of cases. Donepezil has been tried in certain cases.[7]
- *Alcoholism*: Alcohol intake has a profound influence on cognitive decline, especially among those above 65 years of age. The effect mostly takes a J-shaped curve. Alcohol-related dementia can occur either due to direct alcohol-related damage or due to potentially other causes that cause reversible cognitive damage. They include thiamine deficiency, chronic liver disease, seizures, traumatic brain injury, and other concurrent substance abuse disorders. The brain structures that are predominantly affected are prefrontal and motor cortex. These affected areas experience shrinkage with regular alcohol use but on cessation of drinking there may be an improvement in cognition function.[7]
- *Tumors or space-occupying lesions (SOL)*: Certain tumors and SOL or even subdural hematomas cause cognitive decline, so their prompt recognition is important. Removal of such agents can cause its reversibility **(Fig. 2)**.
- *Miscellaneous causes*: Rarer reversible causes of dementia may also warrant consideration when supported by history and examination, including transient epileptic amnesia. Transient epileptic amnesia is associated with acute and transient memory disruptions lasting minutes (typically <1 hour) that are often accompanied by fluctuations in attention and amnesia. Although the symptomatic expression may lead to an initial diagnosis of transient global amnesia, the frequency of attacks (recurrent attacks occurring a median of 12 times per year) and brief duration (median duration 30–60 minutes) commonly distinguish patients with transient epileptic amnesia. EEG may be helpful in establishing the diagnosis of transient epileptic amnesia, with epileptiform abnormalities or nonspecific focal slow waves detected in many affected patients.

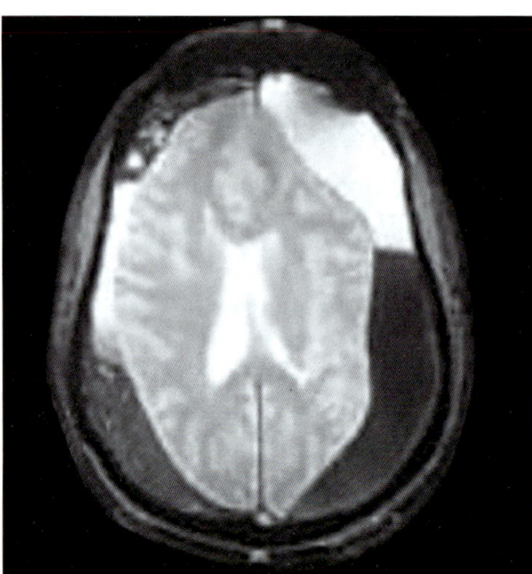

FIG. 2: Magnetic resonance imaging (MRI) brain with gradient echo (GRE) sequencing showing bilateral acute on a chronic subdural hematoma in a patient on dabigatran presenting with 3-week history of rapid cognitive decline. There was no history of trauma.
Courtesy: Dr Annapurna Patwari, consultant radiologist, Kolkata, India.

HIGH-RISK EXPOSURES

Careful screening for high-risk medications (including over-the-counter medications), drugs, and toxins is imperative when making a new diagnosis of dementia. Narcotic, benzodiazepine, and anticholinergic medications are common precipitants of cognitive decline. Patients with other active health issues like chronic liver disease or chronic kidney disease may be particularly vulnerable to the cognition-impairing effects of medications. Anticholinergic medications and drugs that have certain anticholinergic effects like first-generation antipsychotics are very problematic in patients with AD. This is because there is associated degeneration of basal forebrain cells, which produce the neurotransmitter acetylcholine. These medications may even contribute to the progression of neurodegenerative pathology raising the question whether we should use these drugs in demented patients. Several tools are there that help us to identify drugs that can be potentially more harmful for cognition, one of them is the American Geriatrics Society (AGS) 2023 updated Beers criteria.[8]

Excessive alcohol consumption leads to Wernicke encephalopathy (WE) due to depletion of vitamin B1 (thiamine). Those patients with an active or recent history of alcohol abuse should be considered at risk for the acute and chronic sequelae of WE. Thiamine is an essential vitamin critical to glucose metabolism, which is an integral part of brain function and brain metabolism. Without thiamine, glucose is metabolized via anaerobic pathways. This leads to intracellular acidosis, mostly of periventricular structures like thalami, mammillary bodies, and oculomotor nuclei. These lead to cardinal manifestations of WE like altered mental status, ocular abnormalities, and gait dysfunction. If promptly recognized, the life-threatening effects of thiamine deficiency may be prevented by administering high doses of parenteral thiamine. It is especially important to know that thiamine is to be replenished before refeeding or even parenteral administration of glucose-containing fluids. This is because of the fact that loading with carbohydrates shall increase the consumption of already depleted thiamine. This shall worsen the clinical manifestations of WE. If overlooked and untreated, the consequences of thiamine deficiency may become irreversible. This can lead to death or severe cognitive impairment in the form of Korsakoff amnestic syndrome.

HISTORY OF HIGH-RISK BEHAVIOR

History of high-risk behavior like multiple sexual partners or use of intravenous (IV) drugs increases the risk of certain infections, as in a study by Chandra et al.[9] showed neurocysticercosis as one of the most common infections to cause dementia. Other infections that can cause infection-related dementia, especially in tropical countries, are tuberculosis, Whipple's disease, syphilis, herpes simplex encephalitis, and subacute sclerosing panencephalitis (SSPE). Neurosyphilis is a great masquerade of diseases in such conditions. Clinical findings like trombone tongue, if sought properly, can clinch the diagnosis.

UNEXPLAINED/UNANTICIPATED FINDINGS ON THE NEUROLOGIC EXAMINATION

The insidious onset and slow progression of short-term memory deficits in an older patient most commonly denote a diagnosis of symptomatic AD. However, the neurologic examination should be largely normal in patients with amnestic AD because the motor and sensory cortices are spared by neuropathology in AD. So, if there are subtle motor signs, they warrant the consideration of atypical AD and most importantly reversible diseases. The detection of progressive memory loss, gait apraxia, and urinary incontinence may be associated with a diagnosis of normal pressure hydrocephalus (NPH), justifying further evaluation. NPH may occur even with the presence of one or two features of the triad. It is not necessary that all features must be present at the same time. NPH is a reversible subcortical dementia. Any dementing illness with motor features should prompt consideration of NPH. If needed, CSF flow study and therapeutic CSF removal trial are to be done.[10]

INCONGRUENT COGNITIVE TESTING

Performance on cognitive testing that is substantially better or worse than expected from the clinical history should trigger investigations for reversible causes of dementia.

Hearing and visual impairment can substantially increase cognition load and worsen dementia. It is unclear if this is a chance association. Hearing impairment is the most common sensory impairment in the population. Impaired hearing leads to social withdrawal, depression, and dementia. Initial screening should focus on the detection of conditions known to compromise the encoding and recall of learned information, resulting in inconsistent or widely fluctuating performance on tasks or subjective symptoms. Even visual impairment can lead to worsening cognition, social withdrawal, and hallucinations like in Charles Bonnet syndrome which can be confused with psychiatric disorder. Behavioral variant frontotemporal dementia (bvFTD) represents an important irreversible cause of incongruent findings on history and test performance. There is a disparity in symptoms and also in objective performance on formal cognitive testing due to the early loss of social judgment and empathy. There is a relative preservation of memory and visuospatial function.[10]

REFERENCES

1. Djukic M, Wedekind D, Franz A, Gremke M, Nau R. Frequency of dementia syndromes with a potentially treatable cause in geriatric in-patients: Analysis of a 1-year interval. Eur Arch Psychiatry Clin Neurosci. 2015;265(5):429-38.
2. Geschwind MD. Rapidly progressive dementia. Continuum (Minneap Minn). 2016;22(2 Dementia):510-37.
3. Hermann P, Zerr I. Rapidly progressive dementias—aetiologies, diagnosis and management. Nat Rev Neurol. 2022;18(6):363-76.
4. Dalmau J, Graus F. Antibody-mediated encephalitis. N Engl J Med. 2018;378(9):840-51.
5. Katsanos AH, Alexiou GA, Fotopoulos AD, Jabbour P, Kyritsis AP, Sioka C. Performance of 18F-FDG, 11C-methionine, and 18F-FET PET for glioma grading: A meta-analysis. Clin Nucl Med. 2019;44(11):864-9.
6. Seth V, Kushwaha S, Verma R, Patel PM, Kiran Gowda R, et al. Autoimmune encephalitis versus Creutzfeldt-Jakob disease in a patient with typical facio-brachial dystonic seizures: A case report with diagnostic challenges. Brain Behav Immun Health. 2021;13:100236.
7. Little MO. Reversible dementias. Clin Geriatr Med. 2018;34(4):537-62.
8. By the 2023 American Geriatrics Society Beers Criteria® Update Expert Panel. American Geriatrics Society 2023 updated AGS Beers Criteria® for potentially inappropriate medication use in older adults. J Am Geriatr Soc. 2023;71(7):2052-81.
9. Chandra SR, Viswanathan LG, Pai AR, Wahatule R, Alladi S. Syndromes of Rapidly Progressive Cognitive Decline-Our Experience. J Neurosci Rural Pract. 2017;8(Suppl 1):S66-71.
10. Day GS. Reversible dementias. Continuum (Minneap Minn). 2019;25(1):234-53.

CHAPTER

6

Alzheimer's Dementia: Clinical Presentations and Advances in Management

Kuntal Biswas, Atanu Biswas

ABSTRACT

Classically, Alzheimer's disease (AD) is seen in persons above 65 years of age with progressive amnestic disorder with subsequent impairment of other cognitive functions. Around one-third patients of AD may present with visuospatial/perceptual dysfunction, language deficits, dysexecutive, behavioral, or corticobasal syndrome. These atypical AD patients usually have younger age of onset and rapid progression. Diagnosis of these atypical AD is difficult due to overlapping clinical features with other diseases and requires careful clinical assessment supplemented by biomarkers support. Drugs targeting amyloid and *tau* are considered to be effective in modifying the disease course. As disease has a long preclinical stage when pathology gradually develops before subjects become symptomatic, early diagnosis with molecular imaging and/or biomarkers is essential. Recent approval of lecanemab, a monoclonal antibody against amyloid protofibrils by the United States Food and Drug Administration (US FDA) for treatment of mild AD, raises hope for successful management of the disease. However, as successful amyloid clearance is not linearly related with clinical improvement, many other targets including oxidative stress, inflammation, mitochondrial dysfunction, etc. and targeting multiple pathomechanisms together could be the effective treatment strategy in future.

Keywords: Alzheimer's disease, Amnestic, Atypical, Lecanemab, Management, Young-onset.

INTRODUCTION

Alzheimer's disease (AD) is the most common cause of dementia in the community across the globe. Pathologically, AD is characterized by the presence of extracellular amyloid plaques comprised of amyloid-β (Aβ) peptide and intracellular neurofibrillary tangles (NFT) comprised of hyperphosphorylated *tau* protein, along with neurodegeneration.[1]

More than a century ago, AD was described in a German lady in her 50s with cognitive and behavioral disorders who had plaques and NFTs in her brain. A disease which was known as presenile dementia for a long without much progress in the understanding became a global concern in last few decades. The concept of AD was later expanded to include senile dementia, affecting patients over the age of 65 years (also known as late-onset AD). The first diagnostic criteria were formulated in 1984, which defined probable AD as a predominantly amnestic disorder in which other cognitive domains could also get affected.[2] It necessitated postmortem biopsy of brain to confirm the diagnosis. This was unique in clinical medicine as the criteria required pathological confirmation for making a definite diagnosis. Most of the studies in 1990s focused AD as amnestic syndrome with imaging findings highlighting atrophy of the hippocampus.[3] Neuropathological findings showed *tau* pathology, which correlated with clinical events, spreads from the transentorhinal region to the hippocampus, the lateral temporal, parietal, and other cortical regions.[4] Studies also showed that incidence of amnestic AD increased with age, substantiating the concept of AD being an amnestic disease affecting the elderly.

Typically, these subjects demonstrate loss of "recent episodic memory" recognized as memory loss "of the hippocampal type."[5] Memory impairment of recent events, unusual repeated omissions, and difficulty in learning new information characterize the first clinical signs of AD. Pathologically, in early stages of AD (Braak stage I–III), NFTs are restricted to medial temporal regions (hippocampal formations, parahippocampal gyrus, and entorhinal cortex) and consequently, episodic memory deficit is the initial and reliable neuropsychological marker of AD. Thereafter, deficits in other cognitive domains such as visuospatial function, language, praxis, and gnosis become evident. This corroborates with the progression of the underlying cerebral lesions into the neocortical association areas (Braak V).

Subsequently, various studies were reported in 1980s and 90s with pathological evidence of AD who had nonamnestic clinical presentation before death. Pathologically, these atypical presentations were associated with different distribution of *tau* pathology (NFTs). Radiologically, these were associated with different atrophy pattern in various cortices with relative sparing the hippocampus. They were collectively defined as hippocampal-sparing variant of AD as compared to limbic-predominant AD with greater involvement of hippocampus.[6] These presentations were collectively termed atypical AD, primary presentations of which include visual and visuospatial, language, frontal executive function, etc. These patients usually have younger age of onset and account for one third of all AD cases with rapid progression of the disease course.[7] Since the early 2000s, there has been increasing recognition and characterization of atypical variants of AD.

Insights were gained from longitudinal studies and it became clear that the disease has a prolonged preclinical phase during which pathology accumulates over 10–20 years, but individuals remain cognitively unimpaired. With the advent of magnetic resonance imaging (MRI), cerebrospinal fluid (CSF) biomarkers and amyloid and *tau* positron emission tomography (PET), the new diagnostic criteria were proposed by the International Working Group (IWG).[8] Subsequently, the National Institute of Aging and Alzheimer's Association (NIA–AA) working groups provided biomarker-based criteria.[9] The new diagnostic algorithm, aptly known as ATN criteria, recognizes the pathological roles of amyloid (A), and *tau* (T) which in turn result into neurodegeneration (N).

Several important developments are included in these criteria. Firstly, it defines AD as a clinicobiological entity, a major shift from McKhann criteria of 1984, which defined the disease as a clinicopathological entity. Secondly, a prolonged preclinical stage is recognized and mild cognitive impairment (MCI) is considered as prodromal AD when supported by biomarkers. Thirdly, atypical presentations are acknowledged and a diagnosis of AD with such atypical presentation can be made if supported by biomarkers.

During the long preclinical phase when brain accumulates AD pathology, individuals remain functionally normal in the community. Once a threshold is reached, symptoms appear, but the subject continues to function normally. Subjective memory complaints are the very early symptoms for typical amnestic form of the disease. For atypical forms, complaints are often missed by the carer and even by the physician, leading to delay in diagnosis. MCI is the phase when persons exhibit impairment in cognitive function in neuropsychological testing, but instrumental activities of daily living (IADL) remain unimpaired. In contrast, impairment of IADL makes a diagnosis of early AD. Assessment of IADL is crucial and care needs to be taken for deciding its impairment in an individual. In Indian societies, elderly are quiet often not allowed to perform complex activities such as shopping, travelling alone, financial transaction, and decision-making, resulting in erroneous impression of preservation of IADL. Biological diagnosis of AD is possible in MCI stage with the help of biomarkers. In India, amyloid and *tau* PET are not available, but CSF-based biomarkers are now launched commercially, although relatives and physicians are not finding these worthy as disease-modifying therapies are yet unavailable in the country.

VISUAL VARIANT OF ALZHEIMER'S DISEASE

Also known as posterior cortical atrophy (PCA), these patients present with early higher-order visual dysfunction with visuospatial and perceptual difficulties with preserved recent episodic memory. They often get a psychiatric diagnosis or are evaluated for ophthalmic cause and even receive cataract surgery before being recognized as having a neurological disease. Difficulties include finding objects even when these are in plain sight, frequent bumping on objects, difficulty in judging distance of a moving car, difficulty in navigating uneven surfaces such as going up and down stairs, accidents while veering out of the lane during driving, difficulty in putting objects together, or dressing. Careful examination reveals features of Bálint syndrome (simultanagnosia, optic ataxia, and oculomotor apraxia) due to bilateral affection of superior parietal lobule or Gerstmann syndrome (left/right disorientation, finger agnosia, dyscalculia, and dysgraphia) due to affection of dominant angular gyrus, with various degrees of limb or constructional or dressing apraxia, suggesting dorsal variant affecting occipitoparietal cortices.[10] The ventral variant is characterized by apperceptive agnosia, prosopagnosia, and sometimes alexia with letter-by-letter reading suggesting affection of occipitotemporal network.[10] In rare caudal variant, patient may have visual field defect or diminished visual acuity. In the early phase, insight and other cognitive domains usually remain preserved. However, attention and working memory deficits are sometimes observed even in early stage. In some patients, myoclonus, dystonia, or extrapyramidal signs may be evident, suggestive of other neuropathologic entities, such as corticobasal degeneration (CBD) or dementia with Lewy bodies (DLB). In around 96% of patients, an underlying AD pathology is described.[11] Neuroimaging reveals atrophy corresponding to the observed clinical syndrome. The classic structural imaging finding is posterior-predominant atrophy with involvement of the visual association cortices and, in the caudal variant, also the primary visual cortex. The pattern of *tau* distribution observed on *tau* PET closely corresponds to the atrophy pattern, whereas amyloid is diffusely distributed throughout the brain. Fluorodeoxyglucose-(FDG)-PET findings consist of posterior-predominant hypometabolism largely matching the *tau* distribution and the brain atrophy.

LANGUAGE VARIANT

Some subjects present with difficulty in communication with anomia and word-finding pauses. When carefully tested, they are found to have trouble with sentence repetition and phonological sounds' errors with mispronouncing words (phonemic paraphasias) and circumlocution. Some of these patients meet the criteria of logopenic variant of primary progressive aphasia (PPA), although in majority of these subjects, presence of other cognitive dysfunction such as amnesia and executive dysfunction preclude a diagnosis of PPA. Of logopenic variant PPA cases, 86–90% are due to AD, compared to only 11–16% of cases of semantic dementia, and 15–20% of cases of nonfluent/agrammatic variant PPA.[11]

On testing, these patients show difficulties in confrontation naming, and reduced verbal fluency for both animals and letter, with phonemic paraphasias. Comprehension is reduced, but semantic knowledge and single-word comprehension are usually preserved. Spontaneous speech is relatively fluent, but filler words and circumlocutions are frequent, with normal grammatical speech with no motor speech disorder.

Amyloid deposition in logopenic PPA is diffuse as in PCA, *tau*-PET and FDG-PET show *tau* deposition, and hypometabolism, respectively involving the lateral temporal and temporoparietal cortices of the left side.

DYSEXECUTIVE AND BEHAVIORAL VARIANTS

Relatively rare presentation of AD with only 2% of cases can have dysexecutive and behavioral variants.[12] Predominant symptoms of core executive dysfunctions including deficits in working memory, planning, judgment, impairment of cognitive flexibility, cognitive inhibitory control, difficulty in multitasking, etc., very early in the disease course without recent episodic memory deficit signifies this variant. These patients are often confused with behavioral variant of frontotemporal dementia (bvFTD). Even the atrophy pattern in MRI does not help in differentiating. Lack of marked behavioral symptoms and personality changes help in differentiating dysexecutive variant of AD from patients of bvFTD.

Behavioral variant AD has remarkable similarities with bvFTD with change of personality, lack of empathy, disinhibition, and disregard of social and societal norms, apathy, obsessive-compulsive behaviors, and also rarely hyperorality. It is very difficult to differentiate this form of AD from bvFTD clinically. Presence of neuropsychiatric symptoms such as delusions and hallucinations are few points favoring behavioral AD.

As with all atypical AD, amyloid deposition is more diffuse, but structural imaging shows prominent frontal atrophy with relative preservation of medial temporal lobes. In frontal variant AD, *tau* PET reveals prominent *tau* tracer retention in the frontal lobes in addition to the classic medial, inferior and lateral temporal, and lateral parietal distribution.

CORTICOBASAL SYNDROME

Corticobasal syndrome (CBS) is also known as motor or praxic variant of AD. These individuals are dyspraxic, with difficulty in performing motor tasks, pantomime gestures, loss of tool knowledge, or difficulties in using tools despite having no motor or sensory deficits. They also develop asymmetric rigidity, bradykinesia, dystonia, myoclonus, cortical sensory deficits, and rarely alien limb phenomenon. These subjects do not have problem in recent episodic memory, although this may become evident in later years. Neuropsychologically, they have prominent visuoconstructional deficits, anomia, apraxia of speech, and executive dysfunction. Although CBS is most commonly linked with corticobasal degeneration (CBD), a four-repeat *tau*-pathy, neuropathologic studies have reported that 15–54% of cases are due to AD.[13] Distinguishing CBS–CBD from CBS–AD is not straightforward because of significant overlap in clinical presentation. Molecular imaging and CSF biomarker assessments will be helpful in establishing the diagnosis of AD.

NEUROPATHOLOGICAL UNDERPINNING OF ATYPICAL AND TYPICAL ALZHEIMER'S DISEASE

The pattern of cortical *tau* deposition observed in *tau* PET imaging matches with pattern of cortical atrophy and with regional distribution of NFTs in neuropathological studies in patients with atypical AD as well as in young-onset amnestic AD. Distribution of NFTs is correlated with neurodegeneration with resultant cerebral hypometabolism, volume loss, and clinical manifestation.

In late-onset amnestic AD, however, the relationship of *tau* uptake does not correlate with volume loss of medial temporal lobe. Late-onset AD is pathologically heterogeneous, where besides amyloid and *tau*, TDP-43 is implicated in a large proportion of cases, particularly in the oldest old and coexistent vascular pathology is not uncommon.

Atypical AD is a group of disorders with diverse clinical manifestation but pathologically unified by *tau* deposition, a strong marker of the disease. However, clinical homogeneity in typical late-onset amnestic AD is pathologically diverse. Based on these observations, AD is considered as a syndrome with marked clinical as well as pathological heterogeneity.

HOW TO MAKE A DIAGNOSIS OF ATYPICAL ALZHEIMER'S DISEASE?

Clinically, it is challenging to make a diagnosis of atypical AD as features overlap with other diseases. However, a careful elicitation of history of evolution of symptoms, subsequent involvement of other cognitive domains, associated behavioral and psychiatric symptoms, and motor manifestations help in making a clinical diagnosis. As in all degenerative diseases, one-time assessment may be insufficient for diagnostic labeling and follow-up assessment is required to look into the evolution of clinical findings for the diagnosis. Application of molecular PET imaging that can detect β-amyloid and *tau* deposition in the antemortem brain have made the diagnosis of AD in patients with these clinical presentations much easier during life. Evidence of deposition on both β-amyloid and *tau* PET scans provides a biomarker diagnosis of AD.[3] Most patients diagnosed with the visual and language variants of AD at specialist centers have biomarker evidence for AD.[14]

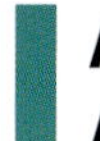

ADVANCES IN MANAGEMENT OF ALZHEIMER'S DISEASE

Currently, single-target drugs such as acetylcholinesterase inhibitors (AChEI) and memantine, an N-methyl D-aspartate (NMDA) receptor antagonist, have been approved, but there is a growing interest in developing multitarget drugs that can address various aspects of AD pathology, including Aβ deposition, *tau* protein phosphorylation, oxidative stress, and mitochondrial autophagy dysfunction, which are currently undergoing clinical trials **(Table 1)**.[15]

Antiamyloid Therapy

Main target of antiamyloid therapies is to reduce Aβ burden in brain and subsequent cognitive improvement.

β-secretase Inhibition

These drugs are formulated to reduce Aβ production by targeting beta-site amyloid precursor protein (APP)-cleaving enzyme 1 (BACE1, also known as β-secretase 1). Verubecestat (MK-8931) was the first in this category to enter phase III trial because of its ability to cross the blood brain barrier (BBB) and improve bioavailability but two phase III clinical trials, EPOCH and APECS, were terminated prematurely after the drug failed to improve cognitive decline in participants and increased adverse events (AE).[16,17] Other drugs were lanabecestat, atabecestat, umibecestat, and elenbecestat. Each of these agent showed some benefits in phase I and II trials, but all of them either failed to show promising effect in phase III trials or had moderate-to-severe adverse effects during study period.[18-21]

γ-secretase inhibition

Semagacestat (LY450139) is a nonselective small-molecule γ secretase inhibitor that targets the same mechanism as that of β-secretase inhibitors. Initially, it showed some efficacy in open-label, randomized crossover phase III clinical trial. Additionally, the drug was well tolerated during the trial and no safety concerns were reported. Later, this trial had to be discontinued due to higher rate of adverse effects, e.g., weight loss, skin malignancy, and infection.[22]

Active Immunization

The first anti-Aβ vaccine (AN1792) demonstrated some success in eliminating Aβ plaques, initially. However, in the phase IIa clinical trial, approximately

TABLE 1: Summary of various drugs and their mechanism of action.

Drug	Classification	Mechanisms	Problem
Monoclonal antibodies	Disease modifying	Target the amyloid protein	Monoclonal antibody has not succeeded because cognitive decline usually does not correlate with amyloid deposition
Gamma (γ)-secretase inhibitors	Disease modifying	Targeting γ-secretase which reduce amyloid production	Neither significant improvement nor worsening after 3 months of treatment. Side effects were reported with higher doses
Tau inhibitors	Disease modifying	Reduces *tau* aggregation and NFT formation	Long treatment failed to show clinically significant improvement
Neurochemical enhancers	Symptomatic	Idalopiridine that inhibits 5-hydroxytryptamine 6 (5-HT6), acts as procholinergic effector	Further study did not show promising results
Miscellaneous	Symptomatic	Affects α-adrenergic and serotonergic receptors, AMPA and NMDA glutamate receptors, and L-type voltage-gated calcium channels	Although phase II trial showed hope, phase III trial did not show promising result

(AMPA: α-amino-3-hydroxy-5-methyl-4-isoxazolepropionic acid; NFT: neurofibrillary tangles; NMDA: N-methyl D-aspartate)

6% of patients with AD treated with AN1792 developed meningoencephalitis, leading to the termination of the trial.[23] Similar fate has been observed with another molecule CAD106 which was discontinued due to serious AE, for example, cognitive impairments, changes in brain volume, and weight loss in participants.[24]

Passive Immunization

Bapineuzumab is a humanized monoclonal antibody developed to target Aβ to reduce its abnormal deposition. In two phase III trials (NCT00575055 and NCT00574132), bapineuzumab did not show any significant improvement of cognitive function and it was associated with amyloid-related imaging abnormalities (ARIA) with effusion or edema (ARIA-E).[25]

Crenezumab and ponezumab, an immunoglobulin G4 (IgG4) and IgG2 monoclonal antibody, respectively, did not show much benefit in phase III clinical trials.[26,27]

On the other hand, gantenerumab is an IgG monoclonal antibody that accelerates the clearance of Aβ plaques through Fc receptor-mediated phagocytosis and showed promising effect in clinical trials. About 1,200 mg dose of gantenerumab could stably clear Aβ plaques and no serious AE were reported after large-volume subcutaneous injection in these studies.[28]

Donanemab is another promising agent that completed phase III trial in 2023. Four studies showed good Aβ clearance and low *tau* accumulation, but there was significant proportion of adverse effects in the form of ARIA and ARIA-E in these studies.[29,30]

Another promising agent aducanumab, a monoclonal antibody that targets both soluble and insoluble Aβ and selectively binds to Aβ, received approval from the United States Food and Drug Administration (US FDA) on June 7, 2021. It was the first new drug for the treatment of AD for 20 years and it is currently under regulatory review in Japan and Europe to assess its safety and tolerability for long-term use. However, like donanemab, this drug can also cause significant incidence of ARIA and ARIA-E.[31] European Medical Agency (EMA) revoked the commercial approval for aducanumab in April 2022 considering the fact that a decrease in brain Aβ aggregates is insufficient as a biomarker to anticipate clinical benefit.[32]

Lecanemab is a monoclonal antibody that recognizes protofibrils and prevents Aβ deposition in AD. It got its accelerated approval from the US FDA in January 2023 and got full approval in July 2023. CLARITY AD, a phase III randomized, controlled clinical trial was done to evaluate efficacy of lecanemab. It was a multicenter, randomized, double-blind, placebo-controlled, parallel-group study that enrolled 1,795 participants with MCI or mild dementia patients with Aβ pathology. Participants were randomized to receive placebo or lecanemab at a dose of 10 mg/kg, once every 2 weeks. Lecanemab demonstrated a statistically and clinically significant reduction of decline from baseline to 18 months on the primary endpoint, the Clinical Dementia Rating Scale Sum of Boxes score, compared to placebo. Lecanemab also demonstrated efficacy on all secondary endpoints, for example, Alzheimer's Disease Assessment Scale Cognitive Subscale 14 and the Alzheimer's Disease Cooperative Study-Activities of Daily Living Scale for Mild Cognitive Impairment.[33] However, like its predecessor lecanemab also showed tendency to cause ARIA and ARIA-E, but serious life-threatening events are very rare.

Anti-*tau* Therapy

The treatment of anti-*tau* drugs mainly includes three targets: Preventing *tau* hyperphosphorylation and aggregation, stabilizing microtubules, and accelerating *tau* clearance.

Glycogen Synthase Kinase-3 Beta Inhibitor

Tideglusib is a thiadiazole which inhibits *glycogen synthase kinase-3 beta* (GSK-3β) irreversibly and reduces *tau* phosphorylation. Double-blind, placebo-controlled phase II trial did not show any clinical efficacy of GSK-3 inhibitors till date.[34]

Lithium has been used in psychiatric diseases for long and it has been found to be an inhibitor of GSK-3, involved in glucose metabolism, cell signaling and proliferation, and glial cell function regulation. Lithium also showed to prevent amyloid formation and *tau* hyperphosphorylation. Although there have been some case reports as well as case control studies showing that lithium can reduce the symptoms of AD but clinically available lithium has serious adverse effects. Further studies are needed to prove its long-term benefit and a safer dose for long-term use.[35]

Tau Aggregation Inhibitor

Methylene blue is also a drug with a long history of use in clinical practice, primarily in methemoglobinemia, and carbon monoxide poisoning. It failed to show clinical benefit for AD in a 24-week phase II study.[36]

Low-dose Leuco-Methylthioninium Bis(Hydromethanesulphonate) (LMTM) is another compound with a higher bioavailability and lower toxicity than methylene blue. In one phase III trial involving mild-to-moderate AD, LMTM failed to show any clinical benefit.[37]

Two agents, TRx-0014 (Rember) (completed phase II trial) and TRx0237 (completed phase III trial) have been studied recently. TRx-0014 did not show any clear clinical benefit, but TRx0237 showed benefit in mild-to-moderate AD patients with improvement in Alzheimer Disease Assessment Scale (ADAS-Cog).[38,39]

Microtubules Stabilization

Davunetide, derived from the neuroprotective fragment of activity-dependent neuroprotective protein (ADNP), is responsible for controlling signaling pathways regulating the cytoskeleton, direct microtubule end-binding protein interaction facilitating microtubule dynamics, and *tau* microtubule interaction at the microtubule end-binding protein site. A placebo-controlled phase I study with amnestic MCI was done showing its safety and tolerability. However, it failed to show any significant efficacy later on.[40]

Active Immunotherapy

AADvac1 is a peptide that contains one of the epitopes of antibody DC8E8. Phase I trial with AADvac1 showed no adverse immune reactions or any microhemorrhages. It also slowed decline in cognitive impairment in phase II trial.[41] However, further studies needed to prove its long-term benefit and safety.

Passive Immunotherapy

Tilavonemab is the humanized anti-*tau* IgG4 antibody, which was found to be safe and tolerable in phase I trials but found nonsignificant efficacy in treating patients with early AD in phase II trials.[42]

Semorinemab is another anti-*tau* antibody that targets maximum binding across different extracellular *tau* species. Till date, two phase I semorinemab studies have been completed with prodromal/probable AD and another with moderate AD patients. Both trials showed improvement in the clinical characteristics of patients with AD.[43] **Flowchart 1** shows the various drugs and their action.

Mitochondrial Targeting Therapy

It has been seen in various studies that coenzyme Q (CoQ) and its synthetic analog, idebenone, can enhance mitochondrial electron transport chain activity, and exhibit antioxidant- and free radical-scavenging activity. However, they have failed to show any promising effect on disease modification.[44]

Peroxisome proliferator-activated receptor (PPAR)-γ agonists such as thiazolidinediones, pioglitazone, and rosiglitazone have been studied and showed improvement in brain functioning. However, clinical trials (REFLECT-2 and REFLECT-3) that have been done on MCI and mild AD patients did not show a statistically significant improvement in cognitive function.[45]

Dimebon showed strong neuroprotective and cognition-enhancing effects in different animal models. Even in phase II clinical trials on human subjects, it showed a strong beneficial effect on cognition in patients with AD. Unfortunately, phase III trial failed to show such promising effects later on.[46]

Idalopirdine is a molecule that inhibits 5-hydroxytryptamine 6 (5-HT6) receptors and consequently enhances the release of acetylcholine, i.e., it acts as procholinergic effector. A phase II study of idalopirdine plus donepezil therapy showed a significant improvement in cognitive performance, such as in ADAS-Cog and Mini-Mental State Examination (MMSE) scores, but phase III development programs for idalopirdine showed no statistically significant efficacy.[47]

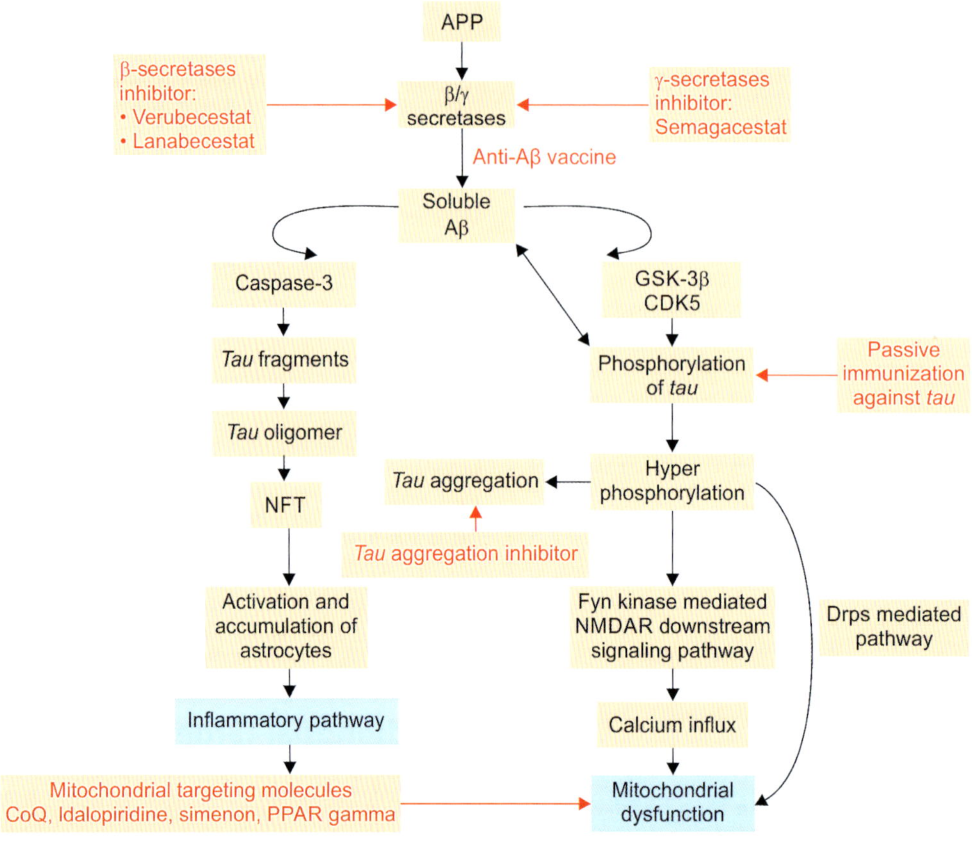

FLOWCHART 1: Correlation between Aβ and *tau* pathology and drugs acting on various levels of this pathway.
(Aβ: amyloid-β; APP: amyloid precursor protein; CDK5: cyclin-dependent kinase 5; CoQ: coenzyme Q; GSK-3β: glycogen synthase kinase-3 beta; NFT: neurofibrillary tangles; NMDAR: N-methyl-D-aspartate receptor; PPAR: peroxisome proliferator-activated receptor)

CONCLUSION

The clinical spectrum of AD has expanded over time. While typical late-onset amnestic form is the most common, it is pathologically diverse. On the contrary, nonamnestic forms and young-onset amnestic variety, considered as atypical forms are now included in NIA-AA diagnostic criteria and are clinically heterogeneous but harbor *tau* pathology in clinically relevant brain areas along with widespread amyloid pathology in brain. The atypical variants constitute one third of all AD cases and are difficult to diagnose due to overlap with other diseases. Biomarkers will help clinicians to make a diagnosis of AD in these atypical forms.

Amyloid and *tau* proteins play orchestrated role in AD where amyloid acts as trigger and *tau* as bullet. Although these two proteins play key roles in the pathogenesis, treatments targeting amyloid or *tau* alone did not produce satisfactory results. Recent success of antiamyloid therapies supports the role of amyloid in the pathogenesis, offers hope for a better life of AD sufferers, and also raises many questions. That removal of amyloid from the brain alone is not sufficient for clinical benefit, demand search for therapies targeting other pathways. Various inflammatory and mitochondrial pathways are also involved in this complex nature of the disease. Such complexity should be addressed in disease management for better treatment outcomes. The multi-target-directed ligands (MTDLs) approach is one of the most promising therapeutic interventions of future for these types of complex multifactorial diseases.[48,49] This strategy targets system's biology pathways rather than selectively targeting individual proteins or drug targets, i.e., drugs and/or technologies designed to interact with more than one target involved in the pathogenesis of a defined disease, going beyond the "one-molecule, one-target" system.[50]

REFERENCES

1. McDade EM. Alzheimer disease. Continuum (Minneap Minn). 2022;28:648-75.
2. McKhann G, Drachman D, Folstein M, Katzman R, Price D, Stadlan EM. Clinical diagnosis of Alzheimer's disease: report of the NINCDS-ADRDA work group under the auspices of Department of Health and Human Services Task Force on Alzheimer's disease. Neurology. 1984;34:939-44.
3. Jack CR Jr, Petersen RC, O'Brien PC, Tangalos EG. MR-based hippocampal volumetry in the diagnosis of Alzheimer's disease. Neurology. 1992;42:183-8.
4. Braak H, Braak E. Neuropathological stageing of Alzheimer-related changes. Acta Neuropathol. 1991;82:239-59.
5. Dubois B, Picard G, Sarazin M. Early detection of Alzheimer's disease: new diagnostic criteria. Dialogues Clin Neurosci. 2009;11(2):135-9.
6. Murray ME, Graff-Radford NR, Ross OA, Petersen RC, Duara R, Dickson DW. Neuropathologically defined subtypes of Alzheimer's disease with distinct clinical characteristics: a retrospective study. Lancet Neurol. 2011;10:785-96.
7. Koedam EL, Lauffer V, van der Vlies AE, van der Flier WM, Scheltens P, Pijnenburg YA. Early-versus late-onset Alzheimer's disease: more than age alone. J Alzheimers Dis. 2010;19:1401-8.
8. Dubois B, Feldman HH, Jacova C, Hampel H, Molinuevo JL, Blennow K, et al. Advancing research diagnostic criteria for Alzheimer's disease: the IWG-2 criteria. Lancet Neurol. 2014;13:614-29.
9. McKhann GM, Knopman DS, Chertkow H, Hyman BT, Jack CR Jr, Kawas CH, et al. The diagnosis of dementia due to Alzheimer's disease: recommendations from the National Institute on Aging–Alzheimer's Association workgroups on diagnostic guidelines for Alzheimer's disease. Alzheimers Dement. 2011; 7:263-9.
10. Crutch SJ, Schott JM, Rabinovici GD, Murray M, Snowden JS, van der Flier WM, et al. Consensus classification of posterior cortical atrophy. Alzheimers Dement. 2017;13(8):870-84.
11. Ossenkoppele R, Jansen WJ, Rabinovici GD, Knol DL, van der Flier WM, van Berckel BN, et al. Prevalence of amyloid PET positivity in dementia syndromes: a meta-analysis. JAMA. 2015;313(19):1939-49.
12. Snowden JS, Stopford CL, Julien CL, Thompson JC, Davidson Y, Gibbons L, et al. Cognitive phenotypes in Alzheimer's disease and genetic risk. Cortex. 2007;43(7):835-45.
13. Townley RA, Graff-Radford J, Mantyh WG, Botha H, Polsinelli AJ, Przybelski SA, et al. Progressive dysexecutive syndrome due to Alzheimer's disease: a description of 55 cases and comparison to other phenotypes. Brain Commun. 2020;2(1):fcaa068.
14. Singh NA, Graff-Radford J, Machulda M, Carlos AF, Schwarz CG, Senjem ML, et al. Atypical Alzheimer's disease: new insights into an overlapping spectrum between the language and visual variants. Alzheimer's Association international conference. Alzheimers Dement. 2023;19:658-70.
15. Athar T, Al Balushi K, Khan SA. Recent advances on drug development and emerging therapeutic agents for Alzheimer's disease. Mol Biol Rep. 2021;48:5629-45.
16. Doggrell SA. Lessons that can be learnt from the failure of verubecestat in. Alzheimer's disease. Expert Opin Pharmacother. 2019;20:2095-9.
17. Egan MF, Mukai Y, Voss T, Kost J, Stone J, Furtek C, et al. Further analyses of the safety of verubecestat in the phase 3 EPOCH trial of mild-to-moderate Alzheimer's disease. Alzheimers Res Ther. 2019;11:68.
18. Wessels AM, Tariot PN, Zimmer JA, Selzler KJ, Bragg SM, Andersen SW, et al. Efficacy and safety of Lanabecestat for treatment of early and mild Alzheimer Disease: the AMARANTH and DAYBREAK-ALZ randomized clinical trials. JAMA Neurol. 2020;77:199-209.
19. Sperling R, Henley D, Aisen PS, Raman R, Donohue MC, Ernstrom K, et al. Findings of efficacy, safety, and biomarker outcomes of atabecestat in preclinical alzheimer disease: a truncated randomized phase 2b/3 clinical trial. JAMA Neurol. 2021;78: 293-301.
20. Vormfelde SV, Pezous N, Lefevre G, Kolly C, Neumann U, Jordaan P, et al. A pooled analysis of three randomized phase I/IIa clinical trials confirms absence of clinically relevant effect on the QTc interval by Umibecestat. Clin Transl Sci. 2020;13: 1316-26.
21. Miranda A, Montiel E, Ulrich H, Paz C. Selective secretase targeting for Alzheimer's disease therapy. J Alzheimers Dis. 2021;81:1-17.
22. Doody RS, Raman R, Farlow M, Iwatsubo T, Vellas B, Joffe S, et al. A phase 3 trial of semagacestat for treatment of Alzheimer's disease. N Engl J Med. 2013;369:341-50.
23. Nicoll JAR, Buckland GR, Harrison CH, Page A, Harris S, Love S, et al. Persistent neuropathological effects 14 years following amyloid-beta immunization in Alzheimer's disease. Brain. 2019; 142:2113-26.
24. Ohtake Y, Kong W, Hussain R, Horiuchi M, Tremblay ML, Ganea D, et al. Protein tyrosine phosphatase σ regulates autoimmune encephalomyelitis development. Brain Behav Immun. 2017; 65:111-24.
25. Salloway S, Sperling R, Fox NC, Blennow K, Klunk W, Raskind M, et al. Two phase 3 trials of bapineuzumab in mild-to-moderate Alzheimer's disease. N Engl J Med. 2014;370:322-33.
26. Ostrowitzki S, Bittner T, Sink KM, Mackey H, Rabe C, Honig LS, et al. Evaluating the safety and efficacy of crenezumab vs placebo in adults with early alzheimer disease: two phase 3 randomized placebo-controlled trials. JAMA Neurol. 2022;79: 1113-21.
27. Landen JW, Andreasen N, Cronenberger CL, Schwartz PF, Borjesson Hanson A, Ostlund H, et al. Ponezumab in mild-to-moderate Alzheimer's disease: randomized phase II PET-PIB study. Alzheimers Dement. 2017;3:393-401.
28. Portron A, Jordan P, Draper K, Muenzer C, Dickerson D, van Iersel T, et al. A phase I study to assess the effect of speed of injection on pain, tolerability, and pharmacokinetics after high-volume subcutaneous administration of gantenerumab in healthy volunteers. Clin Ther. 2020;42:108-20.e1.
29. Mintun MA, Lo AC, Duggan Evans C, Wessels AM, Ardayfio PA, Andersen SW, et al. Donanemab in early Alzheimer's disease. N Engl J Med. 2021;384:1691-704.
30. Shcherbinin S, Evans CD, Lu M, Andersen SW, Pontecorvo MJ, Willis BA, et al. Association of amyloid reduction after Donanemab treatment with tau pathology and clinical outcomes: the TRAILBLAZER-ALZ randomized clinical trial. JAMA Neurol. 2022;79:1015-24.
31. Dhillon S. Aducanumab: first approval. Drugs. 2021;81:1437-43.
32. Lovestone S, Boada M, Dubois B, Hull M, Rinne JO, Huppertz HJ, et al. A phase II trial of tideglusib in Alzheimer's disease. J Alzheimers Dis. 2015;45:75-88.

33. Center for Drug Evaluation and Research. U.S. Food and Drug Administration (FDA). (2023). Summary Review. [online] Available from https://www.accessdata.fda.gov/drugsatfda_docs/summary_review/2023/761269Orig1s000SumR.pdf [Last accessed July, 2024].
34. European Medicines Agency. (2022). Aduhelm. [online] Available from https://www.ema.europa.eu/en/medicines/human/withdrawn-applications/aduhelm [Last accessed July, 2024].
35. Luca A, Luca M. Lithium in Alzheimer's disease: from prevention to treatment. Psychogeriatrics. 2023;23:204-5.
36. Tucker D, Lu Y, Zhang Q. From mitochondrial function to neuroprotection—an emerging role for methylene blue. Mol Neurobiol. 2018;55:5137-53.
37. Seripa D, Solfrizzi V, Imbimbo BP, Daniele A, Santamato A, Lozupone M, et al. Tau-directed approaches for the treatment of Alzheimer's disease: focus on leuco-methylthioninium. Expert Rev Neurother. 2016;16:259-77.
38. Wischik CM, Staff RT, Wischik DJ, Bentham P, Murray AD, Storey JM, et al. Tau aggregation inhibitor therapy: an exploratory phase 2 study in mild or moderate Alzheimer's disease. J Alzheimers Dis. 2015;44:705-20.
39. Gauthier S, Feldman HH, Schneider LS, Wilcock GK, Frisoni GB, Hardlund JH, et al. Efficacy and safety of tau-aggregation inhibitor therapy in patients with mild or moderate Alzheimer's disease: a randomised, controlled, double-blind, parallel-arm, phase 3 trial. Lancet. 2016;388:2873-84.
40. Morimoto BH, Schmechel D, Hirman J, Blackwell A, Keith J, Gold M. A double-blind, placebo-controlled, ascending-dose, randomized study to evaluate the safety, tolerability and effects on cognition of AL-108 after 12 weeks of intranasal administration in subjects with mild cognitive impairment. Dement Geriatr Cogn Disord. 2013;35:325-36.
41. Novak P, Schmidt R, Kontsekova E, Kovacech B, Smolek T, Katina S, et al. FUNDAMANT: an interventional 72-week phase 1 follow-up study of AADvac1, an active immunotherapy against tau protein pathology in Alzheimer's disease. Alzheimers Res Ther. 2018;10:108.
42. Florian H, Wang D, Arnold SE, Boada M, Guo Q, Jin Z, et al. Tilavonemab in early Alzheimer's disease: results from a phase 2, randomized, double-blind study. Brain. 2023;146:2275-84.
43. Teng E, Manser PT, Pickthorn K, Brunstein F, Blendstrup M, Sanabria Bohorquez S, et al. Safety and efficacy of semorinemab in individuals with prodromal to mild alzheimer disease: a randomized clinical trial. JAMA Neurol. 2022;79:758-67.
44. Salloway S, Farlow M, McDade E, Clifford DB, Wang G, Llibre-Guerra JJ, et al. A trial of gantenerumab or solanezumab in dominantly inherited Alzheimer's disease. Nat Med. 2021;27:1187-96.
45. Shevtsova EF, Maltsev AV, Vinogradova DV, Shevtsov PN, Bachurin SO. Mitochondria as a promising target for developing novel agents for treating Alzheimer's disease. Med Res Rev. 2021;41:803-27.
46. MacKay J, Harnett S, Machado P. (2010). Pfizer and Medivation announce results from two phase 3 studies in Dimebon (Latrepirdine*) Alzheimer's disease clinical development program. [online] Available from https://www.pfizer.com/news/press-release/press-release-detail/pfizer_and_medivation_announce_results_from_two_phase_3_studies_in_dimebon_latrepirdine_alzheimer_s_disease_clinical_development_program [Last accessed July, 2024].
47. Peng Y, Jin H, Xue YH, Chen Q, Yao SY, Du MQ, et al. Current and future therapeutic strategies for Alzheimer's disease: an overview of drug development bottlenecks. Front Aging Neurosci. 2023;15:1206572.
48. Oset-Gasque MJ, Marco-Contelles J. Alzheimer's Disease, the "One-Molecule, One-Target" Paradigm, and the Multitarget Directed Ligand Approach. ACS Chem Neurosci. 2018;9:401-3.
49. Agis-Torres A, Sölhuber M, Fernandez M, Sanchez-Montero JM. Multi-Target-Directed Ligands and other Therapeutic Strategies in the Search of a Real Solution for Alzheimer's Disease. Curr Neuropharmacol. 2014;12:2-36.
50. Benek O, Korabecny J, Soukup O. A perspective on multi-target drugs for Alzheimer's disease. Trends Pharmacol Sci. 2020;41:434-45.

CHAPTER 7

Spectrum of Mild Cognitive Impairment Subtypes and Outcome Predictors

Asish Vijayaraghavan, Saranya B Gomathy, Ramshekhar N Menon

ABSTRACT

Mild cognitive impairment (MCI) is defined as a condition characterized by a subtle decline in cognitive abilities beyond what is expected for age or educational background, without significant functional impairment. It is a heterogeneous condition with various subtypes, etiologies, and outcomes. Notwithstanding the etiological and neuropsychological subtypes, a significant proportion of individuals can progress to dementia within a relatively short period (variable across studies which show 2–25% annual conversion to Alzheimer's disease). However, many people with MCI remain stable, experience slow deterioration, and a surprising number even show spontaneous improvement over time. This chapter explores the spectrum of MCI subtypes and identifies predictors of outcome. Classification of MCI subtypes, including amnestic and nonamnestic MCI or single- and multidomain classification schema, is discussed alongside relevant biomarkers and neuropsychological assessment tools. Additionally, we highlight the challenges and pitfalls in diagnosing MCI, including the subjective nature of cognitive assessment, the lack of consensus on diagnostic criteria, and the variability in progression rates among individuals with MCI. Understanding the spectrum of MCI subtypes, employing a multimodal approach that incorporates blood, cerebrospinal fluid (CSF), and imaging biomarkers and neuropsychological evaluation can help identify predictors of outcome. These are crucial for early detection, intervention, and the development of targeted therapies aimed at preventing or delaying the progression to dementia.

Keywords: MCI, Subtypes, Neuropsychology, Biomarkers, Dementia conversion.

INTRODUCTION

Mild cognitive impairment (MCI) is a broad concept which potentially describes a prodromal and transitional phase from normal cognitive function to dementia.[1] The entity is viewed as a potential target for interventions designed to delay progression to dementia. Petersen et al. proposed the initial clinical criteria for MCI which focused primarily on the amnestic subtype [amnestic MCI (aMCI)].[2] Later, broader definitions incorporating amnestic and nonamnestic components of MCI were formulated.[3,4] Subsequently, the National Institute on Aging–Alzheimer's Association (NIA-AA) workgroups, American Psychiatric Association, and other organizations proposed various criteria and guidelines for MCI diagnosis.[5]

PREVALENCE OF MILD COGNITIVE IMPAIRMENT

A large number of epidemiologic studies have been conducted in the last two decades to estimate the prevalence of MCI in general population. There has been great variability in the prevalence figures because of the differences in methodology of neuropsychological evaluation and MCI criteria used. Many international studies have been performed involving several thousand participants and these tend to estimate the overall prevalence of MCI in the 12–18% range in persons >60 years of age. **Table 1** shows the prevalence figures of MCI in many national and international population-based studies along with the risk factors. A review of incidence

TABLE 1: Prevalence estimates of MCI in population-based studies.[6]

Study	Reference	N	Age (years)	Prevalence (overall %)	Design and criteria for MCI	Risk factors for MCI identified
CHS Cognition study, USA	Lopez et al. 2003	1,690	≥75	22	Prospective, multiethnic cohort, predominantly urban setting	Depression, psychiatric medications, Parkinson's disease, multiple system atrophy, metabolic encephalopathy
Kolkata, India	Das et al. 2007	745	≥50	14.9	Cross-sectional design. Systematic random sampling of households in urban setting. aMCI criteria and multiple domain subtypes identified	Educational attainment, diabetes, and hypertension identified as risk factors for both subtypes
ILSA, Italy	Di Carlo et al. 2007	2,830	65–84	16.1	• Population-based, prospective, community-dwelling cohort • Amnestic and multidomain MCI	Previous stroke and impairment in instrumental ADLs
3C, France	Artero et al. 2008	6,892	≥65	42.0	Population-based, community dwelling; revised published MCI consensus criteria	• *Men*: ApoE4 allele, stroke, low education, age, loss of IADL • *Women*: IADL loss, ApoE4 allele, subclinical depression, anticholinergic use, age
Manhattan, USA	Manly et al. 2008	2,364	≥65	21.8	• Prospective, population-based, multi-ethnic cohort • MCI criteria, urban setting	MCI with impairment in memory and at least one other domain had increased risk for progression to AD
Rochester, USA	Petersen et al. 2010	1,969	70–89	14.8	Population-based, published MCI criteria	Male gender, age, ApoE3/E4 allele, never married—prevalence increased
CSBA, Italy	Ravaglia et al. 2008	1,016	≥65	7.7	Longitudinal cohort, population based; amnestic and nonamnestic MCI	Poor education, older age
Tone Town, Japan	Sasaki et al. 2009	1,888	≥65	18.9	Cross-sectional study; standard MCI criteria	Presence of ApoE4 allele
HNR, Germany	Dlugaj et al. 2010	4,145	50–80	7.8	Prospective study, MCI-original and MCI-modified criteria	Older age, lower education
South Korea, Korea	Kim et al. 2011	1,673	≥65	24.1	Prospective study, amnestic and nonamnestic MCI (single and multidomain)	Older age, male gender, lower education, illiteracy, smoking, and history of head trauma or depression were associated with increased risk; alcohol use and moderately intense exercise were associated with reduced dementia risk
10/66 Dementia Research Group; Latin America, China, India	Sosa AL et al. 2012	15,376	65+	0.8% in China, 4.3% in India	Cross-sectional survey; Mayo Clinic aMCI criteria	Male gender
Swedish GÅS population study, Sweden	Overton et al. 2019	3,752	60–81	5.13–29.9%	Participants were randomly selected in four waves from rural and urban areas of Sweden; expanded Mayo clinic criteria for MCI was employed	Age
CHARLS, China	Feng Qin et al. 2022	3,768	≥60	22.24%	Cross-sectional study; MMSE was used to look for cognitive impairment	South west China, unmarried, sleep duration >90 minutes, depression

Continued

Continued

Study	Reference	N	Age (years)	Prevalence (overall %)	Design and criteria for MCI	Risk factors for MCI identified
India	Patel RM et al. 2018	560	≥50	25%	Community-based, cross-sectional study in rural and urban field areas of a medical college; patients screened using Gujarati MMSE version	≥60 years of age, illiteracy
India	Iype T et al. 2023	366	≥65	18.6%	Community-based cross-sectional study; MCI diagnosed using the criteria by European Alzheimer's Disease Consortium	≥70 years of age, illiteracy

(ADLs: activities of daily living; ApoE4: apolipoprotein E4; CHARLS: China Health and Retirement Longitudinal Study; CHS: Cardiovascular Health Study; CSBA: Conselice Study of Brain Ageing; GÅS: Good Aging in Skåne; IADL: instrumental ADL; HNR: Heinz Nixdorf Recall; ILSA: Italian Longitudinal Study of Aging; aMCI: amnestic mild cognitive impairment; MCI: mild cognitive impairment; MMSE: Mini–Mental State Examination)

and prevalence studies provides valuable insights into the heterogeneity of demographic and modifiable risk factors for the development of MCI. However, future studies of biomarker-based risk stratification are likely to impact these figures in longitudinal cohorts.

INCIDENCE RATES AND MILD COGNITIVE IMPAIRMENT RISK FACTORS

In contrast to prevalence studies, there are fewer studies on MCI incidence rates. There is a wide range of incidence rates (per 1,000 person years) from 5.1 to 168.[7,8] A few studies only reported estimates of incident aMCI, which ranged from 10 to 14.[9,10] The key risk factors for MCI described from these studies included older age, low education, and apolipoprotein E (ApoE) ε4 allele. In addition, cardiovascular disease (type 2 diabetes), Black and Hispanic ethnicity, subjective memory complaints, and stroke have also been associated with incident MCI.

RATES OF MILD COGNITIVE IMPAIRMENT PROGRESSION TO DEMENTIA AND PROGRESSION PREDICTORS

The annual risk of developing dementia in the elderly general population is around 1–2%, patients with MCI have a 10–15% annual risk. In population-based studies of MCI, the annual risk of developing dementia is around 5–10%.[11] **Table 2** gives the rates of progression from MCI to dementia and the predictors of progression across various international longitudinal studies.[12]

UPDATED CLASSIFICATION CRITERIA FOR MILD COGNITIVE IMPAIRMENT

The term "MCI" has been around for nearly four decades, first appearing in the literature when researchers at the New York University categorized stage 3 of the Global Deterioration Scale as this entity.[13] A 1999 Mayo Clinic study identified participants in their community aging program who reported memory concerns exceeding typical age-related decline.[14]

Originally, the Mayo Clinic criteria aimed to identify the earliest memory-related symptoms of Alzheimer's disease (AD). However, these criteria proved limiting as not all cases of forgetfulness progressed to AD and not everyone with MCI experienced solely memory problems. These tests required a decline in episodic memory with a score of at least 1.5 standard deviations (SD) below the average (mean) to be considered indicative of MCI. However, this approach overlooked potential impairments in other cognitive domains.

To address this, the Key Symposium in Stockholm (2003) led to the development of broader criteria published in 2004.[2,4] The specific recommendations for the general MCI criteria included the following: (1) The person has neither normal nor developed dementia; (2) there is evidence of cognitive deterioration shown by either objectively measured decline over time and/or subjective report of decline by self and/or informant in conjunction with objective cognitive deficits; and (3) activities of daily living are preserved and complex instrumental functions are either intact or minimally impaired. The criteria divided principal cognitive impairment into amnestic, single nonmemory domains, or involving multiple cognitive domains. Each of these clinical presentations can have multiple etiologies such as degenerative, vascular, metabolic, traumatic, psychiatric, or others **(Table 3)**.

TABLE 2: Rates of progression of MCI to dementia across longitudinal studies.[12]

Study	Reference	MCI cases, follow-up period	Progression to dementia frequency	Predictors of progression	Reversion rate
Italian Longitudinal Study on Aging, Italy	Solfrizzi, 2004	Prevalent MCI 72; 3.5 years	20.8%	Stroke	37.5%
3 Cities Study, France	Artero, 2008	Prevalent MCI 2,882; 4 years	6.6% incident dementia; 56.5% stable MCI	ApoE4 allele, stroke, low education, impaired IADL, older age, hypertension, diabetes, subclinical depression	37%; men likely to revert more compared to women
Aging, Demographics and Memory Study, USA	Plassman, 2008	Prevalent MCI 180; 1.4 years	16.7% progression to dementia; 63.8% stable MCI	Older age, low education, women	19.6%
Conselice Study of Brain Aging, Italy	Ravaglia, 2008	Prevalent MCI 60; 3.8 years	41.7% progressed; 65% stable MCI	Older age, ApoE4 allele, women, low education, lower MMSE, aMCI, multidomain MCI	35%
Cache County Study of Memory Health and Aging, USA	Peters, 2012	Prevalent CIND 230; 3.3 years	37% progressed; 63% stable MCI	Older age, ApoE4 allele, lower MMSE, high CDR sum, neuropsychiatric features	–
Pittsburgh Cardiovascular Health Study, USA	Lopez, 2012	Prevalent and incident MCI 3,020; 2.5 years	27.6% progressed; 39.5% stable MCI	Not reported	16%
Mayo Clinic Study of Aging, USA	Roberts RO, 2012	MCI cases: 478 (282 prevalent, 196 incident); 2.5 years	27.6% progressed, 39.5% stable MCI	Women, aMCI, multidomain MCI	35.2%
Indian Study	Poulose, 2023	MCI cases 95; ≥2 years	22.2% progressed	Multidomain MCI; lower baseline list recognition, lower immediate logical memory and high perseverative error scores on set shifting	–

(aMCI: amnestic mild cognitive impairment; ApoE4: apolipoprotein E4; CDR: Clinical Dementia Rating; CIND: cognitive impairment no dementia; IADL: instrumental activities of daily living; MCI: mild cognitive impairment; MMSE: Mini–Mental State Examination)

TABLE 3: Etiology of various subtypes of MCI.

Etiology	Amnestic MCI Single domain	Amnestic MCI Multi-domain	Non-amnestic MCI Single domain	Nonamnestic MCI Multi-domain
Degenerative	AD	AD	FTD including aphasic subtypes, AD, PSP, PDD, degenerative ataxias	DLB, AD, FTD, PDD, PSP, dysmyelinating disorders, normal pressure hydrocephalus
Vascular	Strategic infarct VCI	VCI	VCI	VCI
Psychiatric	Depression	Depression	Depression, FTD phenocopy	Depression, FTD phenocopy
Systemic/ structural	Endocrine/toxic/ SOL	Metabolic/toxic/endocrine/ SOL tumors, B12 deficiency	Metabolic/endocrine/SOL tumors, brain-sagging syndrome	Metabolic/toxic/SOL

(AD: Alzheimer's disease; FTD: frontotemporal dementia; DLB: diffuse Lewy body dementia; MCI: mild cognitive impairment; PDD: Parkinson's disease dementia; PSP: progressive supranuclear palsy; SOL: space-occupying lesion; VCI: vascular cognitive impairment)

These new criteria achieved two key goals: (1) Expanding the classification beyond memory, and (2) acknowledging that MCI could stem from various causes, not just AD. The Key Symposium's characterization of MCI further led to the distinction between aMCI and nonamnestic MCI (naMCI). This differentiation arose because these clinical presentations seemed to be linked to different underlying cause and potentially have varying long-term outcomes.

In 2011, seeking to include the entire Alzheimer's spectrum, the NIA-AA developed new criteria.[5] These criteria largely preserved the core of the Key Symposium

Criteria for MCI due to AD but made some diagnostic features clearer. Additionally, they incorporated biomarkers to refine the underlying etiology and potentially predict future outcomes which has now evolved into the Amyloid/Tau/Neurodegeneration (A/T/N) framework **(Box 1)**.[15] Notably, the NIA-AA criteria did not distinguish between aMCI and naMCI. Additionally, criteria have been formulated for subjects. 50 years of age with behavioral or personality changes for >6 months (decreased motivation, affective dysregulation, poor impulse control, social inappropriateness, or abnormal perception or thought content) with or without objective evidence of MCI, who may require follow-up for evolution into dementia. These can be labeled as mild behavioral impairment (MBI).[16] If no such issues are noted, the condition can be labeled as subjective cognitive impairment (SCI) with reassurance and follow-up advisable **(Flowchart 1)**.

Concurrently, the Diagnostic and Statistical Manual of Mental Disorders, Fifth Edition (DSM-5) introduced

BOX 1 **Biomarkers in MCI due to AD (A/T/N framework).[15]**

A: Aggregated Aβ or associated pathologic state
- Low cerebrospinal fluid amyloid-beta (Aβ42)
- Positive PET amyloid imaging

T: Aggregated tau (neurofibrillary tangles) or associated pathologic state
- p-tau181
- p-tau217, tau: Aβ42 ratio in CSF, tau PET

N: Neurodegeneration or neuronal injury
- Expanding role for plasma NfL and GFAP
- Decreased metabolism in the parietal and temporal cortical lobe on 18-flurodeoxyglucose PET
- Atrophic change on MRI in temporal (medial, lateral, and basal) and medial parietal cortical lobe
- CSF total-tau

(Aβ: amyloid beta; AD: Alzheimer's disease; CSF: cerebrospinal fluid; GFAP: glial fibrillary acidic protein; MCI: mild cognitive impairment; MRI: magnetic resonance imaging; NfL: neurofilament light chains; PET: positron emission tomography)

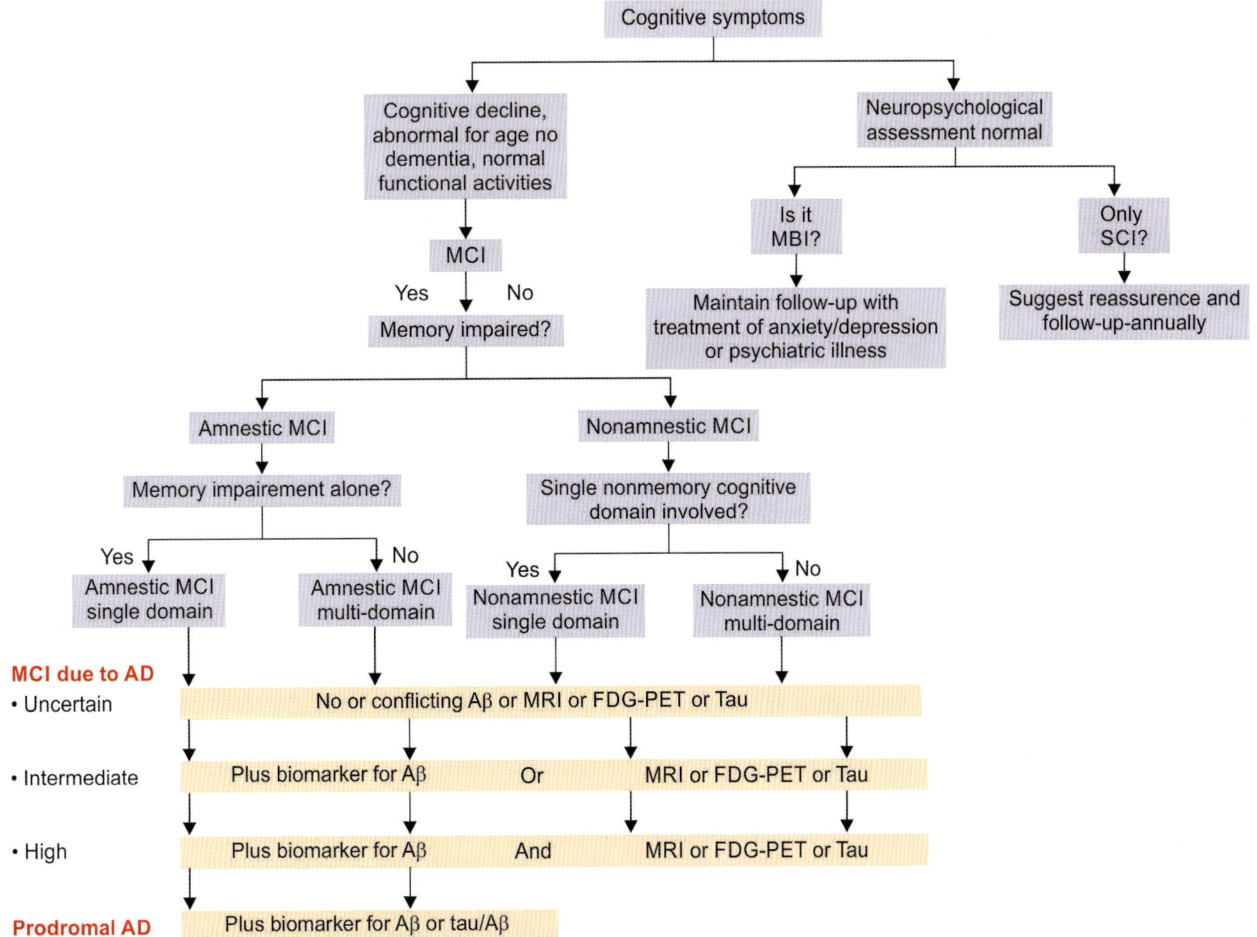

FLOWCHART 1: Consensus approach to the diagnostic spectrum of MCI.

(Aβ: amyloid beta; AD: Alzheimer's disease; FDG-PET: fluorodeoxyglucose positron emission tomography; MCI: mild cognitive impairment; MBI: mild behavioral impairment; MRI: magnetic resonance imaging; SCI: subjective cognitive impairment)

a new category—mild neurocognitive disorder. This predementia phase closely resembles the Key Symposium Criteria for MCI. Similar to the NIA-AA framework, the DSM-5 suggests incorporating specific features to potentially subclassify the clinical presentation based on underlying pathology. Notably, the mild neurocognitive disorder due to AD category aligns significantly with the NIA-AA's classification of MCI due to AD. The concept of prodromal AD, representing the earliest symptomatic stages of AD, emerged over time based on accumulating research.[17] Proponents of this concept suggested that a particular form of aMCI combined with biomarkers for amyloid or both amyloid and tau pathology represented the earliest symptomatic phase of the AD process.[17]

Hence, four distinctive subtypes are defined based on the number of cognitive domains affected: Single and multidomain aMCI and naMCI, respectively, with an etiology-specific approach are mandatory after delineating the cognitive phenotype.[13] Subjects with behavioral or personality changes such as due to depression or FTD phenocopy without objective demonstration of cognitive impairment on testing can be labeled as MBI.[16]

BIOMARKERS FOR RISK STRATIFICATION IN MILD COGNITIVE IMPAIRMENT

Blood Biomarkers in Mild Cognitive Impairment

Blood-based biomarkers are promising diagnostic tools for identifying AD in its prodromal stages, including MCI. They are anticipated to be utilized as screening tools for patients presenting with cognitive complaints. Broadly speaking, a biomarker is a measurable indicator of a biological state or pathological condition. The neuropathological signature of AD, including amyloid-beta (Aβ) plaques, neurofibrillary tangles (NFT), and neurodegeneration, can be detected by quantifying specific proteins [Aβ42, Aβ40, total tau (t-tau), and phosphorylated tau 181 (p-tau181)] in cerebrospinal fluid (CSF). In AD, researchers have validated CSF biomarkers for Aβ plaque pathology (a reduced CSF Aβ42 concentration or CSF Aβ42/40 ratio due to selective retention of the 42 amino acid form of Aβ in plaque-laden brain tissue), as well as disordered neuronal tau metabolism associated with neurodegeneration and tangle pathology (increased secretion of both T-tau and P-tau into the CSF).[18] Taken together, these biomarkers demonstrate 85–95% sensitivity and specificity for AD, applicable in both the MCI and dementia stages of the disease. Recent technological advances, characterized by extremely high sensitivity, have facilitated the reliable quantification of core AD proteins in peripheral blood. This advancement can potentially reduce the necessity for lumbar punctures during patient monitoring and screening.

In blood, p-tau181 has demonstrated the ability to differentiate between Aβ-positive (Aβ+) and Aβ-negative (Aβ–) MCI patients, as determined by the gold standard amyloid PET imaging. Additionally, p-tau at threonine 217 (p-tau217) consistently demonstrates high performance in differentiating AD from other neurodegenerative disorders and in detecting AD pathology in patients with MCI.[19] Notably, p-tau217 exhibits larger-fold changes compared to p-tau181 and p-tau231, often achieving high discrimination with area under the curve (AUC) exceeding 90%.[20] Additionally, p-tau217 demonstrates a unique longitudinal trajectory, showing increases associated with worsening brain atrophy and declining cognitive performance in individuals with elevated Aβ pathology. A recent study showed that a commercially available plasma p-tau217 immunoassay accurately identified biological AD, comparable to CSF biomarkers, with consistent cutoffs across cohorts.[18]

Blood neurofilament light chains (NfL), a marker of neurodegeneration, has garnered significant evidence supporting its value across various neurodegenerative disorders. It correlates with longitudinal measures of disease severity and has been utilized as a measure of the efficacy of disease-modifying treatments. Finally, glial fibrillary acidic protein (GFAP), a marker of reactive astrogliosis, has shown a correlation with Aβ burden in MCI patients similar to that of p-tau181. NfL, GFAP, and p-tau181 demonstrated good diagnostic accuracy to identify progression to AD dementia, which improved when combined. Estimation of GFAP and p-tau181 were highly correlated with CSF Aβ42 levels.[21]

Imaging Biomarkers for Cognitive Decline in Mild Cognitive Impairment

Magnetic Resonance Imaging

Structural changes on MRI provide early dementia prediction, especially when combined with other measures.[22] aMCI is characterized by MRI volumetric reduction in medial temporal lobe structures, where hippocampal volume (HCV) is correlated with Aβ-associated memory decline. MCI subjects who show MRI and/or CSF biomarker abnormalities are at increased risk for cognitive decline and progression to AD. Hippocampal atrophy rate in MCI predicts the rate of conversion to AD.[23] Reduced cortical thickness was the other finding noted in presymptomatic persons who eventually developed AD.[24] In MCI subjects who have abnormalities on both CSF and MRI, versus only one of those, there is a four times higher risk to progress to AD within <2 years. Studies have found that the volume of CA1 and subiculum were more closely associated than total HCV with conversion to MCI-AD.[25] Multimodality imaging incorporating volumetry, tensor imaging, and spectroscopy has shown high sensitivity–specificity for imaging MCI at risk.[26] Perfusion MRI and alteration in resting state functional connectivity have also been identified in predicting conversion from MCI to AD.[27]

Molecular Imaging Biomarkers

Molecular imaging uses tracers whose in vivo uptake patterns and pharmacokinetics indicate and quantify the presence or activity of specific receptors, transporters, enzymes, and metabolic pathways. Currently, positron emission tomography (PET) and single-photon emission computed tomography (SPECT), which both use radiolabeled tracers, are the molecular imaging techniques used for dementia imaging.[28]

- *[^{18}F] Fluorodeoxyglucose (FDG) PET*: Regional uptake and retention of the PET tracer in the brain provides a measure of brain glucose metabolism. Sensitivity of this technique for diagnosing early AD is approximately 90%, though the specificity for distinguishing it from other dementias is lower (71–73%).[29,30]
- *Amyloid imaging*: Abnormal aggregation of Aβ is the hallmark pathology in AD and it plays the central role in its pathogenesis. Multiple amyloid imaging modalities have been invented including Pittsburgh compound B (PiB), florbetapir, flutemetamol, and florbetaben. These agents bind to the fibrillary form of Aβ protein which is found in the amyloid plaques. A joint report from the Society of Nuclear Medicine and Molecular Imaging and Alzheimer's Association has issued appropriate use criteria for amyloid PET.[29]

  It may be employed in the following scenarios: (1) Progressive or persistent unexplained MCI; (2) atypical course or mixed presentation in patients meeting core clinical criteria for AD; (3) early age of onset of progressive dementia, typically <65 years of age; and (4) prior to inclusion in monoclonal antiamyloid antibody-based therapeutic intervention trials.
- *Tau PET*: Flortaucipir tracers are currently employed in the context of AD. Tau PET studies have shown that tau deposition seems to follow the staging pattern given by Braak, suggesting tau spreads from entorhinal cortex (Braak I/II) to inferolateral temporal and medial parietal lobes (Braak III/IV) and finally the neocortex (Braak V/VI). In cognitively normal persons, tau seems to be associated with regional atrophy and hypometabolism and subtle cognitive deficits. Tau PET can identify prodromal AD. This imaging modality was employed in research and is now entering the clinical domain.[29]
- *Synaptic vesicle glycoprotein 2A (SV2A) PET*: Loss of synaptic density in hippocampus and medial temporal lobe underlies the deleterious amnestic presentation of AD. Synaptic density changes can be visualized in vivo using the SV2A PET imaging. Scan protocols are yet to be determined.[29]

ELUCIDATING THE NEUROPSYCHOLOGICAL SPECTRUM OF MILD COGNITIVE IMPAIRMENT (CASES 1 TO 3)

Instruments vary in sensitivity and specificity. Hence, a patient meeting MCI criteria with one instrument may not do so with another. Also, the degree of memory test dysfunction is not absolutely defined and the 1.5 SD value commonly used refers to group, not individual performances. For naMCI, there is even less clarity on which cognitive domains to assess and how. Hence, it would be reasonable and helpful to be able to achieve guidelines that clearly identify as to how many tests in each domain should be used to establish MCI subtypes. Neuropsychological tests should complement clinical assessment, be brief to avoid elderly fatigue, and ideally assess multiple functional domains. Assessment should include tests that evaluate performance in cognitive domains other than memory, such as attention/executive function, language, perception, and visuoperceptual/visuoconstructional functions. Self-administered, computerized tests could also offer a solution.[31]

The *Montreal Cognitive Assessment (MoCA) and Addenbrooke's Cognitive Examination III (ACE-III)* are recommended as good screening instruments in MCI with Indian studies in multiple languages, validating their utility with high sensitivity and specificity (94% and 90%, respectively, for ACE-III[32] and 90% and 92%, respectively, for MoCA[33]).

The *Mini-Mental Status Examination (MMSE)* and the *Clinical Dementia Rating (CDR)* Scale are not recommended as screening tools for MCI because of their limitations in detecting early cognitive dysfunction accurately. A meta-analysis indicated that the MoCA's accuracy for detecting MCI at the cutoff point of 24/25 had a sensitivity of 80.48% and specificity of 81.19% as opposed to the MMSE which at the cutoff point of 27/28 (given the impairment in three-word recall) had a sensitivity of 66.34% and specificity of 72.94%.[34] Clinical judgment, including considerations of premorbid functioning such as intellectual capacity and occupational status, remains essential in MCI diagnosis.

Addenbrooke's Cognitive Examination recall scores in regional languages have been found to be an effective screening tool for identifying patients with suspected aMCI.[35] Recently, validated tools such as the *Indian Council of Medical Research (ICMR)-Neurocognitive Tool Box (MUDRA)* with multidomain emphasis harmonized

CASE 1: MCI DUE TO FOCAL CORTICAL DEGENERATION

A 72-year-old practicing orthodontist experienced memory impairment for the past 2 years. Initially, he had difficulty recollecting names of distant relatives, which progressed over the past 2 months to the point of being unable to recognize them altogether. While he failed to recognize students, he was able to identify family members and close relatives. He has become withdrawn at social gatherings over the past 6 months, expressing, *"I find it difficult to recognize the people I meet. I know the face but cannot recall who they are; can't able to name them."* Despite these challenges, he managed his dental clinic well, albeit with a reduced workload. He handles financial transactions and pays bills regularly, though he occasionally forgets shopping items. His behavior exhibits mild irritability, which he attributes to his memory issues with no signs of depression noted. There are no evident visuospatial, executive, language, or praxis issues. He remains independent for all activities of daily living (ADLs), with a clinical dementia rating (CDR) of 0.5.

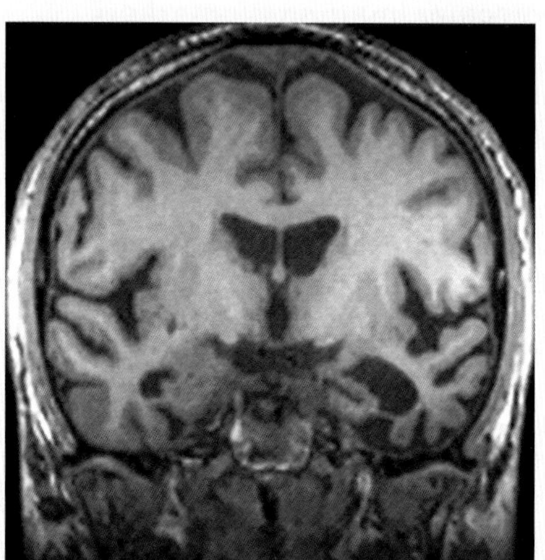

Cognitive scores: ACE score 87/100 [just above mild cognitive impairment (MCI) cutoff score for age and education], memory—registration 18/21; recall 7/10; Weschler Memory Scale–visual subset delayed recall score 4/41; and semantic battery 38/55.

Warrington recognition memory test for faces 13/25 (apperceptive prosopagnosia); volumetric MRI scan (radiological convention—asymmetric cortical atrophy involving right temporal lobe and fusiform gyri—consistent with right temporal variant semantic dementia.

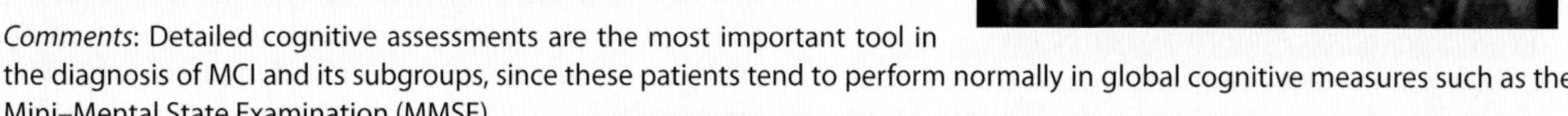

Comments: Detailed cognitive assessments are the most important tool in the diagnosis of MCI and its subgroups, since these patients tend to perform normally in global cognitive measures such as the Mini–Mental State Examination (MMSE).

CASE 2: MCI REVERTED TO NORMAL COGNITION-MILD BEHAVIORAL IMPAIRMENT (MBI)

A 65-year-old woman with 14 years of education presented for evaluation with a 3-year history of cognitive decline. She had symptoms such as feeling of worthlessness, apathy, anxiety, crying spells, suicidal ideation, insomnia, and loss of appetite, resulting in a weight loss of 6 kg over 1 year. Additionally, she experienced short-term memory problems and difficulty managing her finances and medication regimen. However, the effects of her cognitive problems on her ADL were difficult to determine, since she did not do much at home because of her low mood and lack of motivation. The patient had a medical history significant for breast cancer (treated with mastectomy), coronary artery disease, glaucoma, and arthritis but no previous history of depression or other psychiatric illnesses. She was prescribed sertraline 25 mg/day for her depressive symptoms 3 months ago. Her laboratory test results were normal and a brain MRI showed mild atrophy with no infarcts or white matter lesions. During examination, the patient appeared tearful and exhibited minimal bradykinesia. Her MMSE score was 24 (1/3 recall and 1/5 in attention subtests). She could not complete the clock-drawing test and her verbal fluency for animals was 7. Her Hamilton Depression Rating Scale score was 20, meeting criteria for major depression. Due to the severity of her depression, her sertraline dosage was gradually increased to 150 mg/day. A follow-up examination was conducted 6 months later, during which she had been stable on sertraline 150 mg/day for a month. Her MMSE score had improved to 30, her clock-drawing test was normal and verbal fluency for animals was 12. Her Hamilton Depression Rating Scale score had decreased to 5, indicating full remission of major depression.

Comment: This case highlights the development of late-life major depression, which significantly impacted the patient's cognition and ability to perform instrumental ADL. Initially, she presented with the memory plus other cognitive domain subtype of MCI. Following treatment with antidepressant medication, both her cognition and depressive symptoms improved and she returned to normal functioning. This case serves as an illustration that late-life mood disorders can manifest as an MCI syndrome and with appropriate treatment, patients can achieve full recovery. However, it is crucial to closely monitor both the symptoms of depression and its treatment, as there is a risk of symptom recurrence. Annual cognitive evaluations are also recommended, as depressed mood has been identified as a risk factor for incident AD.

CASE 3: MCI CONVERTOR TO AD

A 65-year-old physiatrist with 21 years of formal education presented with a 1-year history of progressive memory problems impacting his job performance. Although his colleagues had not noticed any issues and his wife had not reported cognitive problems at home, he was concerned. He had recently been diagnosed with hypertension and he denied any symptoms of major depression. His neurologic examination was normal, with a MMSE score of 29/30, although he did forget the floor of the doctor's office during the orientation subtest. Additionally, his clock-drawing test results were normal and he showed good verbal fluency for animals.[11] Laboratory tests and brain MRI showed no abnormalities. Due to his concerns about progressive memory problems, he underwent a comprehensive neuropsychological assessment, which revealed impaired memory functions on Rey Auditory Verbal Learning and delayed recall components with commission errors, as well as impaired paragraph learning on Weschler Memory Verbal subset scores falling <mean-1.5 SD for his age and education level. However, his language, visuospatial, and visuoconstructional functions were normal, consistent with aMCI.

Eight years later, the patient retired due to worsening cognition. His wife noticed problems in his instrumental ADL, such as forgetting to pay bills and getting lost while driving. His MMSE score dropped to 24/30 and a detailed neuropsychological assessment confirmed multidomain involvement in memory, executive as well as early visuospatial affliction. MRI volumetry at baseline and 8 years of follow-up confirmed baseline atrophy in posterior cingulate and precuneus with progressive hippocampal atrophy.

Comment: This highly educated man noticed cognitive decline affecting his work performance, although initially, his wife and colleagues did not observe any issues. A brief neuropsychological evaluation at the neurologist's office was within normal limits. However, a detailed neuropsychological evaluation at baseline demonstrated impaired learning and recall suggestive of episodic verbal memory deficits. This case highlights two important aspects of MCI clinical diagnosis: (1) Bedside screening tools may struggle to detect the syndrome, especially in highly educated individuals, and (2) Additional cognitive evaluations are crucial not only for detecting impaired cognitive domains during the MCI stage but also to enable the clinician to follow the longitudinal trajectory.

across five Indian languages demonstrated a sensitivity of 81.1% and a specificity of 88.8% for diagnosis of all-cause MCI, with a high specificity for diagnosis of vascular subtype of MCI given the cohort recruited in that study.[36] This enables clinician and researchers to select tests across domains to enhance objective diagnosis of neuropsychological impairments in MCI subtypes.

An overall CDR score of 0.5 masks the diverse functional status of individuals, as some with MCI exhibit extensive brain pathology, poorer episodic memory, and executive functions, increasing their risk of developing dementia.[37] Thus, relying solely on global CDR scores appears inadequate for MCI detection, although the emphasis on CDR-sum of boxes (CDR-SB) has gained prominence in randomized controlled studies.

PROBLEMS AND PITFALLS IN NEUROPSYCHOLOGICAL DIAGNOSIS OF MILD COGNITIVE IMPAIRMENT

Mild cognitive impairment is not a single entity and encompasses a range of causes affecting different cognitive domains, making identifying a precise cause challenging. Furthermore, distinguishing between the normal cognitive decline associated with aging and the potentially more serious decline of MCI presents a significant hurdle. Symptoms of MCI, such as forgetfulness, can overlap with those of stress, anxiety, or depression as seen with FTD phenocopies, necessitating a nuanced approach to rule out these factors. Persistent challenges surrounding MCI include determining whether the syndrome exhibits stability or fluctuates, understanding specific causes and risk factors, and elucidating the successive stages of its progression.

While assessing a patient's ability to perform activities of daily living (ADLs) is crucial for diagnosing MCI and differentiating it from dementia, this approach has limitations. Issues remain regarding the definition of ADLs, the level of complexity assessed (instrumental vs. basic activities), and the need to consider individual factors such as age and education. Individual and caregiver perceptions may also vary. Additionally, the relationship between cognitive decline and activities of daily living (ADLs) impairment may vary across different MCI subtypes.

The Petersen/Winblad conventional criteria set a threshold of 1.5 SD below the mean, along with the criterion of a single test failure per cognitive domain. In contrast, the Jak/Bondi criteria focus on a 1.0 SD below the mean, coupled with incorrect performance in two or more tests per cognitive domain.[38] Generally, any diagnostic criteria should be able to detect all cases, from severe to mild. However, this becomes challenging with MCI. When considering cognitive test performance as a continuum, a criterion that decisively identifies a disorder (e.g., using 2.0 SD) likely detects dementia rather than MCI. Thus, emphasis should be on identifying mild cases, which complicates selecting a cutoff point. Studies suggest that using stricter cutoff points (e.g., -1.5 or -2 SD) sacrifices sensitivity for specificity, while a cutoff of -1 SD offers a better balance between sensitivity and specificity. Applying neuropsychological cutoffs can thus be challenging in the clinical context.

In addition to establishing a specific and sensitive cutoff point for detecting changes in neuropsychological test performance indicative of MCI, it is crucial to employ scales or standardized data tailored for older adults. These should consider not only age but also educational and cultural background and the demographic to which they belong. Educational attainment significantly influences the interpretation of neuropsychological test results; thus, it is imperative to incorporate it into standardized data. A score on a test may indicate a deficit, depending on the individual's age and level of education, which are not discernible solely through cutoff points or SD. Researchers at the Mayo Clinic have dedicated over a decade to developing specific standardized data for the neuropsychological assessment of older adults through programs such as Mayo's Older Americans Normative Studies (MOANS) and Mayo's Older African American Normative Studies (MOAANS).[39,40] Social isolation, loneliness, and less participation in leisure activities seem to be important risk factors associated with the progression from normal cognition to MCI and these can influence neuropsychological test performance even if clinically significant anxiety and depression are excluded.

DISTINCTIVE ENTITIES

Operationalized diagnostic criteria for probable and possible *MCI with Lewy bodies*, enhanced by availability of biomarkers such as SPECT or PET scan are published.[41] The problems in diagnosing *MCI in Parkinson's disease (PD)* include assessment of functioning in ADL and differentiating cognitive effects from motor impairment. Other problems are presence of comorbid nonmotor features such as depression, anxiety, apathy, psychosis, fatigue, and sleep disturbances and their impact on cognition and during neuropsychological tests. Motor demands of some of the neuropsychological tests may also affect the outcome. *Vascular MCI (VaMCI)* includes four subtypes as in MCI—amnestic, amnestic plus other domains, nonamnestic single domain, and nonamnestic multiple domain. Presentation-wise, VaMCI should be based on the assumption of a stepwise (as following stroke) or insidious decline in cognitive function [as in CADASIL or cerebral amyloid angiopathy or subcortical ischemic vascular cognitive impairment (VCI) presenting as vascular Parkinsonism or "motoric cognitive risk syndrome"].[42,43]

PROBLEMS IN TREATMENT

The treatment approach for MCI needs clarity. Attempting to treat it like early-stage AD with drugs such as cholinesterase inhibitors has failed because they only address symptoms. While disease-modifying therapies targeting brain amyloid and tau may change this in the future, for now, clinicians should recognize the variability of MCI and aim for specific diagnoses to tailor treatment accordingly.

PROBLEMS IN DISCLOSING DIAGNOSIS TO PATIENTS

While some individuals may rapidly progress to dementia (with a conversion rate of 2–25% annually to AD), many remain stable, deteriorate slowly, or even show spontaneous improvement. This underscores the challenge of relying solely on complaints or symptoms for diagnosis. Identifying those at a prodromal stage of dementia will likely require identifying biological markers, as significant AD changes can occur in the brain before symptoms appear. While factors such as ApoE4, neuroimaging, and neuropsychological testing may offer some insight into propensity for progression, there are no definitive indicators of conversion. Consequently, prognostic uncertainty in MCI persists longer than in AD or other dementias. This ambiguity raises important considerations about whether the diagnosis should be disclosed to the individual. The utility of blood, CSF, and PET biomarkers in accordance within the A/T/N framework are likely to reduce diagnostic uncertainty in future.

CONCLUSION

More data is needed to determine if disclosing an MCI diagnosis leads to increased fears and feelings of helplessness or aids in preparation for the future. Best practice guidelines are likely to evolve in future for disclosing the diagnosis of MCI due to a degenerative etiology, amalgamating clinical judgment with neuropsychological imaging and blood/CSF biomarkers after clear multicenter data including from low-middle-income countries are available. This is of particular relevance with regard to occupational, financial, or inheritance decisions as well as social functioning and caregiving of elderly persons at risk and ratification of privileges such as driving or travel among others.

REFERENCES

1. Petersen RC, Caracciolo B, Brayne C, Gauthier S, Jelic V, Fratiglioni L. Mild cognitive impairment: a concept in evolution. J Intern Med. 2014;275(3):214-28.
2. Petersen RC. Mild cognitive impairment as a diagnostic entity. J Intern Med. 2004;256(3):183-94.
3. Petersen RC, Doody R, Kurz A, Mohs RC, Morris JC, Rabins PV, et al. Current Concepts in Mild Cognitive Impairment. Arch Neurol. 2001;58(12):1985.
4. Winblad B, Palmer K, Kivipelto M, Jelic V, Fratiglioni L, Wahlund LO, et al. Mild cognitive impairment – beyond controversies, towards a consensus: report of the International Working Group on Mild Cognitive Impairment. J Intern Med. 2004;256(3):240-6.
5. Albert MS, DeKosky ST, Dickson D, Dubois B, Feldman HH, Fox NC, et al. The diagnosis of mild cognitive impairment due to Alzheimer's disease: Recommendations from the National Institute on Aging-Alzheimer's Association workgroups on diagnostic guidelines for Alzheimer's disease. Alzheimers Dement. 2011;7(3):270-9.
6. Song WX, Wu WW, Zhao YY, Xu HL, Chen GC, Jin SY, et al. Evidence from a meta-analysis and systematic review reveals the global prevalence of mild cognitive impairment. Front Aging Neurosci. 2023;15:1227112.
7. Palmer K, Bäckman L, Winblad B, Fratiglioni L. Mild Cognitive Impairment in the General Population: Occurrence and Progression to Alzheimer Disease. Am J Geriatr Psychiatry. 2008;16(7):603-11.
8. Larrieu S, Letenneur L, Orgogozo JM, Fabrigoule C, Amieva H, Le Carret N, et al. Incidence and outcome of mild cognitive impairment in a population-based prospective cohort. Neurology. 2002;59(10):1594-9.
9. Caracciolo B, Palmer K, Monastero R, Winblad B, Bäckman L, Fratiglioni L. Occurrence of cognitive impairment and dementia in the community: A 9-year-long prospective study. Neurology. 2008;70(19 part 2):1778-85.
10. Rosenberg PB, Lyketsos C. Mild cognitive impairment: searching for the prodrome of Alzheimer's disease. World Psychiatry. 2008;7(2):72-8.
11. Manly JJ, Jones RN, Langa KM, Ryan LH, Levine DA, McCammon R, et al. Estimating the Prevalence of Dementia and Mild Cognitive Impairment in the US: The 2016 Health and Retirement Study Harmonized Cognitive Assessment Protocol Project. JAMA Neurol. 2022;79(12):1242-9.
12. Parnetti L, Chipi E, Salvadori N, D'Andrea K, Eusebi P. Prevalence and risk of progression of preclinical Alzheimer's disease stages: a systematic review and meta-analysis. Alzheimers Res Ther. 2019;11(1):7.
13. Reisberg B, Ferris SH, De Leon MJ, Franssen ESE, Kluger A, Mir P, et al. Stage-specific behavioral, cognitive, and in vivo changes in community residing subjects with age-associated memory impairment and primary degenerative dementia of the Alzheimer type. Drug Dev Res. 1988;15(2-3):101-14.
14. Petersen RC, Smith GE, Waring SC, Ivnik RJ, Tangalos EG, Kokmen E. Mild Cognitive Impairment: Clinical Characterization and Outcome. Arch Neurol. 1999;56(3):303.
15. Van Der Flier WM, Scheltens P. The ATN Framework—Moving Preclinical Alzheimer Disease to Clinical Relevance. JAMA Neurol. 2022;79(10):968.
16. Ismail Z, Agüera-Ortiz L, Brodaty H, Cieslak A, Cummings J, Fischer CE, et al.; NPS Professional Interest Area of the International Society of to Advance Alzheimer's Research and Treatment (NPS-PIA of ISTAART). The Mild Behavioral Impairment Checklist (MBI-C): A Rating Scale for Neuropsychiatric Symptoms in Pre-Dementia Populations. J Alzheimers Dis. 2017;56(3):929-38.
17. Dubois B, Feldman HH, Jacova C, Hampel H, Molinuevo JL, Blennow K, et al. Advancing research diagnostic criteria for Alzheimer's disease: the IWG-2 criteria. Lancet Neurol. 2014;13(6):614-29.
18. Ashton NJ, Brum WS, Di Molfetta G, Benedet AL, Arslan B, Jonaitis E, et al. Diagnostic Accuracy of a Plasma Phosphorylated Tau 217 Immunoassay for Alzheimer Disease Pathology. JAMA Neurol. 2024;81(3):255.
19. Janelidze S, Bali D, Ashton NJ, Barthélemy NR, Vanbrabant J, Stoops E, et al. Head-to-head comparison of 10 plasma phospho-tau assays in prodromal Alzheimer's disease. Brain. 2023;146(4):1592-601.
20. Thijssen EH, La Joie R, Strom A, Fonseca C, Iaccarino L, Wolf A, et al. Plasma phosphorylated tau 217 and phosphorylated tau 181 as biomarkers in Alzheimer's disease and frontotemporal lobar degeneration: a retrospective diagnostic performance study. Lancet Neurol. 2021;20(9):739-52.
21. Silva-Spínola A, Lima M, Leitão MJ, Bernardes C, Durães J, Duro D, et al. Blood biomarkers in mild cognitive impairment patients: Relationship between analytes and progression to Alzheimer disease dementia. Eur J Neurol. 2023;30(6):1565-73.
22. McConathy J, Sheline YI. Imaging Biomarkers Associated With Cognitive Decline: A Review. Biol Psychiatry. 2015;77(8):685-92.
23. Schuff N, Woerner N, Boreta L, Kornfield T, Shaw LM, Trojanowski JQ, et al. MRI of hippocampal volume loss in early Alzheimer's disease in relation to ApoE genotype and biomarkers. Brain. 2008;132(4):1067-77.
24. Sabuncu MR. The Dynamics of Cortical and Hippocampal Atrophy in Alzheimer Disease. Arch Neurol. 2011;68(8):1040.
25. Apostolova LG, Dutton RA, Dinov ID, Hayashi KM, Toga AW, Cummings JL, et al. Conversion of Mild Cognitive Impairment to Alzheimer Disease Predicted by Hippocampal Atrophy Maps. Arch Neurol. 2006;63(5):693.
26. Sheelakumari R, Sarma S, Kesavadas C, Thomas B, Sasi D, Sarath L, et al. Multimodality neuroimaging in mild cognitive impairment: A cross-sectional comparison study. Ann Indian Acad Neurol. 2018;21(2):133.
27. Soman S, Raghavan S, Rajesh P, Varma R, Mohanan N, Ramachandran S, et al. Relationship between cerebral perfusion on Arterial Spin Labeling (ASL) MRI with brain volumetry and cognitive performance in mild cognitive impairment and dementia due to Alzheimer's disease. Ann Indian Acad Neurol. 2021;24(4):559.
28. Mosconi L. Brain glucose metabolism in the early and specific diagnosis of Alzheimer's disease: FDG-PET studies in MCI and AD. Eur J Nucl Med Mol Imaging. 2005;32(4):486-510.
29. Johnson KA, Minoshima S, Bohnen NI, Donohoe KJ, Foster NL, Herscovitch P, et al. Appropriate use criteria for amyloid PET: A report of the Amyloid Imaging Task Force, the Society of Nuclear Medicine and Molecular Imaging, and the Alzheimer's Association. Alzheimers Dement. 2013;9(1):e1-16.
30. Jagust W, Reed B, Mungas D, Ellis W, DeCarli C. What does fluorodeoxyglucose PET imaging add to a clinical diagnosis of dementia? Neurology. 2007;69(9):871-7.
31. Aharonson V, Korczyn AD. Human–computer interaction in the administration and analysis of neuropsychological tests. Comput Methods Programs Biomed. 2004;73(1):43-53.

32. Mekala S, Paplikar A, Mioshi E, Kaul S, Divyaraj G, Coughlan G, et al. Dementia Diagnosis in Seven Languages: The Addenbrooke's Cognitive Examination-III in India. Arch Clin Neuropsychol. 2020;35(5):528-38.
33. Kaul S, Paplikar A, Varghese F, Alladi S, Sharma M, Dhaliwal RS, et al. MoCA in five Indian languages: A brief screening tool to diagnose dementia and MCI in a linguistically diverse setting. Int J Geriatr Psychiatry. 2022;37(10).
34. Ciesielska N, Sokołowski R, Mazur E, Podhorecka M, Polak-Szabela A, Kędziora-Kornatowska K. Is the Montreal Cognitive Assessment (MoCA) test better suited than the Mini-Mental State Examination (MMSE) in mild cognitive impairment (MCI) detection among people aged over 60? Meta-analysis. Psychiatr Pol. 2016;50(5):1039-52.
35. Menon R, Lekha V, Justus S, Sarma Ps, Mathuranath P. A pilot study on utility of Malayalam version of Addenbrooke⊠s Cognitive Examination in detection of amnestic mild cognitive impairment: A critical insight into utility of learning and recall measures. Ann Indian Acad Neurol. 2014;17(4):420.
36. Menon RN, Varghese F, Paplikar A, Mekala S, Alladi S, Sharma M, et al. Validation of Indian Council of Medical Research Neurocognitive Tool Box in Diagnosis of Mild Cognitive Impairment in India: Lessons from a Harmonization Process in a Linguistically Diverse Society. Dement Geriatr Cogn Disord. 2020;49(4):355-64.
37. Woolf C, Slavin MJ, Draper B, Thomassen F, Kochan NA, Reppermund S, et al. Can the Clinical Dementia Rating Scale Identify Mild Cognitive Impairment and Predict Cognitive and Functional Decline? Dement Geriatr Cogn Disord. 2016;41(5-6):292-302.
38. Bondi MW, Edmonds EC, Jak AJ, Clark LR, Delano-Wood L, McDonald CR, et al. Neuropsychological Criteria for Mild Cognitive Impairment Improves Diagnostic Precision, Biomarker Associations, and Progression Rates. J Alzheimers Dis. 2014;42(1):275-89.
39. Steinberg BA, Bieliauskas LA, Smith GE, Ivnik RJ, Malec JF. Mayo's Older Americans Normative Studies: Age- and IQ-Adjusted Norms for the Auditory Verbal Learning Test and the Visual Spatial Learning Test. Clin Neuropsychol. 2005;19(3-4):464-523.
40. Lucas JA, Ivnik RJ, Willis FB, Ferman TJ, Smith GE, Parfitt FC, et al. Mayo's Older African Americans Normative Studies: Normative Data for Commonly Used Clinical Neuropsychological Measures. Clin Neuropsychol. 2005;19(2):162-83.
41. McKeith IG, Ferman TJ, Thomas AJ, Blanc F, Boeve BF, Fujishiro H, et al. Research criteria for the diagnosis of prodromal dementia with Lewy bodies. Neurology. 2020;94(17):743-55.
42. Gorelick PB, Scuteri A, Black SE, DeCarli C, Greenberg SM, Iadecola C, et al. Vascular Contributions to Cognitive Impairment and Dementia: A Statement for Healthcare Professionals From the American Heart Association/American Stroke Association. Stroke. 2011;42(9):2672-713.
43. Verghese J, Wang C, Lipton RB, Holtzer R. Motoric cognitive risk syndrome and the risk of dementia. J Gerontol A Biol Sci Med Sci. 2013;68(4):412-8.

CHAPTER

8

Frontotemporal Dementia Spectrum Disorders

Sonali Bhattad, Ratnavalli Ellajosyula

ABSTRACT

Frontotemporal dementia (FTD) spectrum disorders are characterized by behavioral, language, and executive dysfunction. FTD is more frequent than recognized and a common cause of young-onset dementia (<65 years) but notably seen in older individuals as well. Although the behavior and the language variants are traditionally emphasized, the motor overlap syndromes are equally common. Signs and symptoms of FTD phenotypes emerge due to the specific patterns of brain networks affected by frontotemporal lobar degeneration (FTLD). This degeneration is associated with the aggregation of various pathological proteins, primarily, tau, transactive response DNA binding protein of 43 (TDP-43), and occasionally, fused in sarcoma (FUS) in sporadic and genetic cases. Delays in diagnosing FTD syndromes are due to low awareness by the family, insufficient knowledge among clinicians, and lack of resources. FTD results in a substantial caregiver burden with individual and societal consequences. Currently, available treatments offer only symptomatic benefits. Nonpharmacological measures are more critical for managing behaviors and possibly slowing the progression. We have made excellent progress in our understanding of FTD. Breakthroughs in underlying molecular mechanisms, genetics, and diagnostic biomarkers are the current driving forces for developing potential disease-modifying therapies. This chapter will address epidemiology, genetics, clinical phenotypes, diagnosis, neuropathology, biomarkers, and management of FTD spectrum disorders.

Keywords: Frontotemporal dementia, Primary progressive aphasia, Nonfluent aphasia, Semantic aphasia, Motor neuron disease, Progressive supranuclear palsy, Corticobasal syndrome.

INTRODUCTION[1-3]

Frontotemporal dementia (FTD) is a progressive neurodegenerative disorder and probably the most common young-onset dementia (YOD). It is characterized by early personality and behavioral changes, language impairment, executive dysfunction, or motor manifestations. Major FTD clinical phenotypes include the behavioral variant (bvFTD), semantic and nonfluent variants of a primary progressive aphasia (svPPA and nfvPPA), and the overlap syndrome, which has three subtypes: FTD associated with motor neuron disease (FTD-MND) or amyotrophic lateral sclerosis (FTD-ALS), FTD-corticobasal syndrome (CBS), and FTD-progressive supranuclear palsy (PSP). There is, thus, substantial clinical heterogeneity, so patients with FTD are of tremendous interest to psychiatrists, geriatricians, speech pathologists, neuropsychologists, neurologists, and dementia, neuromuscular and movement disorder specialists. About 20–25% of individuals with FTD carry a specific mutation linked to a particular underlying pathology.[4]

EPIDEMIOLOGY

Contrary to the belief that it is a rare disease, FTD is one of the most common causes of YOD. An early study from Cambridgeshire, UK, found the prevalence of early-onset Alzheimer's disease (AD) and FTD to be the same, i.e., 15 persons/100,000 population in the 45–64-year age group.[5] A recent study from 9 European countries estimated the annual incidence rate of FTD to be 2.36 cases/100,000 person-years. There was a progressive increase in FTD incidence across ages, reaching its peak at 71 years, and was higher in men than women (2.84 vs.

1.91).[6] BvFTD was the commonest phenotype, and FTD-ALS was uncommon. Thus, several studies highlight that FTD is more common than recognized, and diagnosis should be considered at any age.[3,6,7] FTD-MND has the shortest median survival of 2–3 years, while the median survival is 9–10 years for bvFTD and nfvPPA, and 12 years for svPPA.[7] Currently, the only confirmed risk factors for FTD are mutations in specific genes. Lower education and heart disease were more common in sporadic FTD than familial FTD (f-FTD) in a study from Finland and Italy.[8]

GENETICS OF FRONTOTEMPORAL DEMENTIA[4,9,10]

About a third of FTD cases are genetic (f-FTD) and the rest are sporadic. BvFTD is significantly more heritable than PPA, and nfvPPA is more likely familial than svPPA. The most common genetic mutations are expansions in chromosome 9 open reading frame 72 (C9orf72), followed by the progranulin (GRN) and the microtubule-associated protein tau (MAPT) genes with autosomal dominant inheritance **(Fig. 1)**. Others are rare and account for ~5% of f-FTD. Salient features of the common mutations are given in **Table 1**. Age at onset is highly variable even within families and several

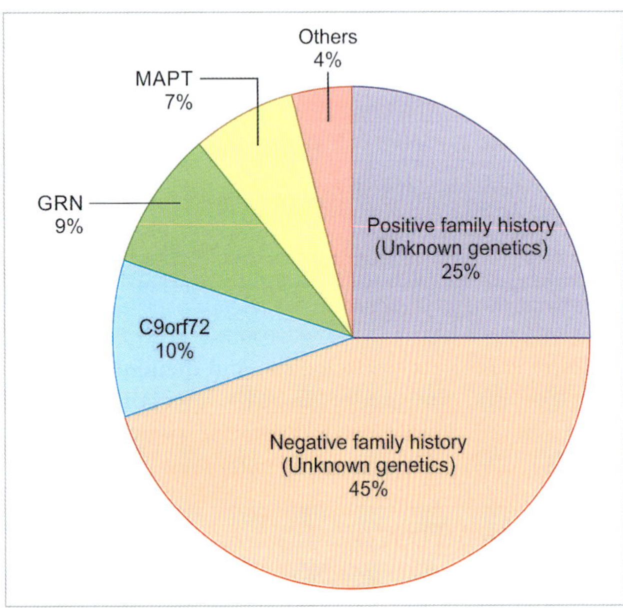

FIG. 1: Genetics of the frontotemporal dementia (FTD) spectrum disorders.[4,9,10]

(C9orf72: chromosome 9 open reading frame 72; GRN: progranulin; MAPT: microtubule-associated protein tau)

Note: Other mutations include valosin-containing protein (VCP), charged multivesicular body protein 2B (CHMP2B), TAR-DNA binding protein (TARDBP), fused in sarcoma (FUS), sequestosome 1 (SQSTM1), coiled-coil-helix-coiled-coil-helix (CHCHD10), TANK-binding kinase 1 (TBK1), optineurin gene (OPTN), cyclin F (CCNF), and T-cell restricted intracellular antigen 1 (TIA1).

genetic modifiers have been identified. Some individuals with f-FTD lack known underlying mutations, and the modified Goldman score helps estimate familial aggregation. Earlier studies from India have failed to find any mutation in FTD, except for one GRN mutation.[11] However, C9orf72 mutations were reported in 10.7% of familial ALS.[12]

Early parental deaths, failure to recognize symptoms by family, and undiagnosed individuals may all appear as apparent negative family history. In 10% of C9orf72 mutation carriers, family history may be absent. Genetic testing with a multigene panel using next-generation sequencing (NGS) to identify the common mutations is recommended for all bvFTD patients, regardless of family history, as mutations are found in about 10% of sporadic bvFTD cases.[4] Genetic testing should also be considered for other FTD phenotypes with a strong family history and to identify possible GRN mutations in mixed PPA subtypes. In patients whose NGS failed to identify a mutation, whole exome sequencing looking for rarer genes **(Fig. 1)** is an option. In clinical settings, it is more prudent to use an individualized approach with appropriate pre and postcounseling of the family, as disease-modifying treatments are not yet available. International genetic cohorts like the Genetic FTD Initiative (GENFI), the Advancement in Research and Treatment in FTLD (ARTFL), and the Longitudinal Evaluation of Familial FTD Subjects (LEFFTDS) Consortium collaborate utilizing shared datasets to improve presymptomatic diagnosis, develop biomarkers, and conduct clinical trials.[3]

CLINICAL PHENOTYPES AND CLASSIFICATION[1,3,13,14]

The primary clinical syndromes are **(Fig. 2 and Table 2)**:

- bvFTD
- Language variant
  - svPPA/semantic dementia (SD)
  - nfvPPA
- *FTD overlap syndrome*: FTD-MND/ALS, FTD-PSP, and FTD-CBS

It is important to emphasize that these clinical phenotypes may not be distinct, and patients usually have overlapping features. Thus, a bvFTD patient has very often associated Parkinsonism or semantic deficits, and a patient with SD has behavioral changes as well.[1-3]

Behavioral Variant Frontotemporal Dementia [1-3,13,15]

Behavioral variant FTD is the most common FTD syndrome characterized by early changes in personality

TABLE 1: Salient features of common genetic mutations in frontotemporal dementia (FTD).[4,9,10]

Salient features	**Genetic mutation**		
	MAPT	***GRN***	***C9orf72***
Age at onset (years)	Mean 49 Range 17–82	Mean 61 Range 25–90	Mean 58 Range 20–91
Penetrance	Full	Incomplete	Variable (increases as age advances with anticipation)
Molecular pathology	Tau	TDP-43 type A	TDP-43 type A or B
Common clinical phenotypes	bvFTD	bvFTD	• bvFTD + psychosis • ALS • FTD-ALS
Less common clinical phenotypes	• PSP • CBS • svPPA • nfvPPA	• Mixed aphasia • CBS • Amnestic syndrome	• nfvPPA • svPPA
Rare clinical phenotypes	• ALS • FTD-ALS	• FTD-ALS • ALS	• CBS • PSP
Magnetic resonance imaging (MRI)	*Often symmetric* • Frontal and temporal lobe atrophy • Characteristic medial temporal lobe and striatal atrophy	*Asymmetric* • Frontal and temporal lobe atrophy • Characteristic parietal lobe atrophy • White matter changes	*Symmetric* • Atrophy in dorsal frontal and temporal regions, insula, occipital, thalamus (medial pulvinar), and cerebellum
Network affected	Default mode	Frontoparietal	Salience and medial pulvinar
Life expectancy (years)	Mean 9 Range 0–45	Mean 7 Range 0–27	Mean 6 Range 0–36

(ALS: amyotrophic lateral sclerosis; bvFTD: behavioral variant frontotemporal dementia; CBS: corticobasal syndrome; C9orf72: chromosome 9 open reading frame72; GRN: progranulin; MAPT: microtubule-associated protein tau; nfvPPA: nonfluent variant PPA; PPA: primary progressive aphasia; PSP: progressive supranuclear palsy; svPPA: semantic variant PPA; TDP-43: TAR DNA-binding protein 43)

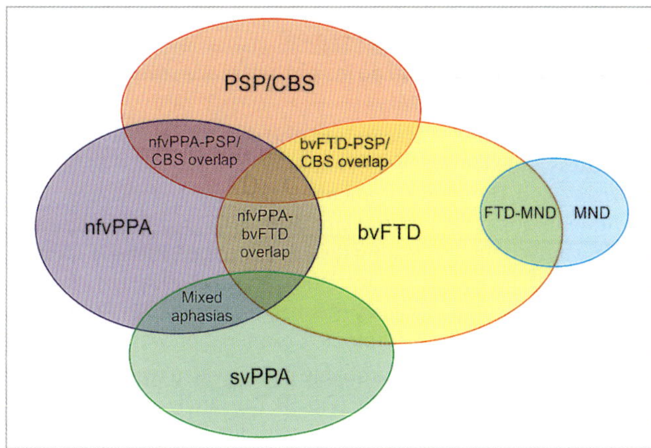

FIG. 2: Phenotypic spectrum of frontotemporal dementia (FTD).[1-3,13,14,24-26]

(bvFTD: behavioral variant FTD; CBS: corticobasal syndrome; MND: motor neuron disease; nfvPPA: nonfluent variant PPA; PPA: primary progressive aphasia; PSP: progressive supranuclear palsy; svPPA: semantic variant PPA)

and behavior. The syndrome may be preceded by a long phase of subclinical behavioral changes, often without cognitive impairment. Apathy is very common, characterized by a decreased drive to move (motor) or a loss of desire and emotional indifference to engage in goal-directed activity leading to social withdrawal (cognitive). Repetitive, stereotyped behaviors are frequent, ranging from simple mannerisms (e.g., tapping) to complex behaviors (e.g., collecting plastic bottle caps, and counting rituals). Socially inappropriate behaviors, loss of sympathy and empathy, overeating, food fads, or a preference for sweet foods are distinctive. Social cognition, the ability to interpret social cues and respond appropriately, which includes emotion recognition, mentalizing (theory of mind), and empathy, is impaired in FTD, resulting in inappropriate social behaviors.[16] The International consensus criteria for bvFTD highlights early deficits in social functioning **(Table 2)**.[13] Prominent anxiety and other mood disturbances or psychotic symptoms, including delusions and hallucinations, may be more common than suspected. The latter are reported more often in association with C9orf72 mutations. In the absence of associated motor manifestations and dysphasia, 30–50% of patients with bvFTD can be misdiagnosed as schizophrenia,

TABLE 2: Diagnostic criteria for the three variants of frontotemporal dementia (FTD).[13,14]

bvFTD clinical diagnosis	svPPA clinical diagnosis	nfvPPA clinical diagnosis
Any three of the following (1–6):	*Both core features must be present:*	*One core feature must be present:*
1. Early disinhibition	1. Impaired confrontational naming	1. Agrammatism
2. Early apathy	2. Impaired single-word comprehension	2. Effortful speech with apraxia of speech
3. Loss of empathy	*Any three of the following:*	*Any two of the following:*
4. Stereotypies	1. Impaired object knowledge	1. Impaired comprehension of syntactically complex sentences
5. Hyperorality and dietary changes	2. Surface dyslexia/dysgraphia	2. Spared single-word comprehension
6. *Neuropsychological profile*: Executive dysfunction with relative sparing of episodic memory and visuospatial functions	3. Spared repetition 4. Spared speech production	3. Spared object knowledge

Probable: Clinical diagnosis + MRI—frontal and/or anterior temporal atrophy (bvFTD), predominant anterior temporal lobe atrophy (svPPA), left posterior frontal-insular atrophy (nfvPPA) *OR* hypoperfusion/hypometabolism on positron emission tomography (PET) in the same regions.

Definite: Clinical diagnosis + Pathology-proven frontotemporal lobar degeneration (FTLD) *OR* positive pathogenic mutation.

**Possible*: Only clinical diagnosis.

(bvFTD: behavioral variant FTD; nfvPPA: nonfluent variant PPA; PPA: primary progressive aphasia; svPPA: semantic variant PPA)

depression, or bipolar disorders and may never come to the attention of a neurologist.[17,18] The Neuropsychiatric International Consortium for FTD (NIC-FTD) has suggested recommendations to differentiate primary psychiatric disease from bvFTD.[19] Executive dysfunction is a core feature of bvFTD and includes difficulties with planning, poor judgment, and problem-solving. Although significant episodic memory impairment is considered an exclusion, it can be impaired, particularly in presymptomatic MAPT and, occasionally, C9orf72 carriers. Memory deficits correlate with medial temporal and prefrontal atrophy, depending on whether consolidation or retrieval impairment is predominant.[4] Perceptual and spatial skills are typically intact but may be affected by inattention and executive dysfunction. Parkinsonism and dysphasia may be seen in later stages or sometimes precede the behavioral symptoms. An illustrative case vignette with MRI is provided in **Box 1 and Figure 3**. Clinical symptoms of bvFTD without progression or atrophy on MRI is called *"FTD-phenocopy"*. This is still not fully understood, but some patients appear to be C9orf72 mutation carriers.

BOX 1 Illustrative case history of a young patient with behavioral variant frontotemporal dementia (bvFTD).

Patient A: 42 years male; engineer; 17-years' education; and spoke 4 languages

- The patient presented with behavioral and personality changes for 3 years, which worsened over 6 months. Since the coronavirus disease (COVID), he had become dull, apathetic, and withdrawn. He changed several jobs and stopped working for the last 3 months. He was socially inappropriate and was eating more sweets. He used to go for a 5-minute walk 10–15 times a day and was disorganized and unable to complete any task. There was no family history. He was initially treated by a psychiatrist for 6 months, who diagnosed him with depression and prescribed escitalopram, olanzapine, and lithium. There was no improvement
- On examination, he had no insight and made several inappropriate comments
- ("Are you married?", "Is your husband dead?"). He was restless and inattentive. Orientation and visuospatial skills were good. The clinical dementia rating scale was 0.5 and Addenbrooke's cognitive examination (ACE) score was 90/100. Neuropsychological testing revealed impaired verbal learning and recall, working memory deficit, and executive dysfunction [reduced phonemic fluency (Kannada—'pa'-7 vs. animals-16) and impaired trails]. Neurological examination was normal
- He was diagnosed with probable bvFTD with a typical clinical picture and compatible MRI **(Fig. 3)**. The family was counseled, and olanzapine and lithium were withdrawn. Escitalopram was continued, and several activities and physical exercises were suggested

Language Variant Frontotemporal Dementia

Semantic Variant Primary Progressive Aphasia[3,14,15,20]

Semantic variant primary progressive aphasia more commonly referred to as SD, is estimated to account for one-third of all cases of FTD, with an average age at symptom onset of 64 years. SD is typically sporadic, and a positive family history is seen in <5% of patients. In SD, there is a progressive breakdown of semantic memory, which results in a loss of concepts and vocabulary. Patients present with word-finding difficulties and have lost the meaning of words. As the disease progresses, patients have difficulty understanding conversation, speech appears empty, and frequently use "this" or

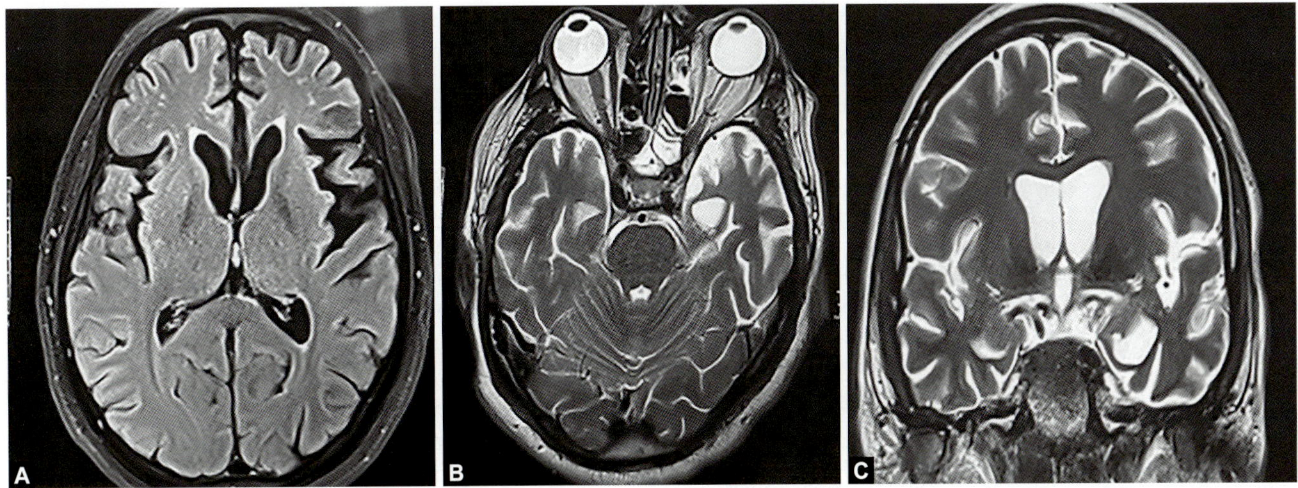

FIGS. 3A TO C: MRI fluid-attenuated inversion recovery (FLAIR) axial (A); T2 axial (B); and coronal (C) in patient A—bilateral frontotemporal atrophy left >right.

"that" for most object names. Grammar and syntax are usually spared. Object recognition is also impaired in auditory and visual modalities, suggesting a breakdown in conceptual knowledge and emphasizing that SD is more than a language disorder.

Surface dyslexia or dysgraphia is an overregularization phenomenon, i.e., a tendency to regularize irregular words (pint pronounced like mint). Most Indian languages have transparent orthographies, so surface dyslexia is not seen, which may be true for other languages, highlighting the drawbacks in the diagnostic criteria.[21] Striking loss of L2 was reported in a case series of bilingual patients with SD from South India.[22] This suggests that less proficient or later acquired languages are more vulnerable to neurodegeneration. Different languages in a bilingual appear to share a common semantic network in the brain. More worldwide research is needed on languages (other than English) to understand how a particular language or script influences symptoms of dysphasia.[21]

The concept of the right temporal variant of FTD (rtvFTD) is controversial. Studies indicate that these patients have prominent prosopagnosia and episodic memory impairment. In addition to the usual behavioral changes, depression, somatic complaints, and mental slowness may be distinguished.[23]

Nonfluent Variant Primary Progressive Aphasia[3,14,15]

Patients present in the age of early 60s, at an older age compared to those with bvFTD or SD, with equal sex distribution. Speech is slow and effortful with reduced fluency, often accompanied by simplified syntax and grammatical errors. Single-word comprehension is usually preserved, but there may be difficulty in understanding syntax. Repetition is largely preserved. Articulation errors may emerge if there is a component of apraxia of speech (AOS). Episodic memory, visuospatial function, attention, and executive functions are usually normal.

Frontotemporal Dementia Overlap Syndrome[1-3,24-26]

Frontotemporal dementia-PSP and FTD-CBS are common subtypes encountered in clinical practice. Patients with Parkinsonism should be evaluated for behavioral changes, dysphasia, and cognitive impairment to make a diagnosis of FTD overlap syndrome rather than restrict our focus to the usual phenotypes of "pure PSP" or "pure CBS". The PSP and CBS overlaps are classified as PSP-frontal and PSP-speech and language disorder within the PSP criteria and as frontal behavioral-spatial syndrome within the CBS criteria. Axial rigidity is more common than appendicular rigidity in FTD-PSP, and tremor is less common. About 10–15% of FTD patients develop MND, usually in association with bvFTD followed by nfvPPA and rarely svPPA. Similarly, 15% of MND patients meet FTD criteria, while 50–70% exhibit milder cognitive and behavioral abnormalities. Fasciculations are more prominently seen rather than motor weakness.

NEUROIMAGING[1-4,13,14,24-26]

Magnetic resonance imaging (MRI) is a critical component in the diagnostic workup of FTD patients, as each FTD subtype is associated with a specific pattern of atrophy **(Tables 1 and 3)**. T1 axial and coronal images to

TABLE 3: Magnetic resonance imaging (MRI) findings in frontotemporal dementia (FTD) variants.[1-3,13,14,24-26]

Frontotemporal dementia (FTD) variant	Key radiological features
Behavioral variant FTD	• Symmetric or asymmetric bilateral prefrontal and/or anterior temporal lobe atrophy • *Additional areas*: Atrophy of anterior cingulate, insula, orbital and medial frontal lobe, and temporal pole • *Core feature*: Degeneration of basal and limbic networks; sparing of posterior structures
Semantic variant primary progressive aphasia	• *Asymmetric atrophy*: Anterior temporal lobes and the fusiform gyrus, usually the left • *Classical feature*: "Knife-blade" appearance due to marked destruction in the amygdala, anterior hippocampus, and fusiform gyrus • Rostral–caudal gradient of hippocampal atrophy
Nonfluent variant primary progressive aphasia	• Asymmetric atrophy of dominant posterior-inferior frontal gyrus • *Additional areas*: Atrophy of insula, supplementary motor area, premotor cortex, and basal ganglia
Progressive supranuclear palsy	Midbrain and superior cerebellar peduncle atrophy ("hummingbird sign" or "Mickey Mouse sign") on sagittal T1 MRI
Corticobasal syndrome	Asymmetrical cortical atrophy, prominent in the perirolandic region and posterior frontal and parietal lobes, contralateral to the clinically more affected side

evaluate the temporal lobe and sagittal images to visualize the brainstem (to look for PSP features) are essential. Gray matter atrophy and hypometabolism may emerge a decade or more before symptoms in mutation carriers. Fludeoxyglucose-18-positron emission tomography (FDG-PET) can be used in inconclusive cases where MRI is equivocal and to rule out AD but is expensive and prone to interpretation errors.

DIAGNOSIS[1-3,15]

Diagnosing FTD is challenging because subtle early personality changes may not be recognized by the family, and they may be considered normal for the culture, background, or ethnicity.[21] Even in the best centers, there is usually a 1–2-year delay in diagnosing FTD. In a study from a memory clinic in urban South India, substantial delay was observed in the diagnosis of FTD compared to other dementias (median of 36 months in FTD vs. 18 months for vascular dementia).[27] Early diagnosis of bvFTD hinges on a reliable history from a family member. A detailed family history of three generations should be obtained, asking for symptoms/diagnosis of FTD, MND, Parkinsonism, dementia, psychiatric disorders, autism, and dyslexia in the first-degree relatives. Even a diagnosis of Parkinson's disease or AD in a family member should not preclude the diagnosis of FTD, as some genetic variants can have these phenotypes **(Table 1)**. A multi-domain cognitive assessment supplements the clinical interview and neurological examination. In particular, working memory (serial subtraction or days of week backward), phonemic and category fluency (words beginning with "pa", animals in one minute), naming, and recognition of pictures are crucial. Attention should be paid to the scores and the overall approach and demeanor, which may be more informative. Poor performance on a test may not indicate a domain impairment as amotivation, inattention, impulsivity, retrieval deficits, perseveration, and intrusions may all affect performance.

Loss of insight, lack of spontaneous conversation, or disinhibition (inappropriate jocularity or remarks to the doctor or staff) may point to the diagnosis. Patients may be restless and exhibit various motor stereotypies (e.g., finger tapping). Cortical sensory deficits, apraxia, abnormalities in extraocular movements, amyotrophy, fasciculations, bradykinesia, rigidity, and slowness of gait should be looked for which may aid in subtyping FTD. Buccofacial apraxia or stuttering may suggest nonfluent aphasia. Single-word comprehension tested by defining an object (e.g., "What is a lemon?") and inability to name and recognize (failure to point to a cat among an array of animal pictures) are characteristic findings of svPPA. The repeat and point test, where patients have to repeat ten nouns (usually a tool or an animal) and then select the corresponding picture from an array of six similar options, is a simple and quick measure to use in the clinic to differentiate SD and nfvPPA. Patients with SD exhibit pointing impairment, while those with nfvPPA show no deficits in pointing but are impaired in repetition.[28]

NEUROPSYCHOLOGICAL TESTING[1-3,15]

Neuropsychological testing is beneficial to differentiate FTD from vascular dementia, other degenerative dementias, and primary psychiatric disorders. It is also helpful in patients with atypical symptoms or normal imaging and in monitoring progression. The test battery should include social cognition tests (the faux pas, humor interpretation, Ekman 60 Faces Test, and others).[16,21] A normal or atypical neuropsychological profile does not rule out FTD, and a typical bvFTD profile may not be specific.

DIAGNOSTIC WORKUP

It is important to exclude treatable and reversible dementias. Serology for neurosyphilis, human immunodeficiency virus (HIV), and vasculitis is a must. Exclude autoimmune and paraneoplastic encephalitis, especially if there are fluctuations, rapid progression, shorter duration of illness (<2 years), or inconsistent findings. MRI is an essential component of the workup. Cerebrospinal fluid (CSF) analysis can be done to rule out infections, where appropriate, and to test AD biomarkers. Plasma biomarkers for AD may be particularly useful to exclude AD.

FRONTOTEMPORAL DEMENTIA MIMICS[1-3,15,19, 29-32]

Several disorders can masquerade as FTD; the more important and clinically relevant to our setting along with the differentiating pointers are presented briefly in **Table 4**. Differences are relative and not absolute; in uncertain cases, close follow-up and selective investigations may be necessary. Several studies have shown an overlap between autoimmune diseases and neurodegenerative diseases, particularly FTD. Therefore, it is prudent to rule out autoimmune disorders before labeling a patient as FTD with the caveat that a patient may have both.

TABLE 4: Features to differentiate mimics from behavioral variant frontotemporal dementia (bvFTD).[1-3, 15,19,29-32]

Mimics	Differentiating features
Primary psychiatric diseases	• Absence of dysphasia and neurological signs • Social cognition impairment is more severe in bvFTD • No focal or asymmetric atrophy on MRI • Normal PET favors psychiatric disease but hypometabolism does not exclude it • Negative genetic mutations • Biomarkers (serum or CSF NfL in future)
Vascular dementia (strategic infarcts)	• Presence of focal neurological signs • Sudden onset; progression is unusual • Presence of vascular risk factors • *MRI*: Infarcts and white matter changes
Frontal/dysexecutive variant AD	• Early memory deficits in AD; impaired social cognition (faux pas and sarcasm) in bvFTD • Depression, irritability, and agitation are more common in AD. Hyperorality is more common in bvFTD • *MRI*: Symmetric diffuse atrophy or more prominent in medial temporal or parietal • CSF/plasma biomarkers specific for AD
Spontaneous intracranial hypotension	• Headache in 90% • *MRI*: Absence of frontotemporal atrophy. Severe brain sagging of the brainstem, and bilateral temporal lobe herniation. Pachymeningeal contrast enhancement • Spinal imaging can detect a CSF leak • Complete recovery after treating the CSF leak
Neurosyphilis	• Subacute onset and faster progression • Syphilis serology and abnormal CSF • Associated AR pupil, areflexia • MRI—can show frontal and temporal atrophy. Features of chronic meningitis and infarcts • Partial recovery with antibiotic treatment
Vitamin B12 deficiency	• Anemia, neuropathy, glossitis, and vegetarian diet • Low serum vitamin B12 levels • Reversibility with vitamin B12 replacement • *MRI*: Diffuse atrophy or white matter changes; no focal atrophy
Autoimmune encephalitis	• Seizures, chorea, myoclonus, and hyponatremia • Rapid progression and fluctuating course • CSF abnormalities, if present • Absence of frontotemporal atrophy on MRI • Abnormal EEG • Significant improvement with treatment

(AD: Alzheimer's disease; CSF: cerebrospinal fluid; EEG: electroencephalogram; MRI: magnetic resonance imaging; NfL: neurofilament light chain; PET: positron emission tomography)

NEUROPATHOLOGY[1-3,15,33]

Frontotemporal lobar degeneration is an umbrella term for the neuropathology of FTD spectrum disorders with atrophy in the frontal, temporal lobes, and striatum with neuronal loss, gliosis, and microvacuolar changes. On a molecular basis, FTLD is classified into three types based on the protein component of abnormal inclusions and its distribution: FTLD-tau is characterized by abnormal tau deposition, FTLD-TDP by TDP-43, and FTLD-FET (FUS protein–Ewing sarcoma–TAF15) by FUS. Tau or TDP-43 pathology accounts for most cases of FTLD, while FET accounts for 10%. Abnormal deposition of TDP-43 affects neuronal development and synaptic function while hyperphosphorylated tau disrupts axonal transport. FUS proteins have a role in DNA and RNA metabolism. Each FTLD pathology can be associated with more than one clinical syndrome, and each clinical syndrome may be associated with different FTLD subtypes in different individuals. bvFTD is linked to various underlying pathologies, including tau, TDP-43, and FET; nfvPPA with speech apraxia to tau and nfvPPA with agrammatism to TDP-43, while svPPA is associated with TDP-43 type C. FTD-MND is associated with TDP pathology subtype 4 and occasionally with FTLD-FET. The most common subtypes of FTLD-tau are Pick's disease, CBS, and PSP. Microscopically, Pick bodies are the pathological hallmark of Pick's disease. Similarly, tau pathology is seen in MAPT, TDP-43 A typically in GRN, and TDP-43 A or B in C9orf72 mutations **(Fig. 4)**. Very young onset (<40 years), negative family history, obsessions, hyperorality, hypersexuality, and ritualistic behaviors with striking caudate atrophy are seen in FUS pathology.

Degeneration begins within epicenters—anterior cingulate and frontoinsular cortex in bvFTD, inferior frontal gyrus in nfvPPA, inferomedial temporal pole in SD, perirolandic cortex in CBS, and dorsal midbrain tegmentum in PSP. These epicenters often contain specialized neurons with heightened vulnerability to early pathological processes. For example, in ALS, upper motor neurons show early vulnerability to TDP-43 pathobiology. There is early loss of von Economo neurons in layer V of the anterior cingulate and frontal-insular cortex in bvFTD, which are thought to play a central part in integrating cortical and subcortical networks.

FLUID BIOMARKERS IN FRONTOTEMPORAL DEMENTIA[3,4,34]

Fluid biomarkers in CSF, serum, or plasma are essential to provide objective indicators of biological processes and treatment responses. However, no biomarkers have been approved for FTD diagnosis and treatment. **Table 5** shows emerging biomarkers in FTD and their significance.

MANAGEMENT OF FRONTOTEMPORAL DEMENTIA[1-3,35]

The impact of FTD and related disorders is profound. It may lead to devastating consequences, including divorce, loss of job and income, sexual indiscretion, gambling, excessive spending, financial losses, and tragic accidents. The caregiver burden is enormous, with a decline in caregiver's health and psychological well-being

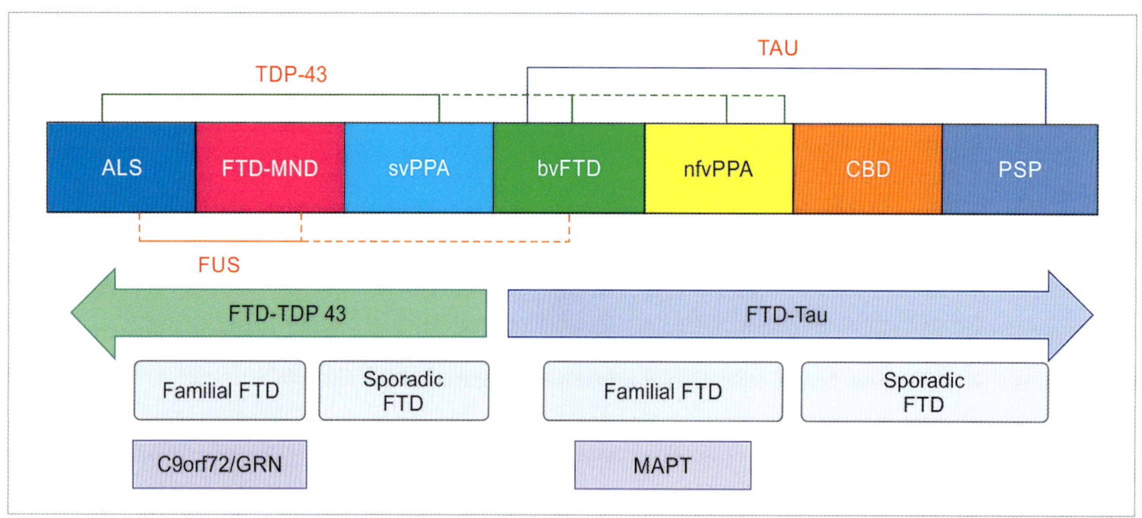

FIG. 4: Clinico–pathological–genetic spectrum of frontotemporal dementia (FTD).[1-3,15,33]

(ALS: amyotrophic lateral sclerosis; bvFTD: behavioral variant FTD; CBD: corticobasal syndrome; C9orf72: chromosome 9 open reading frame 72; FUS: fused in sarcoma protein; GRN: progranulin; MAPT: microtubule-associated protein tau; MND: motor neuron disease; nfvPPA: nonfluent variant PPA; PSP: progressive supranuclear palsy; svPPA: semantic variant PPA; PPA: primary progressive aphasia; TDP-43: TAR DNA-binding protein 43)

TABLE 5: Biomarkers in frontotemporal dementia (FTD).[3,4,34]

Emerging biomarkers	Significance
Progranulin	Decreased levels of progranulin in CSF and blood in GRN mutation carriers
Poly (GP)-dipeptide repeat proteins	• Increased in presymptomatic and symptomatic stages of C9orf72-related FTD-ALS • Marker of treatment response in ASO therapy trials
Serum and CSF Neurofilament light chain (NfL)	• Intensity of neurodegeneration • Highest levels in C9orf 72-ALS and lowest in MAPT carriers • Predicts progression and survival in genetic FTD Not specific for FTD
GFAP to NfL183 ratio	Distinguishes between FTD-tau and FTD-TDP, but replication studies are required for confirming validity

(AD: Alzheimer's disease; AR pupil: Argyll Robertson pupil; bvFTD: behavioral variant FTD; CSF: cerebrospinal fluid; EEG: electroencephalogram; MRI: magnetic resonance imaging; NfL: neurofilament light chain; PET: positron emission tomography; ALS: amyotrophic lateral sclerosis; ASO: antisense oligonucleotide; CSF: cerebrospinal fluid; C9orf72: chromosome 9 open reading frame 72; GFAP: Glial fibrillary acidic protein; GRN: progranulin; MAPT: microtubule-associated protein tau)

and an increase in caregiver's health-related costs. In the absence of disease-modifying treatment, behavioral management remains central.

Nonpharmacological Interventions

Behavioral therapies for bvFTD and speech and language therapy for PPA patients may offer benefits in conjunction with cognitive rehabilitation. Providing incentives for apathetic patients, identifying triggers for agitation, and distraction techniques such as squishy balls for compulsive behaviors are helpful. Physical exercises, music, art, pet therapy, games, puzzles, and control of vascular risk factors can reduce agitation, improve quality of life, and potentially slow the rate of cognitive decline. A few case series have shown that repetitive transcranial magnetic stimulation and transcranial direct current stimulation improve language function in PPA and troublesome behaviors in bvFTD.

Pharmacological Treatment

Treatment is individualized, largely symptomatic, targeted at a distressing or disruptive behavior, and requires a multidisciplinary approach, with a team of psychiatrists, psychologists, and neurologists working with the family. Uncontrolled trials and observation studies have shown that trazodone and selective serotonin reuptake inhibitors (SSRIs) control aggression, disinhibition, and repetitive behaviors. Among the atypical antipsychotics, quetiapine is preferred for its lower risk of extrapyramidal side effects. Antiepileptics have also been tried for hypomania, disinhibition, and food cravings (topiramate) with variable success, but tolerance is an issue. It is best to avoid valproate as it can cause Parkinsonism and lead to weight gain. Intranasal oxytocin appeared to be efficacious in improving empathy. However, cholinesterase inhibitors and memantine are not helpful and should be avoided due to their potential to worsen neuropsychiatric symptoms.

Disease-modifying Treatment

Disease-modification treatment focuses on targeting pathological proteins like tau or TDP-43. Therapy targeting tau may include tau aggregation inhibitors, microtubule-stabilizing drugs, tau-targeted immunotherapy, and tau vaccines. Antisense oligonucleotide therapy (ASO) can be helpful in decreasing levels of potentially harmful C9orf72 mRNAs. Progranulin replacement therapy is being considered a potential treatment for GRN mutations. We await further developments in this crucial field.

CAREGIVER BURDEN AND SUPPORT

As already discussed, the caregiver burden is significant, and providing an ear to the caregiver is essential. Behavioral changes, rather than the disability level, are closely tied to caregiver distress. Strategies should include providing information about the disease and progression, nonpharmacological interventions, and psychosocial support. Caregiver networks and local and national dementia chapters can be useful. An enrichment program called "Cogworks", an initiative by the Cognitive Neurology Clinic in Bengaluru, uses physical exercise, movement therapy, art, games, baking, gardening, and dancing to improve troublesome behaviors and enhance the quality of life for individuals with dementia and their caregivers.

CONCLUSION

Frontotemporal dementia research has made tremendous progress, particularly in forming large international genetic cohorts with a better understanding of molecular pathology. A concerted effort is required for Indian researchers to join these global endeavors to delineate the genetics, risk factors, and clinical phenotypes of FTD and to enter clinical trials and prevention initiatives. FTD research aims to find an effective treatment for the disease and understand brain functions better. Longitudinal studies of both sporadic and f-FTD using new radioligands in molecular PET imaging, newer techniques of MRI, optic coherence tomography, and fluid biomarkers will pave the way forward. In addition, automated analysis of digitized speech samples, computer-based batteries of cognitive assessments, eye tracking wearables, and autonomic variables to detect subtle language, executive, and social cognition impairments will be valuable to diagnose presymptomatic FTD. Using artificial intelligence and machine learning to extract patterns from large-scale longitudinal data sets of multimodal biomarkers is now a reality. The next decade of FTD research will be a game-changer and exciting.

REFERENCES

1. Sivasathiaseelan H, Marshall CR, Agustus JL, Benhamou E, Bond RL, van Leeuwen JEP, et al. Frontotemporal Dementia: A Clinical Review. Semin Neurol. 2019;39(2):251-63.
2. Boeve BF, Boxer AL, Kumfor F, Pijnenburg Y, Rohrer JD. Advances and controversies in frontotemporal dementia: Diagnosis, biomarkers, and therapeutic considerations. Lancet Neurol. 2022;21(3):258-72.
3. Grossman M, Seeley WW, Boxer AL, Hillis AE, Knopman DS, Ljubenov PA, et al. Frontotemporal lobar degeneration. Nat Rev Dis Primers. 2023;9(1):40.
4. Greaves CV, Rohrer JD. An update on genetic frontotemporal dementia. J Neurol. 2019;266(8):2075-86.
5. Ellajosyula R, Brayne C, Dawson K, Hodges JR. The prevalence of frontotemporal dementia. Neurology. 2002;58(11):1615-21.
6. Logroscino G, Piccininni M, Graff C, Hardiman O, Ludolph AC, Moreno F, et al. Incidence of syndromes associated with frontotemporal lobar degeneration in 9 European Countries. JAMA Neurol. 2023;80(3):279-86.
7. Coyle-Gilchrist IT, Dick KM, Patterson K, Vázquez Rodríquez P, Wehmann E, Wilcox A, et al. Prevalence, characteristics, and survival of frontotemporal lobar degeneration syndromes. Neurology. 2016;86(18):1736-43.
8. Soppela H, Katisko K, Gadola Y, Krüger J, Hartikainen P, Alberici A, et al. Modifiable potential risk factors in familial and sporadic frontotemporal dementia. Ann Clin Transl Neurol. 2022;9(8):1195-205.
9. Moore KM, Nicholas J, Grossman M, McMillan CT, Irwin DJ, Massimo L, et al. Age at symptom onset and death and disease duration in genetic frontotemporal dementia: An international retrospective cohort study. Lancet Neurol. 2020;19(2): 145-56.
10. Wagner M, Lorenz G, Volk AE, Brunet T, Edbauer D, Berutti R, et al. Clinico-genetic findings in 509 frontotemporal dementia patients. Mol Psychiatry. 2021;26(10):5824-32.
11. Aswathy PM, Jairani PS, Raghavan SK, Verghese J, Gopala S, Srinivas P, et al. Progranulin mutation analysis: Identification of one novel mutation in exon 12 associated with frontotemporal dementia. Neurobiol Aging. 2016;39:218.
12. Shamim U, Ambawat S, Singh J, Thomas A, Pradeep-Chandra-Reddy C, Suroliya V, et al. C9orf72 hexanucleotide repeat expansion in Indian patients with ALS: A common founder and its geographical predilection. Neurobiol Aging. 2020;88:156.
13. Rascovsky K, Hodges JR, Knopman D, Mendez MF, Kramer JH, Neuhaus J, et al. Sensitivity of revised diagnostic criteria for the behavioural variant of frontotemporal dementia. 2011; 134(9):2456-77.
14. Gorno-Tempini ML, Hillis AE, Weintraub S, Kertesz A, Mendez M, Cappa SF, et al. Classification of primary progressive aphasia and its variants. Neurology. 2011;76:1006-14.
15. Snowden JS. Changing perspectives on frontotemporal dementia: A review. J Neuropsychol. 2023;17(2):211-34.
16. Henry JD, von Hippel W, Molenberghs P, Lee T, Sachdev PS. Clinical assessment of social cognitive function in neurological disorders. Nat Rev Neurol. 2016;12(1):28-39.
17. Woolley JD, Khan BK, Murthy NK, Miller BL, Rankin KP. The diagnostic challenge of psychiatric symptoms in neurodegenerative disease: Rates of and risk factors for prior psychiatric diagnosis in patients with early neurodegenerative disease. J Clin Psychiatry. 2011;72(2):126-33.
18. Waldö ML, Gustafson L, Passant U, Englund E. Psychotic symptoms in frontotemporal dementia: A diagnostic dilemma? Int Psychogeriatr. 2015;27:531-9.
19. Ducharme S, Dols A, Laforce R, Devenney E, Kumfor F, van den Stock J, Dallaire-Théroux C, et al. Recommendations to distinguish behavioural variant frontotemporal dementia from psychiatric disorders. Brain. 2020;143(6):1632-50.
20. Landin-Romero R, Tan R, Hodges JR, Kumfor F. An update on semantic dementia: Genetics, imaging, and pathology. Alzheimers Res Ther. 2016;8(1):52-60.
21. Franzen S, Nuytemans K, Bourdage R, Caramelli P, Ellajosyula R, Finger E, et al. Gaps in clinical research in frontotemporal dementia: A call for diversity and disparities-focused research. Alzheimers Dement. 2023;19(12):5817-36.
22. Ellajosyula R, Narayanan J, Patterson K. Striking loss of second language in bilingual patients with semantic dementia. J Neurol. 2020;267(2):551-60.
23. Ulugut Erkoyun H, Groot C, Heilbron R, Nelissen A, van Rossum J, Jutten R, et al. A clinical-radiological framework of the right temporal variant of frontotemporal dementia. Brain. 2020: 143(9);2831-43.
24. Armstrong MJ, Litvan I, Lang AE, Bak TH, Bhatia KP, Borroni B, et al. Criteria for the diagnosis of corticobasal degeneration. Neurology. 2013;80(5):496-503.
25. Burrell JR, Halliday GM, Kril JJ, Ittner LM, Götz J, Kiernan MC, et al. The frontotemporal dementia-motor neuron disease continuum. Lancet. 2016;388(10047):919-31.
26. Höglinger GU, Respondek G, Stamelou M, Kurz C, Josephs KA, Lang AE, et al. Clinical diagnosis of progressive supranuclear palsy: The movement disorder society criteria. Mov Disord. 2017;32:853-64.
27. Ellajosyula R, Narayanan J, Hegde S, Kamath V, Murgod U, Easwaran V, et al. Delay in the diagnosis of dementia in urban India: Role of dementia subtype and age at onset. Int J Geriatr Psychiatry. 2022;37(12):1-8.
28. Hodges JR, Martinos M, Woollams AM, Patterson K, Adlam AL. Repeat and Point: Differentiating semantic dementia from progressive non-fluent aphasia. Cortex. 2008;44(9):1265-70.
29. Musa G, Slachevsky A, Muñoz-Neira C, Méndez-Orellana C, Villagra R, González-Billault C, et al. Alzheimer's disease or behavioral variant frontotemporal dementia? Review of key points toward an accurate clinical and neuropsychological diagnosis. J Alzheimers Dis. 2020;73(3):833-48.

30. Caroppo P, Villa C, Del Sole A, Bernardi G, Carradori S, Tiraboschi P, et al. Neurosyphilis mimicking behavioral variant of frontotemporal dementia in a 59-year-old man. Cogn Behav Neurol. 2022;35(2):140-6.
31. Lashkarivand A, Eide PK. Brain sagging dementia–Diagnosis, treatment, and outcome: A review. Neurology. 2022;98:798-805.
32. Bastiaansen AEM, van Steenhoven RW, Te Vaarwerk ES, van der Flier WM, Teunissen C, de Graaff E, et al. Antibodies associated with autoimmune encephalitis in patients with presumed neurodegenerative dementia. Neurol Neuroimmunol Neuroinflamm. 2023;10(5):e200137.
33. Mackenzie IRA, Neumann M. Molecular neuropathology of frontotemporal dementia: Insights into disease mechanisms from postmortem studies. J Neurochem. 2016;138:54-70.
34. Swift IJ, Sogorb-Esteve A, Heller C, Synofzik M, Otto M, Graff C, et al. Fluid biomarkers in frontotemporal dementia: Past, present and future. J Neurol Neurosurg Psychiatry. 2021;92(2): 204-15.
35. Guimet MN, Zapata-Restrepo LM, Miller BL. Advances in treatment of frontotemporal dementia. J Neuropsychiatry Clin Neurosci. 2022;34(4):316-27.

CHAPTER

9

Vascular Cognitive Impairment

PT Alexander, Ravi Prakash Singh, Suvarna Alladi, Subhash Kaul

ABSTRACT

Vascular cognitive impairment (VCI) and dementia are a spectrum of disorders characterized by cognitive impairment or dementia that occurs due to cerebral parenchymal insult secondary to vascular etiology. VCI is a heterogeneous entity that is a result of several pathophysiological mechanisms. Recurring strokes, a strategically located single infarct, small vessel disease (SVD) resulting in subcortical infarcts or white matter disease, microhemorrhages and macrohemorrhages, and chronic hypoperfusion are the well-established underlying mechanisms. Newly identified vascular mechanisms that contribute to VCI include microinfarcts, enlarged perivascular spaces (PVS), impaired cerebral autoregulation, blood–brain barrier (BBB) dysfunction, and neurovascular decoupling. Modifiable vascular risk factors such as hypertension, diabetes, and obesity in a background of nonmodifiable risk factors like age, genetic, and environmental factors, lead to subclinical vascular pathologies, giving rise to the pathobiological hallmarks of VCI, namely, impaired cerebral blood flow (CBF), BBB permeability and network dysfunction. The recent Vascular Impairment of Cognition Classification Consensus Study (VICCCS) criteria classified VCI into mild VCI and major VCI [vascular dementia (VaD)], and VaD into four subtypes: (1) Poststroke dementia (PSD), (2) subcortical ischemic vascular dementia, (3) multi-infarct dementia, and (4) mixed dementia. The role of biomarkers, including quantitative imaging markers and clinically applicable fluid biomarkers, is on the brink of expansion and is transitioning from the bench to the bedside. Management should focus on prevention by controlling risk factors, pharmacological measures, rehabilitation, and caregiver support systems.

Keywords: Vascular cognitive impairment and dementia, Vascular dementia, Multi-infarct dementia (MiD), Small vessel disease, Cerebral amyloid angiopathy (CAA), White matter hyperintensities (WMH), Stroke.

INTRODUCTION

Vascular cognitive impairment (VCI) and dementia are a spectrum of disorders characterized by cognitive impairment or dementia that occurs due to cerebral parenchymal insult secondary to vascular etiology.

History

The origin of descriptions of VCI can be traced back to Sir Thomas Willis in the 17th century, who compiled the first case series of post apoplexy (stroke) dementia, describing a spectrum of clinical presentations including "dullness of mind and forgetfulness" with hemiplegia, the cause attributed to "cerebral congestion"—an explanation that held for the next two centuries, till the introduction of the sphygmomanometer and recognition of arterial hypertension as the likely etiology. Toward the 20th century, Otto Binswanger described chronic progressive subcortical encephalopathy and Alois Alzheimer characterized arteriosclerotic brain atrophy and distinguished clinicopathological variants among VCI. Although "lacunes" were described by Amédée Dechambre and its pathogenesis was postulated by Maxime Durand-Fardel in the 19th century, it was Miller Fisher et al. who published observations on lacunes in the 1960s and described the clinical "stepwise progression" characteristic of vascular dementia.[1]

The advent of neuroimaging with computed tomography (CT) and magnetic resonance imaging (MRI) allowed in vivo identification of vascular brain pathologies, which aided in replacing the term "cerebral arteriosclerosis" with "multi-infarct dementia" in 1974,[2] and coining the term "leukoaraiosis" in 1987,[3] by Hachinski et al. In the same year, Fazekas et al. proposed the white matter hyperintensities (WMH) grading system,[4] while small vessel disease (SVD) imaging standardization was brought about by the STRIVE (STandards for ReportIng Vascular changes on nEuroimaging) guidelines in 2013 by Wardlaw et al.[5]

EPIDEMIOLOGY

Vascular cognitive impairment is considered the second leading cause of dementia and accounts for nearly a one-third of dementia in low-and-middle-income countries (LMICs), which includes India.[6] A meta-analysis reported pooled prevalence for VCI was 116 per 10,000 persons.[7] The Rush Religious Orders Study and Memory and Aging Project showed that 88% of autopsied brains of people with dementia had evidence of cerebrovascular disease along with another neurodegenerative pathology.[8]

Two-thirds of stroke patients have varying degrees of cognitive impairment.[9] Approximately one in ten patients have dementia before stroke, whereas one in ten develop dementia within a year of their first stroke.[10] A study from Kolkata reported that 20% survivors of stroke developed poststroke cognitive impairment (PSCI).[11] A hospital based study from Mumbai showed PSCI in 31.7%.[12] Another study from Mumbai reported that up to two-thirds suffered from PSCI.[13] Cognitive evaluation of patients in the Hyderabad Stroke and Memory Clinic Registry, demonstrated that around 74% were found to have PSCI after 3 months of the stroke.[9]

ETIOPATHOGENETIC MECHANISMS IN VASCULAR COGNITIVE IMPAIRMENT

Vascular cognitive impairment is heterogeneous and a result of several pathophysiological mechanisms. Recurring strokes that lead to multiple large or small vessel infarcts, a strategically located single infarct, SVD resulting in subcortical infarcts or white matter disease, microhemorrhages and macrohemorrhages, and chronic hypoperfusion are the well-established underlying mechanisms. Newly identified vascular mechanisms that contribute to VCI include micro-infarcts, enlarged perivascular spaces (PVS), impaired cerebral autoregulation, blood-brain barrier (BBB) dysfunction, and neurovascular decoupling.

Large Artery Infarcts

Large infarcts (>10 mm) are associated with large-vessel extracranial or intracranial atherosclerosis and cardiac disease and pose risk for poststroke dementia (PSD)[10] or multi-infarct dementia. Atherosclerosis of large- and medium-sized arteries is characterized by deposition of fibrous elements and lipoprotein in the intimal lining beneath injured endothelial cells and involvement of lymphocytes and macrophages in plaque formation.[14] Large artery occlusion by cardiac emboli by cardiac emboli or thrombosis leads to infarcts involving superficial cortical grey and underlying subcortical white matter, disrupting networks, resulting in stepwise progression of symptoms or multi-infarct dementia or PSD.[15]

Cerebral Small Vessel Disease

Cerebral SVD occurs due to pathological changes in cerebral perforating arterioles and is associated with a wide heterogeneity in brain pathologies. SVD is considered to be the most prevalent mechanism underlying VCI and cognitive deficits of varying severity are consistently associated with arteriosclerosis and resultant SVD. The pathophysiological consequences of SVD affect the neurovascular unit leading to impaired cerebral blood flow regulation, altered BBB permeability, microvascular stiffening and luminal narrowing, causing cerebral microinfarcts, lacunar infarcts, enlarged PVS, white matter demyelination, micro- and macrohemorrhages, and secondary neuronal degeneration.[16,17] Arteriosclerosis and SVD affect subcortical areas, mainly frontal white matter, basal ganglia and thalamus, that are crucial for different aspects of cognitive functions. Cognitive impairment is a result of disturbances in brain networks involved in attention, executive function, language, or memory.[15]

Neurovascular Unit Dysfunction

The neurovascular unit (NVU) is a concept integral to the mechanism of VCI, which explains the coupling of cerebral blood flow (CBF) with neural activity **(Fig. 1)**. The NVU is a complex structure comprising specialized endothelial cells of the BBB covered by the basal lamina, associated neurons, pericytes, microglia, astrocytes, and extracellular matrix. NVU dysfunction results in various brain pathologies, including VCI.[18] Vascular risk factors lead to subclinical vascular pathologies giving rise to the pathobiological hallmarks of VCI, namely, CBF and network dysfunction **(Flowchart 1)**. These changes can potentially be countered by addressing vascular risk factors and lifestyle modifications that enhance cognitive reserve and resilience.[8]

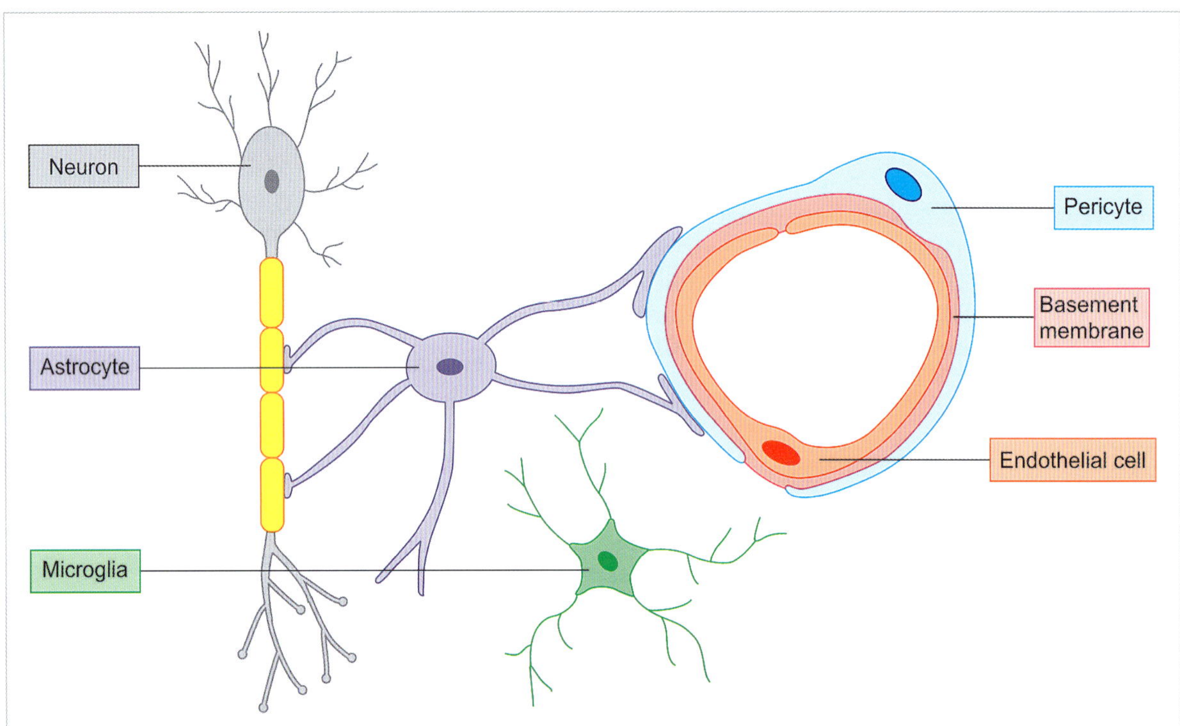

FIG. 1: The neurovascular unit.[15]

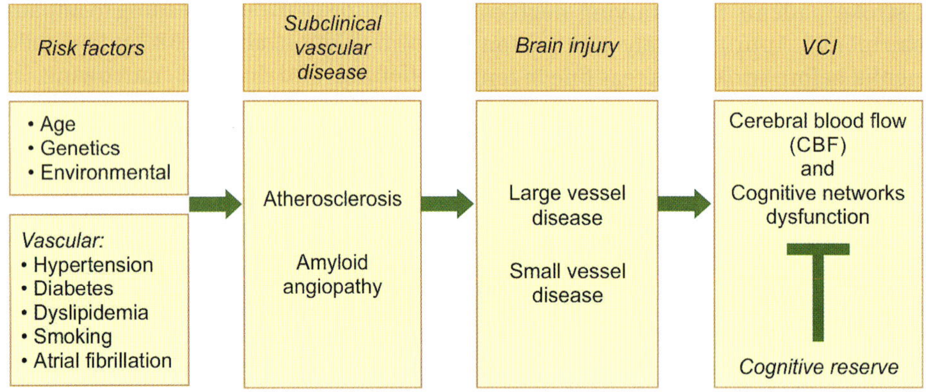

FLOWCHART 1: Mechanism of vascular cognitive impairment (VCI).[8,15]

Endothelial Dysfunction, Altered Blood–Brain Barrier Permeability, and Inflammation

Cerebral endothelial cells are prone to the effects of hypoperfusion. During inflammation and oxidative stress, there is an impairment of the endothelial nitric oxide synthase (eNOS) pathway, causing reduced nitric oxide (NO) production leading to endothelial dysfunction. This alters BBB permeability and neurons are then exposed to toxins, causing disruption of neurovascular trophic coupling, thereby worsening cerebral hypoperfusion.[19] Elevated cytokine levels, and microglial and astrocyte activation are markers of oxidative stress and inflammation in white matter lesions with VCI. Free radicals and peroxidation products generated during gliosis and oxidative stress lead to loss of white matter integrity.[7] Studies also showed disturbances of cerebral choline acetyltransferase in dementia patients with a history of stroke and loss of cholinergic neurons in the hippocampi and cortices, which correlated with WMH on MRI.[20]

Perivascular Spaces or Virchow–Robin Spaces and the Glymphatic System

The glymphatic system is a perivascular pathway that acts as a drainage system with retrograde, no or low resistance flow draining into cervical lymph nodes and is a cerebral network for clearance of metabolic waste within the brain parenchyma in which cerebrospinal fluid (CSF) is exchanged with interstitial fluid. PVS are potential spaces around the arterioles, capillaries, and venules of the brain involved in the clearance of interstitial fluid and waste products. PVS have a role in maintenance of the cerebral immune system, clearance of interstitial β-amyloid, and exchange of energy substrates.[21] The hypothesis is that breakdown of the BBB and loss of pericytes lead to leakage of interstitial fluid that causes prominent PVS. An increased burden of PVS is noted with SVD and is plausibly related to an increased number of WMH, lacunar infarcts, and microbleeds. Ongoing research will further elucidate the contribution of PVS in the development of VCI and dementia.[22]

Microbleeds

Cerebral microbleeds (CMBs) are very prevalent in VCI and are based on the underlying etiology. CMBs due to SVD are typically present in subcortical regions in patients with hypertensive SVD unlike CMBs in the lobar regions that occur with cerebral amyloid angiopathy (CAA). CMBs indicate prior microscopic hemorrhages and subsequent perivascular hemosiderin deposits that are visualized as punctate hypointense lesions on paramagnetic-sensitive MRI sequences.[23]

Cerebral Amyloid Angiopathy

Cerebral amyloid angiopathy occurs due to the accumulation of β-amyloid in cortical and pial arteries and capillaries, sparing penetrating arterioles that supply deep grey matter, and may be sporadic or genetic. It usually, though not necessarily, presents with intracerebral hemorrhage (ICH). CAA clinically manifests also as transient focal neurological episodes ("amyloid spells") and is associated with a high risk of ICH in future.[8] Cognitive and behavioral symptoms associated with CAA include reduced processing speed, episodic and semantic memory, and executive dysfunction. These symptoms could be caused by CAA-related microinfarction, ischemic white matter demyelination, impaired vascular reactivity, or the cumulative effects of hemorrhages. Hemorrhage-sensitive MRI sequences, such as susceptibility-weighted imaging (SWI) help in diagnosis by demonstration of microbleeds.[24] A hallmark of CAA on neuroimaging is cortical superficial siderosis (cSS), which refers to blood-breakdown products deposited within the subarachnoid space, leptomeninges, and superficial cortex.

RISK FACTORS FOR VASCULAR COGNITIVE IMPAIRMENT

Vascular cognitive impairment represents a preventable form of cognitive impairment since a significant proportion of VCI burden can be reduced by addressing its highly prevalent risk factors, especially in India.[25-27] Hypertension and diabetes rank among the most important risk factors for VCI. Obesity, high body mass index, atrial fibrillation, smoking, alcohol consumption, low vitamin B12, and homocysteine are also important risk factors for VCI. Stroke increases the risk of dementia by up to ninefold and around 60–70% of stroke have cognitive impairment at follow-up. Severity of stroke, dominant infarcts, aphasia, larger infarct volume, recurrent strokes, and family history of stroke increase VCI risk. Additionally, asymptomatic carotid stenosis, peripheral vascular disease, increased intimal medial thickness, and hyperlipidemia also increase the risk. Emerging evidence suggests that environmental factors such as pollution also contribute to VCI risk. The non-modifiable risk factors for vascular dementia include advancing age, male gender, family history, and genetic background.[25,26]

The combined modifiable risk for dementia globally as per the 2020 Lancet Dementia Commission for 12 risk factors was estimated to be 40%.[28] Among the risk factors, hypertension, diabetes, smoking, alcoholism, obesity, and physical inactivity contribute to 12% of modifiable risk for dementia, thereby emphasizing the important contribution of vascular risk to the global burden of dementia **(Table 1)**. The combination of risk factors predicts cognitive decline better than independent ones. In contrast, a greater number of positive cardiovascular health factors is protective against cognitive decline.[8] The cardiovascular risk factors, aging, and incidence of dementia (CAIDE)[29] and Northern Manhattan Study (NOMAS) global vascular risk score (GVRS)[30] scores correlated inversely with the level of global cognition, further lending support to the idea that the more number of vascular risk factors within the individual, the better it predicts cognitive decline.

APPROACH TO THE PATIENT WITH SUSPECTED VASCULAR COGNITIVE IMPAIRMENT

An adequate history and appropriate examination (general, neurological, and cognitive) should lead to clinical localization, which may then be aided with

TABLE 1: Risk and resilience factors for vascular cognitive impairment (VCI).[8,59]

Category	Factors	Level of evidence as prevention strategy
Deleterious	Hypertension	Recommended
	Diabetes/hyperglycemia	Reasonable
	Hypercholesterolemia	Reasonable
	Vascular disease	Reasonable
	Obesity	Reasonable
	Smoking	Reasonable
	Heavy alcohol intake/ abstinence	Reasonable
Resilience	Physical activity	Reasonable
	Education	Reasonable
	Healthy diet	Reasonable
	Cognitive stimulation activities	Reasonable
	Alcohol intake in moderation	Reasonable

necessary neuroimaging to confirm the localization, and then identify the underlying mechanism of cerebrovascular disease subtype to plan further preventive or therapeutic management.

Understanding the initial symptom and charting the progression and recruitment of symptoms is important toward the diagnosis of VCI. An insidious onset and slow progression may suggest subcortical ischemic vascular disease, whereas an acute onset/stepwise progression would favor poststroke/multi-infarct etiology.[15] The distinguishing clinical history with VCI caused by CAA are a slow, progressive cognitive decline [also a feature of Alzheimer's disease (AD)], transient focal neurologic episodes ("amyloid spells"), and sudden-onset focal neurologic deficits due to cortical lobar ICH.[31] Past history of vascular risk factors and family history of cerebrovascular, coronary artery, and peripheral vascular diseases are essential. A strong family history of VCI without vascular risk factors is highly suggestive of genetic etiology [cerebral autosomal-dominant arteriopathy with subcortical infarcts and leukoencephalopathy (CADASIL) and cerebral autosomal-recessive arteriopathy with subcortical infarcts and leukoencephalopathy (CARASIL)], which is important to identify for its implication in future generations.

General and systemic findings suggestive of vascular risk factors including irregular pulse, elevated blood pressure, hypertensive retinopathy, carotid bruit and signs of peripheral vascular disease, and heart failure are important. Focal neurological deficits, including cortical signs, suggest poststroke/multi-infarct disease, whereas features of inattention, mood disturbances, and gait disturbance may point to subcortical ischemic involvement. Cognitive evaluation may reveal impairment based on the location of vascular brain injury.[15] Cognitive assessment should include five core domains: Attention, executive function, memory, language, and visuospatial function.[32] Appropriate cognitive screening tools for patients with VCI include the Addenbrooke's Cognitive Examination (ACE) and the Montreal Cognitive Assessment (MoCA) as they assess all the abovementioned core domains and capture deficits due to vascular brain pathologies more than the mini-mental state examination (MMSE). ACE and MoCA are also more robust for the measurement of executive dysfunction,[33] validated in multiple settings including stroke,[34] and available in multiple languages.[34-36] VCI is likely to demonstrate impairments in processing speed, executive function, and delayed recall of word lists and visual content.[37] For more detailed neuropsychological evaluation, the National Institute of Neurological Disorders and Stroke and the Canadian Stroke Network (NINDS-CSN) harmonization battery,[38] and in the Indian context, the Indian Council of Medical Research (ICMR) neurocognitive toolbox have demonstrated validity in differentiating stroke patients with normal cognition from those with VCI and vascular dementia (VaD).[39] Behavioral disturbances including apathy, irritability, depression, and agitation are also commonly encountered in patients, and patients need to be evaluated systematically for these range of behaviors.

Laboratory investigations should test for vascular risk factors [glycated hemoglobin (HbA1c), lipid profile, and electrocardiogram (ECG)] and reversible causes for cognitive impairment [complete blood counts, metabolic panels, vitamin B12, serum homocysteine, thyroid-stimulating hormone (TSH), workup for syphilis, and autoimmune panels]. Genetic testing in patients with a family history of stroke and dementia needs to be conducted to detect genetic SVD-related syndromes such as CADASIL—due to a mutation in the *NOTCH3* gene on chromosome 19, CARASIL—associated with *HTA1* gene mutation, *COL4A1* gene-related arteriopathy, and Fabry disease caused by mutations of *GLA* gene, among others.

Structural imaging (MRI/CT) should be done to look for focal infarcts in strategic locations, WMH, and generalized atrophy. Metabolic imaging [Positron emission tomography with 2-deoxy-2-[fluorine-18]fluoro-D-glucose (^{18}F-FDG-PET)] may be considered to look for hypometabolism in areas with evidence of vascular brain injury on structural imaging.[15] It is also important to identify the underlying vascular mechanisms, including cardiac disease, to institute treatment to prevent recurrent strokes.[40,41] The use of serum, CSF, and imaging biomarkers for coexistent AD or other neurodegenerative dementias is relevant in patients in whom mixed dementia is being considered, with implications for treatment.[42,43]

BIOMARKERS

Imaging Biomarkers

Imaging biomarkers of cerebrovascular disease are increasingly being recognized as markers of brain health.[44] To harmonize neuroimaging biomarkers of vascular disease, STRIVE1 (2013) and subsequently STRIVE-2 (2023) standardized and categorized features of SVD seen on MRI. The SVD features described include the following:

- *Recent small subcortical infarct:* Evidence on imaging of recent infarct in the territory of one perforating arteriole, with clinical features having a temporal correlation with a lesion occurring in the prior 3 weeks.
- *Lacune:* Ovoid or round (≤15 mm), subcortical, fluid-filled (signal same as CSF) cavity that suggests end tissue damage from recent small subcortical infarct, hemorrhage, or end-stage cavitation within a WMH.
- *WMH:* T2 and fluid-attenuated inversion recovery (T2-FLAIR) hyperintensity in white matter (signal different from CSF) without cavitation.
- *PVS:* Linear, ovoid, or round (depending on slice direction), ≤2 mm, fluid-filled (signal intensity same as CSF in all sequences) space and follows the course of vessel traversing the brain parenchyma through grey or white matter.
- *CMB:* Small (2–5 mm) area of signal void with blooming artifact on susceptibility-weighted imaging/gradient-recalled echo (SWI/GRE) sequence.
- *cSS:* Thin hypointense areas on SWI/GRE, overlying the superficial cortex, either confined to one gyrus and sulcus or, uncommonly, involving several brain regions.
- *Cortical cerebral microinfarct:* Small lesions (≤4 mm), strictly cortical, appear hypointense on T1, hyperintense on FLAIR, and isointense on SWI/GRE.
- *Brain atrophy:* Brain parenchymal volume loss unrelated to any specific focal injury (infarct or trauma).
- *ICH:* This occurs due to SVD in about 85% of cases, including arteriolosclerotic (perforating artery) vasculopathy and CAA—the former is associated with deep ICH, while the latter with peripheral and lobar ICH **(Figs. 2A and B)**.

Parameters using combinations of imaging markers to summarize SVD burden are also being used to harmonize research to prepare cohorts for clinical trials. These include measures such as Summary SVD score, Brain Health Index, BrainAGE, and white matter damage metric.[41] Quantitative imaging markers are being explored for sub-visible tissue damage, lesion-symptom patterns, and subtle abnormalities visible on high-field MRI in VCI.[45,46] These include novel methods such as diffusion tensor imaging, quantitative relaxometry, magnetization transfer ratio, and dynamic contrast-enhanced MRI, among others.

Fluid Biomarkers

The diagnosis of VCI presently relies on clinical features and brain imaging, which offer lower sensitivity and specificity than molecular biomarkers. Identifying clinically useful molecular biomarkers of VCI could improve diagnostic probability. The heterogeneity of VCI warrants use of multiple biomarkers in various combinations.

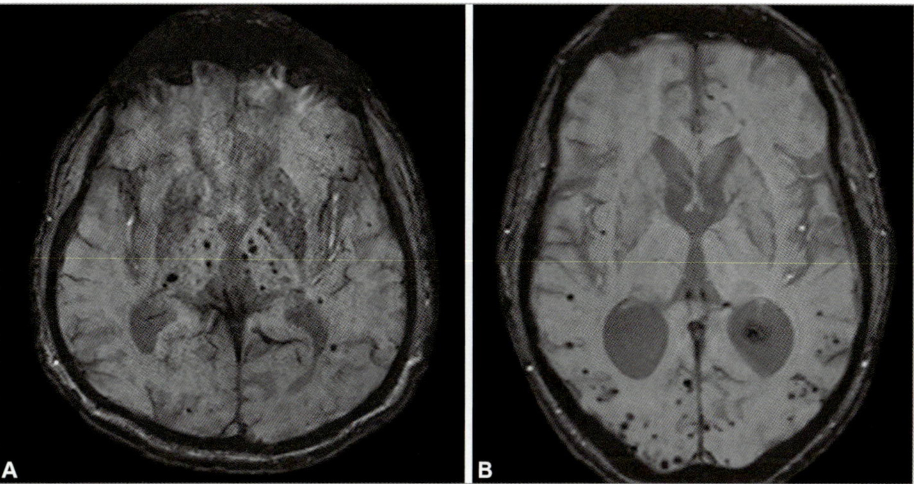

FIGS. 2A AND B: Distinguishing etiology of microbleed [blooming on susceptibility-weighted imaging/gradient-recalled echo (SWI/GRE)] based on location. (A) Hypertensive arteriolosclerosis, deep intracerebral hemorrhage (ICH); (B) Cerebral amyloid angiopathy, lobar ICH.

Molecules relevant to multiple pathophysiological pathways of VCI have potential as clinical biomarkers. Biomarkers of endothelial dysfunction, BBB breakdown, oxidative stress, inflammation, coagulation pathway, and neuronal and glial degeneration are being investigated as potential markers of VCI, to differentiate from healthy controls or other neurodegenerative diseases, or to assess risk, monitor, and prognosticate disease[47,48] **(Table 2)**. Biomarkers for Vascular Contributions to Cognitive Impairment and Dementia (MarkVCID) is a National Institutes of Health (NIH)-funded multisite consortium that is working to analyze, optimize, and validate predictive, diagnostic, target engagement and progression biomarkers of cerebral SVD involved in VCI.[49]

TABLE 2: Potential molecular biomarkers for vascular cognitive impairment (VCI).[48]

Small vessel disease pathophysiology	Biomarkers	
	Serum/plasma	Cerebrospinal fluid
Endothelial dysfunction	ADMA, VCAM-1, PIGF, MR-proADM, ICAM-1	PIGF
BBB breakdown	MMPs (2, 3, 9)	TIMP-1, MMPs (2, 3, 9) sPDGFRβ
	CSF/serum ratio of Albumin MMPs (2, 3, 9)	
Oxidative stress	Lp-PLA2 oxLDL	–
Inflammation	TGF-β, IL-6, IL-18, VEGF-A, VEGF-C	TGF-β, IL-6, LCN2, VEGF-C
Clotting pathway dysfunction	D-dimer, fibrinogen, vWF	–
Neuronal and glial degeneration	GFAP NfL	NfL

(ADMA: asymmetric dimethylarginine; BBB: blood–brain barrier; GFAP: glial fibrillary acidic protein; ICAM: intercellular adhesion molecule; IL: interleukin; LCN2: lipocalin 2; Lp-PLA2: lipoprotein-associated phospholipase A2; MMP: matrix metalloproteinases; MR-proADM: mid-regional pro-adrenomedullin; NfL: neurofilament light chain; oxLDL: oxidized low-density lipoprotein; PIGF: placental growth factor; sPDGFRβ: soluble platelet-derived growth factor receptor-β; TGF: transforming growth factor; TIMP: tissue inhibitors of metalloproteinases; VEGF: vascular endothelial growth factor; VCAM: vascular cell adhesion molecule; vWF: von Willebrand factor)

DIAGNOSIS OF VASCULAR COGNITIVE IMPAIRMENT

The presence of cognitive impairment and its causation due to cerebrovascular disease are required to make a diagnosis of VCI. Over the years, several diagnostic criteria have been developed to diagnose VCI uniformly and reliably **(Table 3)**. The Hachinski ischemic score[50] is a simple clinical tool designed to differentiate between AD and multi-infarct dementia. Later, the State of

TABLE 3: Evolution of nomenclature and diagnostic criteria of vascular cognitive impairment (VCI).[1,8,48]

Year	Terminology	Attribution
1975	Ischemic Score (IS)	Hachinski et al.
1992	Ischemic vascular dementia	• (ADDTC); Chui et al. • The State of California Alzheimer's Disease Diagnostic and Treatment Centers
1992	Vascular dementia	• (ICD-10); World Health Organization (WHO) • International Classification of Diseases 10th revision–Classification of Mental and Behavioural Disorders
1993	Vascular dementia	• (NINDS-AIREN); Román et al. • National Institute for Neurological Diseases and Stroke–Association Internationale pour la Recherche et l'Enseignement en Neurosciences
1994	Vascular dementia	• (DSM- IV); American Psychiatric Association (APA) • Diagnostic and Statistical Manual of Mental Disorders 4th edition
2006	Vascular cognitive impairment	• (NINDS-CSN); Hachinski et al. • National Institute of Neurological Disorders and Stroke–Canadian Stroke Network
2011	Vascular contributions to cognitive impairment and dementia	• (AHA-ASA); Gorelick et al. • American Heart Association-American Stroke Association
2013	Vascular neurocognitive disorder	• (DSM- V); American Psychiatric Association (APA) • Diagnostic and Statistical Manual of Mental Disorders 5th edition
2014	Vascular cognitive disorders (minor and major)	• (VASCOG); Sachdev et al. • International Society for Vascular Behavioural and Cognitive Disorders
2017	Vascular cognitive impairment (mild and major)	• (VICCCS); Skrobot et al. • Vascular Impairment of Cognition Classification Consensus Study

<table>
<tr><th colspan="5">TABLE 4: The Vascular Impairment of Cognition Classification Consensus Study (VICCCS) criteria for VCI.[32]</th></tr>
<tr><th colspan="5">Vascular cognitive impairment and dementia (VCI)</th></tr>
<tr><th>Mild VCI</th><th colspan="4">Major VCI (VaD)</th></tr>
<tr><td rowspan="3">• ≥1 cognitive domain impaired
• ADL not/mildly impaired
• Not subtyped</td><td colspan="4">• ≥1 cognitive domain significantly impaired
• ADL severely impaired
• Four subtypes</td></tr>
<tr><td>Poststroke dementia (PSD)</td><td>Subcortical ischemic vascular dementia (SIVD)</td><td>Multi-infarct dementia (MiD)</td><td>Mixed dementia</td></tr>
<tr><td>• Cognitive decline immediate to within 6 months of stroke
• No reversal of symptoms
• PSD-AD, PSD-LBD, etc.</td><td>• Subcortical
• Small vessel disease (lacunar infarcts and WM lesions)</td><td>• Cortical infarcts
• Large vessel atherosclerosis
• Multiple lesions</td><td>• Combination of VCI with any neurodegenerative disease
• VDI-AD, VCI-LBD, etc.</td></tr>
</table>

(AD: Alzheimer's disease; ADL: activities of daily living; LBD: Lewy body dementia; VaD: vascular dementia; WM: white matter)

California Alzheimer's Disease Diagnostic and Treatment Centers[51] and the National Institute for Neurological Disorders and Stroke-Association Internationale pour la Recherche et l'Enseignement en Neurosciences (NINDS-AIREN) criteria[52] were developed for use in clinical practice and research. The NINDS-CSN developed common standards in diagnosis, epidemiology, imaging, neuropathology, experimental models, genetics, and clinical trials to recommend minimum, common, clinical and research standards for the description and study of VCI.[38] These criteria demonstrate variable sensitivity and specificity and differ in methods that establish the causal relationship to cerebrovascular disease. More recently, in the background of heterogeneity, the International Society for Vascular Behavioural and Cognitive Disorders (VASCOG) group recommends diagnostic criteria under the umbrella term of vascular cognitive disorders (VCD).[53] The continuum of mild impairment to frank dementia can also be harmonized with the Diagnostic and Statistical Manual 5 (DSM-5) criteria. Most recently, the Vascular Impairment of Cognition Classification Consensus Study (VICCCS) criteria[32] classified VCI into mild VCI and major VCI (VaD), and further subtyped VaD into four categories: poststroke dementia, subcortical ischemic vascular dementia, multi-infarct dementia, and mixed dementia **(Table 4)**.

MANAGEMENT OF VASCULAR COGNITIVE IMPAIRMENT

The ideal approach for VCI is prevention by controlling vascular risk factors **(Table 1)**. VCI is unique among dementias as its risk factors are modifiable and it may be delayed in onset and progression, if these are well controlled. In 2017, the American Heart Association (AHA)/American Stroke Association (ASA) defined optimal brain health[54] by seven metrics—untreated blood pressure (BP) <120/80 mm Hg (avoiding hypotension), fasting blood glucose (FBS) <100 mg/dL (avoiding hypoglycemia), total cholesterol <200 mg/dL, body mass index (BMI) <25 kg/m^2, nonsmoker, physical activity, and healthy diet—all together playing a role in preserving cognition.[55] Controlling vascular risk factors and treatment of underlying vascular and stroke mechanisms are the mainstay of secondary prevention and reducing risk of progression of VCI.

Preventive Management

Most studies show that lowering BP is associated with a lower risk of dementia or nonprogression of cognitive decline.[56-58] The SPRINT MIND trial demonstrated the beneficial effects of intensive BP lowering not only on cognition, but also on other vascular markers, including brain volume and WMH.[58] However, in the elderly or those with Fazekas grade 3 WMH due to hypertensive arteriolosclerosis, it is safer to maintain systolic blood pressure (SBP) between 120 and 140 mm Hg. In CAA, BP should ideally be maintained at <120/80 mm Hg, as even slightly elevated BP increases the risk of ICH.[15]

Both traditional (metformin) and newer glucose-lowering drugs such as glucagon-like peptide-1 (GLP-1) analogs, dipeptidyl peptidase-4 (DPP-4) inhibitors, and sodium-glucose cotransporter-2 (SGLT-2) inhibitors were found to be associated with a decreased risk of dementia in people with diabetes mellitus.[59] However, the ACCORD study and a meta-analysis of randomized controlled trials (RCTs) reported no definitive evidence that management of diabetes prevents or slows down cognitive impairment.[8]

Midlife hypercholesterolemia tends to increase the risk of VCI. Early trials with statins, including PROSPER and Heart Protection Study failed to show any benefit on cognitive decline.[60] A benefit of preserving white matter histology was observed in cognitively normal adults with statins, suggestive of potential for VCI prevention. Maintaining normal serum cholesterol levels remains a preventive strategy in VCI.[8]

The management of underlying vascular mechanisms is important to prevent recurrent stroke and involves antiplatelets and, in case of atrial fibrillation or valvular pathologies, anticoagulation.[56,61] Following a lacunar stroke, the phosphodiesterase-3 (PDE-3) inhibitor cilostazol showed reductions in both recurrent stroke and cognitive impairment in the Lacunar Intervention-2 (LACI-2) trial.[62] In patients with atrial fibrillation, warfarin and oral anticoagulants are useful in reducing strokes and slowing cognitive decline. An exception is CAA, where antiplatelet drugs are avoided for primary prevention but can be used for secondary prevention after cardiac procedures.

Multidomain intervention that involves a healthy diet, physical exercise, cognitive training, and vascular risk reduction is protective against cognitive decline. The Finnish Geriatric Intervention Study to Prevent Cognitive Impairment and Disability (FINGER) that enrolled elderly people into a multimodal intervention (exercise, diet, cognitive retraining, and vascular risk monitoring) provided robust evidence of potential for the prevention of VCI.[63] Higher education, physical exercise, bilingualism, and cognitively stimulating lifestyle have been linked to enhancing cognitive resilience and reserve, emphasizing a life-course approach in reducing the risk of vascular dementia.[35,64]

Symptomatic Management

Pharmacological Therapy

Several trials have tested the effect of acetylcholinesterase inhibitors (donepezil and galantamine) and N-methyl-D-aspartate (NMDA) receptor antagonist (memantine), and they are reported of modest benefit in VCI.[15] Development of therapeutic agents in VCI has evolved based on the understanding of pathophysiological mechanisms and advances in diagnosis. The focus from studies on vasodilators (perfusion enhancement), popular in the 1970s and 80s, changed to studies on neurotransmitter modulators or drugs acting via multiple mechanisms[7] **(Table 5)**.

TABLE 5: Therapeutic agents for vascular cognitive impairment (VCI) undergoing clinical trials registered to ClinicalTrials.gov.[7]

Phase of clinical trial	Drug	Mechanism	Target type	Therapeutic purpose
I	Donepezil	Inhibits AChE and increases acetylcholine release	Restores function of cholinergic system in the CNS	Cognitive enhancer
II	Metformin	• Reduces oxidative stress • Reduces inflammation • Reduces endothelial dysfunction • Inhibits AChE activity	• Multitarget • Atherosclerosis	Cognitive enhancer
	N-acetylcysteine	Glutathione precursor	• Antioxidant • Anti-inflammatory	Cognitive enhancer
	BAC	Reduce levels of IL-1β	• Antioxidant • Anti-inflammatory	Cognitive enhancer
	CY6463	Compensates NO deficiency	Improves endothelial and BBB dysfunction	Cognitive enhancer
III	Akatinol memantine	• Antagonizes glutamate toxicity • Neuroprotection	Enhances effect of glutamatergic system	Cognitive enhancer
	Butylphthalide	• Improves oxidative stress • Improves function of cholinergic system in the CNS	• Antioxidant • Anti-inflammatory	Cognitive enhancer
	Pimavanserin	Antipsychotic	BPSD	Reduces relapse of psychotic symptoms
	Prospecta	Unidentified	Unknown	Cognitive enhancer
IV	Paracetamol	Analgesic	BPSD	Treatment of pain-induced depression

(AchE: acetylcholinesterase; BBB: blood–brain barrier; BPSD: behavioral and psychological symptoms of dementia; CNS: central nervous system; IL: interleukin; NO: nitric oxide)

Rehabilitation

Studies on rehabilitation in VCI, namely, Cog-VACCINE study[65] and RehAtt study have shown improvement in cognitive function and increased functional connectivity on functional magnetic resonance imaging (fMRI).[66] Attempts have been made to include training of caregivers in stroke rehabilitation programs in stroke units.[67] Culturally adaptable cognitive stimulation therapies (CSTs) are essential.[68] Home-based care, dependent on their families, is the mainstay in our country for patients with VCI.[27]

Caregiver Support

A support system is essential for caregivers to address their challenges and reduce caregiver burden. Addressing their needs, reducing caregiver distress, and improving coping skills potentially promote VCI patient outcomes.[8]

CONCLUSION

Our understanding of VCI has evolved since the initial descriptions by Sir Thomas Willis four centuries ago, and advances in our knowledge of pathological mechanisms and neuroimaging have enriched our diagnostic prowess. VCI is unique among dementias as its risk factors are modifiable, which is the most appropriate step toward prevention and reducing the risk of progression of the disease. However, the need for early diagnosis and monitoring progression with biomarkers and the development of disease-modifying treatments are the need of the hour. To shed light on the path that lies ahead, we quote Vladimir Hachinski from his paper on redefining vascular dementia and introducing the concept of VCI—*"Our concepts and questions...must be clear, otherwise the answers will be muddled. The problems are immense, but the opportunities are even greater."*[69]

REFERENCES

1. Sveikata L, Assal F. History of vascular cognitive impairment and dementia. In: Bogousslavsky J, Paciaroni M, Hennerici MG, Tatu L (Eds). History of Stroke. Basel: MDPI; 2023. pp. 80-90.
2. Hachinski VC, Lassen NA, Marshall J. Multi-infarct dementia. A cause of mental deterioration in the elderly. Lancet. 1974;2(7874):207-10.
3. Hachinski VC, Potter P, Merskey H. Leuko-araiosis. Arch Neurol. 1987;44(1):21-3.
4. Fazekas F, Chawluk JB, Alavi A, Hurtig HI, Zimmerman RA. MR signal abnormalities at 1.5 T in Alzheimer's dementia and normal aging. AJR Am J Roentgenol. 1987;149(2):351-6.
5. Wardlaw JM, Smith EE, Biessels GJ, Cordonnier C, Fazekas F, Frayne R, et al. Neuroimaging standards for research into small vessel disease and its contribution to ageing and neurodegeneration. Lancet Neurol. 2013;12(8):822-38.
6. Kalaria RN, Maestre GE, Arizaga R, Friedland RP, Galasko D, Hall K, et al. Alzheimer's disease and vascular dementia in developing countries: Prevalence, management, and risk factors. Lancet Neurol. 2008;7(9):812-26.
7. Linh TTD, Hsieh YC, Huang LK, Hu CJ. Clinical trials of new drugs for vascular cognitive impairment and vascular dementia. Int J Mol Sci. 2022;23(19):11067.
8. Rundek T, Tolea M, Ariko T, Fagerli EA, Camargo CJ. Vascular Cognitive Impairment (VCI). Neurotherapeutics. 2022;19(1):68-88.
9. Alladi S, Kaul S, Mekala S. Vascular cognitive impairment: Current concepts and Indian perspective. Ann Indian Acad Neurol. 2010;13(Suppl2):S104-8.
10. Iadecola C, Duering M, Hachinski V, Joutel A, Pendlebury ST, Schneider JA, et al. Vascular cognitive impairment and dementia: JACC Scientific Expert Panel. J Am Coll Cardiol. 2019;73(25):3326-44.
11. Das S, Paul N, Hazra A, Ghosal M, Ray BK, Banerjee TK, et al. Cognitive dysfunction in stroke survivors: A community-based prospective study from Kolkata, India. J Stroke Cerebrovasc Dis. 2013;22(8):1233-42.
12. Mukhopadhyay A, Sundar U, Adwani S, Pandit D. Prevalence of stroke and post-stroke cognitive impairment in the elderly in Dharavi, Mumbai. J Assoc Physicians India. 2012;60:29-32.
13. Sundar U, Adwani S. Post-stroke cognitive impairment at 3 months. Ann Indian Acad Neurol. 2010;13(1):42-6.
14. Lusis AJ. Atherosclerosis. Nature. 2000;407(6801):233-41.
15. Chang Wong E, Chang Chui H. Vascular cognitive impairment and dementia. Continuum (Minneap Minn). 2022;28(3):750-80.
16. Kalaria RN. The pathology and pathophysiology of vascular dementia. Neuropharmacology. 2018;134(Pt B):226-39.
17. Zanon Zotin MC, Sveikata L, Viswanathan A, Yilmaz P. Cerebral small vessel disease and vascular cognitive impairment: From diagnosis to management. Curr Opin Neurol. 2021;34(2):246-57.
18. Iadecola C. The neurovascular unit coming of age: A journey through neurovascular coupling in health and disease. Neuron. 2017;96(1):17-42.
19. Wang F, Cao Y, Ma L, Pei H, Rausch WD, Li H. Dysfunction of cerebrovascular endothelial cells: Prelude to vascular dementia. Front Aging Neurosci. 2018;10:376.
20. Liu Q, Zhu Z, Teipel SJ, Yang J, Xing Y, Tang Y, et al. White matter damage in the cholinergic system contributes to cognitive impairment in subcortical vascular cognitive impairment, no dementia. Front Aging Neurosci. 2017;9:47.
21. Nedergaard M, Goldman SA. Glymphatic failure as a final common pathway to dementia. Science. 2020;370(6512):50-6.
22. Wardlaw JM, Benveniste H, Nedergaard M, Zlokovic BV, Mestre H, Lee H, et al. Perivascular spaces in the brain: Anatomy, physiology and pathology. Nat Rev Neurol. 2020;16(3):137-53.
23. Akoudad S, Wolters FJ, Viswanathan A, de Bruijn RF, van der Lugt A, Hofman A, et al. Association of cerebral microbleeds with cognitive decline and dementia. JAMA Neurol. 2016;73(8):934-43.
24. Biffi A, Greenberg SM. Cerebral amyloid angiopathy: A systematic review. J Clin Neurol. 2011;7(1):1-9.
25. Skoog I. Status of risk factors for vascular dementia. Neuroepidemiology. 1998;17(1):2-9.

26. Smith E. Vascular Cognitive Impairment. Continuum (Minneap Minn). 2016;22(2 Dementia):490-509.
27. Arshad F, MM S, Paplikar A, Rajendran S, Kalkonde Y, Alladi S. Vascular cognitive impairment in India: Challenges and opportunities for prevention and treatment. Cereb Circ Cogn Behav. 2021;3:100034.
28. Rolandi E, Zaccaria D, Vaccaro R, Abbondanza S, Pettinato L, Davin A, et al. Estimating the potential for dementia prevention through modifiable risk factors elimination in the real-world setting: A population-based study. Alzheimers Res Ther. 2020;12(1):94.
29. Tolea MI, Heo J, Chrisphonte S, Galvin JE. A Modified CAIDE Risk Score as a screening tool for cognitive impairment in older adults. J Alzheimers Dis. 2021;82(4):1755-68.
30. Rundek T, Gardener H, Dias Saporta AS, Loewenstein DA, Duara R, Wright CB, et al. Global vascular risk score and CAIDE dementia risk score predict cognitive function in NOMAS. J Alzheimers Dis. 2020;73(3):1221-31.
31. Schrag M, Kirshner H. Neuropsychological effects of cerebral amyloid angiopathy. Curr Neurol Neurosci Rep. 2016;16(8):76.
32. Skrobot OA, Black SE, Chen C, DeCarli C, Erkinjuntti T, Ford GA, et al. Progress toward standardized diagnosis of vascular cognitive impairment: Guidelines from the Vascular Impairment of Cognition Classification Consensus Study. Alzheimers Dement. 2018;14(3):280-92.
33. Pendlebury ST, Cuthbertson FC, Welch SJ, Mehta Z, Rothwell PM. Underestimation of cognitive impairment by Mini-Mental State Examination versus the Montreal Cognitive Assessment in patients with transient ischemic attack and stroke: A population-based study. Stroke. 2010;41(6):1290-3.
34. Pendlebury ST, Mariz J, Bull L, Mehta Z, Rothwell PM. MoCA, ACE-R, and MMSE versus the National Institute of Neurological Disorders and Stroke-Canadian Stroke Network Vascular Cognitive Impairment Harmonization Standards Neuropsychological Battery after TIA and stroke. Stroke. 2012;43(2):464-9.
35. Alladi S, Bak TH, Mekala S, Rajan A, Chaudhuri JR, Mioshi E, et al. Impact of bilingualism on cognitive outcome after stroke. Stroke. 2016;47(1):258-61.
36. Mekala S, Paplikar A, Mioshi E, Kaul S, Divyaraj G, Coughlan G, et al. Dementia diagnosis in seven languages: The Addenbrooke's cognitive examination-III in India. Arch Clin Neuropsychol. 2020;35(5):528-38.
37. Looi JC, Sachdev PS. Differentiation of vascular dementia from AD on neuropsychological tests. Neurology. 1999;53(4):670-8.
38. Hachinski V, Iadecola C, Petersen RC, Breteler MM, Nyenhuis DL, Black SE, et al. National Institute of Neurological Disorders and Stroke–Canadian Stroke Network vascular cognitive impairment harmonization standards. Stroke. 2006;37(9):2220-41.
39. Kaul S, Goyal S, Paplikar A, Varghese F, Alladi S, Menon R, et al. Evaluation of vascular cognitive impairment using the ICMR-Neuro Cognitive Tool Box (ICMR-NCTB) in a stroke cohort from India. Ann Indian Acad Neurol. 2022;25(6):1130-7.
40. Adams HP Jr, Bendixen BH, Kappelle LJ, Biller J, Love BB, Gordon DL, et al. Classification of subtype of acute ischemic stroke. Definitions for use in a multicenter clinical trial. TOAST. Trial of Org 10172 in Acute Stroke Treatment. Stroke. 1993;24(1):35-41.
41. Kaul S, Alladi S, Jabeen SA, Bandaru VCSSR, Ankem U, Mekala S, et al. Intracranial Atherosclerosis is the Most Common Stroke Subtype: Ten-year Data from Hyderabad Stroke Registry (India). Ann Indian Acad Neurol. 2018;21(3):209-13.
42. Mielke MM, Frank RD, Dage JL, Jeromin A, Ashton NJ, Blennow K, et al. Comparison of plasma phosphorylated tau species with amyloid and tau positron emission tomography, neurodegeneration, vascular pathology, and cognitive outcomes. JAMA Neurol. 2021;78(9):1108-17.
43. Wallin A, Alladi S, Black SE, Chen C, Greenberg SM, Gustafson D, et al. What does aducanumab treatment of Alzheimer's disease mean for research on vascular cognitive disorders? Cereb Circ Cogn Behav. 2022;3:100044.
44. Vemuri P, Decarli C, Duering M. Imaging markers of vascular brain health: Quantification, clinical implications, and future directions. Stroke. 2022;53(2):416-26.
45. Duering M, Biessels GJ, Brodtmann A, Chen C, Cordonnier C, de Leeuw FE, et al. Neuroimaging standards for research into small vessel disease—advances since 2013. Lancet Neurol. 2023;22(7):602-18.
46. Clancy U, Kancheva AK, Valdés Hernández MDC, Muñoz Maniega S, Quinn TJ, et al. Imaging Biomarkers of VCI: A Focused Update. Stroke. 2024;55(4):791-800.
47. Winder Z, Sudduth TL, Patel E, Anderson S, Neltner J, Bahrani AA, Abner EL, et al. Endpoints and outcomes: The challenge of biomarker choice for VCI trials. Alzheimers Dement. 2022;18(S6):e060534.
48. Hosoki S, Hansra GK, Jayasena T, Poljak A, Mather KA, Catts VS, et al. Molecular biomarkers for vascular cognitive impairment and dementia. Nat Rev Neurol. 2023;19(12):737-53.
49. Wilcock D, Jicha G, Blacker D, Albert MS, D'Orazio LM, Elahi FM, et al. MarkVCID cerebral small vessel consortium: I. Enrollment, clinical, fluid protocols. Alzheimers Dement. 2021;17(4):704-15.
50. Hachinski VC, Iliff LD, Zilhka E, Du Boulay GH, McAllister VL, Marshall J, et al. Cerebral blood flow in dementia. Arch Neurol. 1975;32(9):632-7.
51. Chui HC, Victoroff JI, Margolin D, Jagust W, Shankle R, Katzman R. Criteria for the diagnosis of ischemic vascular dementia proposed by the State of California Alzheimer's Disease Diagnostic and Treatment Centers. Neurology. 1992;42(3 Pt 1): 473-80.
52. Román GC, Tatemichi TK, Erkinjuntti T, Cummings JL, Masdeu JC, Garcia JH, et al. Vascular dementia: Diagnostic criteria for research studies. Report of the NINDS-AIREN International Workshop. Neurology. 1993;43(2):250-60.
53. Sachdev P, Kalaria R, O'Brien J, Skoog I, Alladi S, Black SE, et al. Diagnostic criteria for vascular cognitive disorders: A VASCOG statement. Alzheimer Dis Assoc Disord. 2014;28(3):206-18.
54. Gorelick PB, Furie KL, Iadecola C, Smith EE, Waddy SP, Lloyd-Jones DM, et al. Defining optimal brain health in adults: A Presidential Advisory from the American Heart Association/American Stroke Association. Stroke. 2017;48(10):e284-303.
55. Thacker EL, Gillett SR, Wadley VG, Unverzagt FW, Judd SE, McClure LA, et al. The American Heart Association Life's Simple 7 and incident cognitive impairment: The REasons for Geographic And Racial Differences in Stroke (REGARDS) study. J Am Heart Assoc. 2014;3(3):e000635.
56. Alexander P, Visagan S, Jawhar S, Kare A, Issa N, Issa R, et al. Antiplatelets and vascular dementia: A systematic review. J Aging Res. 2022;2022:9780067.
57. Forette F, Seux ML, Staessen JA, Thijs L, Babarskiene MR, Babeanu S, et al. The prevention of dementia with antihypertensive treatment: New evidence from the Systolic Hypertension in Europe (Syst-Eur) Study. Arch Intern Med. 2002;162(18): 2046-52.

58. Pajewski NM, Berlowitz DR, Bress AP, Callahan KE, Cheung AK, Fine LJ, et al. Intensive vs standard blood pressure control in adults 80 years or older: A secondary analysis of the Systolic Blood Pressure Intervention Trial. J Am Geriatr Soc. 2020;68(3):496-504.
59. Kalaria RN, Akinyemi RO, Paddick SM, Ihara M. Current perspectives on prevention of vascular cognitive impairment and promotion of vascular brain health. Expert Rev Neurother. 2024;24(1):25-44.
60. Trompet S, van Vliet P, de Craen AJM, Jolles J, Buckley BM, Murphy MB, et al. Pravastatin and cognitive function in the elderly. Results of the PROSPER study. J Neurol. 2010;257(1):85-90.
61. Wong KSL, Wang Y, Leng X, Mao C, Tang J, Bath PM, et al. Early dual versus mono antiplatelet therapy for acute non-cardioembolic ischemic stroke or transient ischemic attack: An updated systematic review and meta-analysis. Circulation. 2013;128(15):1656-66.
62. Wardlaw JM, Woodhouse LJ, Mhlanga II, Oatey K, Heye AK, Bamford J, et al. Isosorbide mononitrate and cilostazol treatment in patients with symptomatic cerebral small vessel disease: The Lacunar Intervention Trial-2 (LACI-2) randomized clinical trial. JAMA Neurol. 2023;80(7):682-92.
63. Ngandu T, Lehtisalo J, Solomon A, Levälahti E, Ahtiluoto S, Antikainen R, et al. A 2-year multidomain intervention of diet, exercise, cognitive training, and vascular risk monitoring versus control to prevent cognitive decline in at-risk elderly people (FINGER): A randomised controlled trial. Lancet. 2015;385(9984):2255-63.
64. Pendlebury ST, Rothwell PM. Prevalence, incidence, and factors associated with pre-stroke and post-stroke dementia: A systematic review and meta-analysis. Lancet Neurol. 2009;8(11):1006-18.
65. Tang Y, Xing Y, Zhu Z, He Y, Li F, Yang J, et al. The effects of 7-week cognitive training in patients with vascular cognitive impairment, no dementia (the Cog-VACCINE study): A randomized controlled trial. Alzheimers Dement. 2019;15(5):605-14.
66. Pantoni L, Poggesi A, Diciotti S, Valenti R, Orsolini S, Della Rocca E, et al. Effect of attention training in mild cognitive impairment patients with subcortical vascular changes: The RehAtt Study. J Alzheimers Dis. 2017;60(2):615-24.
67. Pandian JD, Sudhan P. Stroke epidemiology and stroke care services in India. J Stroke. 2013;15(3):128-34.
68. Raghuraman S, Lakshminarayanan M, Vaitheswaran S, Rangaswamy T. Cognitive stimulation therapy for dementia: Pilot studies of acceptability and feasibility of cultural adaptation for India. Am J Geriatr Psychiatry. 2017;25(9):1029-32.
69. Hachinski V. Vascular dementia: A radical redefinition. Dementia. 1994;5(3-4):130-2.

CHAPTER

10

Dementia and Parkinsonism

Debjyoti Dhar, Ravi Yadav

ABSTRACT

The present chapter offers an overview of a wide range of etiologies linking the continuum of dementia and parkinsonism. This broad spectrum encompasses neurodegenerative conditions comprising synucleinopathies such as Parkinson's disease (PD) with mild cognitive impairment (PD-MCI), PD dementia (PDD), and dementia with Lewy bodies (DLB); tauopathies like progressive supranuclear palsy (PSP) and corticobasal syndrome (CBS). Additionally, we have attempted to provide a narrative description of the neurocognitive profile in genetically-determined early-onset PD (EOPD), disorders involving abnormal metal deposition such as Wilson's disease, neurodegeneration with brain iron accumulation spectrum (NBIA), and metabolic disorders including Fahr's disease and cerebrotendinous xanthomatosis (CTX). The presentation of dementia with parkinsonism is also noteworthy in acquired causes, particularly within the context of rapidly progressive dementia, which includes autoimmune and paraneoplastic causes, infective causes such as human immunodeficiency virus-(HIV)-associated neurocognitive disorders, Whipple's disease, neurosyphilis, and prion diseases. Vascular cognitive impairment with parkinsonism represents another significant aspect of this spectrum. The underlying pathology revolves around abnormal aggregation of proteins such as alpha-synuclein, tau, or amyloid, affecting both cortical and subcortical regions and disrupting neurotransmitter systems. Management focuses on identifying the specific cause and implementing a tailored multidisciplinary approach.

Keywords: Dementia, Parkinsonism, Parkinson's disease, Dementia with Lewy bodies, Progressive supranuclear palsy, Rapidly progressive dementia.

INTRODUCTION

Dementia, currently referred to as a major cognitive disorder by the Diagnostic and Statistical Manual of Mental Disorders, Fifth Edition (DSM-5), is defined as the evidence of significant cognitive decline from a previous level in at least one cognitive domain that includes learning and memory, language, executive functions, complex attention, perceptual motor and social cognition; that interferes with the activities of daily living; not occurring in the context of delirium; and not explained by another mental disorder like major cognitive disorder or schizophrenia. On the other hand, parkinsonism is defined as the presence of both bradykinesia alongside rest tremors or rigidity. A combination of dementia and parkinsonism is seen in a wide spectrum of clinical conditions that range from acquired degenerative to inherited etiologies.[1,2] Not only does cognitive decline significantly contribute to the overall disability and dependency associated with the condition, but it also poses unique challenges in management. Unlike motor symptoms, which are partially amenable to dopaminergic therapies, dementia in parkinsonism often responds poorly to conventional Parkinson's medications. The current review focuses on the diverse etiologies linking these two core neurologic entities and highlights the clinical approach to diagnosis and management.

NEURODEGENERATIVE DISORDERS: SYNUCLEINOPATHIES

Dementia in Parkinson's Disease

Epidemiology

Cognitive dysfunction is widely prevalent among individuals with Parkinson's disease (PD), with dementia affecting 75–90% of cases.[2,3] Cognitive symptoms may manifest at any stage, with 20–30% of patients exhibiting mild cognitive impairment (MCI) upon diagnosis. Bradyphrenia, akin to slowed movement in PD, may not necessarily indicate cognitive decline. The 2012 criteria for PD-related MCI (PD-MCI) serve as a bridge between normal cognition and dementia. Approximately 10–15% of individuals with PD-MCI progress to PD dementia (PDD) annually, although some remain stable or revert to normal cognition over time. Subjective cognitive decline (SCD) also serves as a predictor for dementia progression. A recent study revealed that among individuals with PD who reported SCD at the outset, one third developed PD-MCI and PDD within a 7.5-year time frame.[4]

Risk Factors

Nongenetic

Predictors of PDD include advanced age, male gender, severe motor symptoms, hallucinations, rapid eye movement (REM) sleep behavior disorder, and vascular risk factors such as hypertension and smoking. The role of uric acid in PD-related dementia remains debatable, with some studies suggesting an inverse relationship between urate levels and PD risk. Traumatic brain injury (TBI) may increase the risk of cognitive decline in PD, but definitive conclusions await longitudinal studies. Tobacco smoking is associated with a higher prevalence of PD-MCI and PDD. The impact of exercise on PD cognition is inconclusive, with conflicting findings on the efficacy of aerobic exercise. The Mediterranean diet has drawn interest due to its potential cognitive benefits in neurodegenerative diseases such as Alzheimer's. Lower 25-hydroxyvitamin D levels have been associated with PD, but findings are inconsistent. Limited longitudinal evidence suggests caffeine intake may reduce cognitive decline and lower Alzheimer's disease (AD) risk, though clear evidence is lacking.[2,5]

Genetic Factors

Genetic factors, including *synuclein alpha (SNCA)*, *glucocerebrosidase (GBA)*, and *apolipoprotein E (APOE)* ε4 mutations, contribute to dementia risk in PD, showing overlap with AD and Lewy body dementia (LBD) genetic profiles. On the contrary, *leucine-rich repeat kinase 2* (*LRRK2*) mutations, the primary monogenic cause of PD (affecting 5–7% of familial cases), are associated with a lower cognitive impairment risk compared to other genetic variants.[5,6]

SNCA mutations: A recent analysis based on Movement Disorder Society Genetic mutation (MDSGene) database (www.mdsgene.org) found that 70% of individuals carrying *SNCA* mutations experienced cognitive decline. Moreover, *SNCA* mutation carriers exhibited a shorter duration between the onset of motor symptoms and the onset of dementia, as well as notably younger age at the onset of dementia compared to individuals with sporadic PD. Furthermore, there seems to be a dose-dependent relationship, with 88% of *SNCA* triplication carriers demonstrating cognitive alterations, in contrast to 68% of duplication carriers.

GBA mutations: *GBA* mutations, prevalent among Ashkenazi Jews, were found to be associated with a greater prevalence of nonmotor symptoms, including cognitive decline, olfactory impairment, mood disturbances, and autonomic dysfunction. Studies have shown a 2.4–3.2-fold heightened risk of dementia or cognitive impairment associated with *GBA* mutations. In addition, *GBA* gene mutations are linked to a swifter cognitive decline, as evidenced in recent studies. This effect has been observed for both "severe" (L444P) and "mild" (N370S) GBA mutations.

Microtubule-associated protein tau (*MAPT*) *mutations*: The H1 haplotype of *MAPT*, typically linked to frontotemporal dementia (FTD), is implicated in PDD risk. The association between the H1/H1 genotype and the progression to dementia was upheld during a 10-year follow-up of Cambridgeshire Parkinson's Incidence from GP to Neurologist (CamPaIGN) cohort. However, this association's strength diminished as the disease's duration increased. Monogenic forms of EOPD with early and rapid cognitive impairment include DNAJC6 and PLA2G6. Additionally, ATP13A2, SYNJ1, VPS13C, FBX07, and PTRHD1 are the other EOPDs with prominent cognitive decline. RAB39B and PTRHD1 are associated with intellectual disability. The role of *brain-derived neurotrophic factor* (*BDNF*) and *catechol-O-methyltransferase* (*COMT*) genetic polymorphisms has remained controversial despite several studies.[6]

Cognitive Domains Affected in Parkinson's Disease-related Mild Cognitive Impairment and Parkinson's Disease Dementia

The diverse cognitive profile includes executive and visuospatial difficulties, with variable memory and attention issues. Executive dysfunction, attributed to dopaminergic dysfunction in frontostriatal networks, includes planning and attentional problems. Memory and visuospatial impairments may result from decreased attention and executive function, affecting planning and memory retrieval. Language abilities are typically preserved, but comprehension and verbal fluency deficits may occur. Reduced semantic fluency may signal progression to PDD from PD-MCI. Neuropsychiatric symptoms such as anxiety, depression, and psychosis can complicate diagnosis, underscoring the need for regular screening. Cortical pathology, including Lewy bodies and AD, may underlie visuospatial and language challenges **(Table 1)**.[6,7]

Dementia with Lewy Bodies

Dementia with Lewy bodies ranks as the second most prevalent neurodegenerative dementia after AD representing up to 30% of dementia cases. Co-occurrence of pathology between DLB and AD is frequent, with autopsy studies indicating AD pathology in up to 80% of clinical DLB cases. In contrast, AD copathology is found in only about 30% of PDD cases.[2,8]

Cognitive Domains Affected

Visual hallucinations and cognitive fluctuations are common features of both PDD and DLB, with the latter often showing more frequent and pronounced occurrences, even in the early stages. The key clinical distinction lies in the timing of symptom onset, known as the "1-year rule"—PDD is diagnosed when motor symptoms precede cognitive symptoms by at least 1 year, whereas DLB is diagnosed when motor and cognitive symptoms emerge concurrently or when cognitive symptoms precede motor symptoms. In early DLB, attention, executive function, visuoperceptual abilities, and episodic memory are commonly affected. The involvement of basal nuclei and their interconnected circuits in attentional processes is well-documented. Disruption of attentional processes may contribute to the cognitive fluctuations observed in DLB. These subcortical nuclei also play a vital role in executive functions such as decision-making, planning, mental flexibility, and working memory. Language dysfunction occurs in about 5% of DLB cases, often manifesting as pragmatic issues in spontaneous speech, including incoherence, perseveration, and confabulation. Challenges in lexical access during picture naming may arise from visuoperceptual impairments. DLB patients may also struggle with verbal fluency tasks due to executive dysfunction.[8]

Multiple System Atrophy

Multiple system atrophy belongs to the synucleinopathy group, alongside PD and DLB. Historically, dementia was not considered a common feature of MSA according to diagnostic criteria, despite cognitive impairment being

TABLE 1: Cognitive profile in dementia-associated parkinsonism.

Disorder	Cognitive features	Cognitive scales validated	Pathology
Synucleinopathy			
Parkinson's disease	Bradyphrenia, executive and visuospatial dysfunction	PD-CRS, PANDA, SCOPA-COG, Mattis DRS-2, and MoCA	Amyloid pathology occurs more frequently in the temporal cortex and striatum than in DLB
Dementia with Lewy bodies	Executive and visuospatial dysfunction, cognitive fluctuations	MoCA, letter–number sequencing, digit span (forward and backward), verbal fluency tasks, constructional tasks (e.g., Rey–Osterrieth complex figure copy), and judgment of line orientation	• Amyloid pathology: Entorhinal cortex, amygdala, and putamen more common • Greater prevalence of concurrent AD pathology (fibrillary amyloid plaques and intraneuronal tangles) compared to PDD
Multiple system atrophy	Subtle changes in executive and visuospatial function		Nigral and putaminal degeneration and alterations in striato–pallido–thalamo–cortical circuits
Tauopathy			
Progressive supranuclear palsy	Executive dysfunction, impaired verbal fluency	The FAB may be more sensitive for cognitive screening of patients with PSP than the MoCA or MMSE	Aggregation of tau deposits in the form of tufted astrocytes in the superior frontal and supramarginal gyrus located in the superior temporal lobe
Corticobasal syndrome	Executive dysfunction, impaired social cognition, neglect, aphasia	FAB, MoCA, and MMSE	• 4R-tau and TAR DNA • DNA-binding protein 43 kDa (TDP-43) inclusions and AD pathology

(AD: Alzheimer's disease; DLB: dementia with Lewy bodies; DNA: deoxyribonucleic acid; DRS-2: Dementia Rating Scale-2; FAB: Frontal Assessment Battery; MMSE: Mini–Mental Status Examination; MoCA: Montreal Cognitive Assessment; PANDA: Parkinson Neuropsychometric Dementia Assessment; PD-CRS: Parkinson's Disease–Cognitive Rating Scale; PDD: Parkinson's disease dementia; PSP: progressive supranuclear palsy; SCOPA-COG: SCales for Outcomes in PArkinson's disease-COGnition; TAR: transactive response) present in 22–37% of confirmed neuropathological cases. Moreover, DLB emerged to be the most prevalent clinical misdiagnosis in pathologically confirmed MSA cases. While cognitive deficits in MSA mirror those seen in DLB and PDD, they tend to be less severe overall. Given the subtlety of cognitive changes in MSA, neuropsychological testing may be necessary for accurate detection, as cognitive screening tests may overlook these nuances.[2]

NEURODEGENERATIVE DISORDERS: TAUOPATHIES

Progressive Supranuclear Palsy

In the natural course of PSP, up to 70% develop dementia, with 10% initially presenting with cognitive symptoms. Executive dysfunction prevails alongside motor features such as postural instability and restricted vertical gaze. Memory, language, visuospatial function, and social cognition deficits can also arise. The Frontal Assessment Battery may offer better sensitivity for cognitive screening than the Montreal Cognitive Assessment (MoCA) or Mini-Mental Status Examination (MMSE). Verbal fluency, both lexical and semantic, is notably impaired in PSP, aiding its differentiation from PD with 85% specificity and sensitivity when ≤7 words per minute are produced. PSP exhibits more lexical than semantic fluency deficits, unlike AD, and may overlap with other syndromes such as nonfluent/agrammatic primary progressive aphasia and corticobasal syndrome (CBS).[7,9]

Corticobasal Syndrome

Corticobasal syndrome can stem from underlying pathologies such as corticobasal degeneration, frontotemporal lobar degeneration with transactive response deoxyribonucleic acid (DNA)-binding protein 43 (TDP-43), or AD. Clinically, CBS presents as a combination of limb apraxia, parkinsonism, dystonia, myoclonus, and alien limb phenomenon, making it the most asymmetric of the parkinsonian disorders. While executive dysfunction may be present, CBS typically exhibits more pronounced deficits in language, visuospatial abilities, and social cognition. This includes the effects of interpersonal and affective factors on cognitive processes, such as the expression and perception of emotions and intentions. Recognition deficits in facial emotions may aid in distinguishing CBS. Parietal lobe dysfunction is a prominent feature, leading to potential spatial or visual neglect, impaired praxis, Bálint syndrome (characterized by ocular ataxia, oculomotor apraxia, and simultanagnosia), Gerstmann syndrome (involving left-right confusion, finger agnosia, acalculia, and agraphia), and cortical sensory changes. Language dysfunction is observed in up to one third of CBS patients and it may be the initial symptom, with prevalence increasing over the course of the disease. Symptoms include difficulty with word finding, impaired repetition, agraphia, and apraxia of speech. Neuroimaging often reveals asymmetric parietal atrophy.[2]

Chronic Traumatic Encephalopathy

In recent decades, sports-related TBI has gained attention, initially observed in boxers as "punch drunk" syndrome. The term "dementia pugilistica," or "boxer's dementia," or chronic traumatic encephalopathy (CTE) reflects the understanding that TBI from any source heightens the risk of neurodegenerative disease, originally observed in boxers. Behavioral disturbances encompass aggression and impulsivity, while mood disturbances entail anxiety, apathy, depression, emotional instability, mania, and suicidal tendencies. Cognitive impairments involve difficulties in attention, concentration, executive function, and memory and may lead to dementia. Motor deficits may manifest as ataxia, gait disturbances, and parkinsonism.[10]

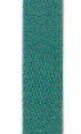

ALZHEIMER'S DEMENTIA WITH EXTRAPYRAMIDAL SYNDROME

Extrapyramidal syndrome (EPS) in the form of parkinsonism has been described in AD cases. The presence of EPS in AD has been linked to impaired functioning of specific cognitive subdomains that comprise attention and visuospatial functions. In patients with AD, parkinsonism has been found to have a strong correlation with the severity of AD. Neuronal loss in the substantia nigra (SN), partly attributable to tau lesions, constitutes a significant pathological basis for EPS in AD. Nonetheless, some cases, both with and without EPS, may exhibit little to no changes in the SN.[11] Additionally, certain genetic forms of AD, particularly those carrying presenilin-1 (PSEN1) mutations, manifest a blend of dementia and parkinsonism. Studies have shown that individuals with clinical parkinsonism among PSEN1 carriers display asymmetric reductions in dopamine transporter positron emission tomography (PET) {N-3-[18F]fluoropropyl-2β-carbomethoxy-3β-4-iodophenyl nortropane (FP-CIT)} uptake in the striatum and exhibit a favorable response to levodopa (L-DOPA) treatment.[1]

HEREDODEGENERATIVE ETIOLOGIES

Complex presentations of early-onset parkinsonism (onset <50 years) with cognitive decline alongside pyramidal symptoms, additional movement disorders such as dystonia or cerebellar features, and psychiatric symptoms indicate evaluation of etiologies such as metal-related disorders, including Wilson's disease (WD) and neurodegeneration with brain iron accumulation (NBIA), degenerative disorders such as juvenile Huntington's disease (JHD), and inherited metabolic disorders (cerebrotendinous xanthomatosis and Fahr's disease) **(Table 2)**.[12,13]

Wilson's Disease

Cognitive issues in WD suggest subcortical involvement, impacting global cognitive tests influenced by motor symptoms. Intelligence test results vary, with some showing verbal and nonverbal deficits. Memory problems resemble Huntington's disease (HD) rather than AD. Executive function and reasoning tests reveal WD patients'

TABLE 2: Profile of early-onset parkinsonism with cognitive impairment.

Disorder	Age at onset	Inheritance	Cognitive decline	Additional motor features	Nonmotor	L-DOPA response	Neuroimaging
Primary EOPD: Monogenic PD							
PARK-ATP13A2	Second to sixth decade	AR	Present	Vertical SGP, slow vertical saccades, pyramidal signs, facial–faucial–finger myoclonus, optic atrophy	Optic atrophy	±	Diffuse atrophy; SWI, GRE, and T2* hypointensity of basal ganglia
PARK-PLA2G6	Third to fourth decade	AR	Present and rapid	Dystonia, psychiatric symptoms, pyramidal signs, limb ataxia	Bulbar involvement and optic atrophy	±	Cerebral and/or cerebellar atrophy; SWI, GRE, and T2* hypointensity of basal ganglia; claval hypertrophy in childhood onset
PARK-SYNJ1	Second to third decade	AR	Present	Dystonia	Epilepsy—infantile onset	+	Diffuse atrophy, T2 WM hyperintensity, or normal brain MRI
PARK-DNAJC6	First to fifth decade	AR	Present and rapid	Rapid progression	Epilepsy with childhood onset, pyramidal signs	+	Mild diffuse atrophy or normal brain MRI
PARK-SNCA	Second to seventh decade	AD	Present	Myoclonus, pyramidal signs	Psychiatric symptoms	+	Normal brain MRI
PARK-VPS13C	Childhood to late adulthood	AR	Early	Pyramidal signs	Autonomic dysfunction	±	Normal brain MRI
PARK-RAB39B	Fourth to seventh decade	XR	Intellectual disability	–		±	CT-hyperdensity and T2 hypointensity of the basal ganglia can be seen and correspond to calcifications
PARK-FBX07	Third to fourth decade	AR	Present	Pyramidal signs, lower limb involvement	Neuropsychiatric manifestations	+	Mild diffuse atrophy or normal brain MRI
PARK-PTRHD1	Third to fourth decade	AD	Intellectual disability	Pyramidal signs	Sensorimotor polyneuropathy, distal amyotrophy	±	Normal brain MRI

Continued

Continued

Disorder	Age at onset	Inheritance	Cognitive decline	Additional motor features	Nonmotor	L-dopa response	Neuroimaging
Parkinsonism in metal-related disorders							
Wilson's disease (ATP7B)	Childhood, adolescence, or early adulthood	AR	Present	Wing-beating tremor, and dystonia	Kayser–Fleischer ring, bulbar signs, and hepatic involvement	±	T2 hyperintensity of putamen and other deep brain nuclei ("giant panda" and "miniature panda" signs)
NBIA (PANK2, PLA2G6, WDR45, C19ORF12, ATP13A2, CP, FTL)	Childhood (PANK2, C19ORF12), adolescence and early adulthood (PLA2G6, ATP13A2, WDR45), or adulthood (CP, FTL)	AR (PANK2, PLA2G6, C19ORF12, ATP13A2, CP), AD (FTL, C19ORF12), XD (WDR45)	Neuro-psychiatric features	Dystonia is predominant, choreoathetosis, pyramidal signs	Developmental delay and visual disturbances	±	WI, GRE, and T2* hypointensity of basal ganglia (eye-of-the-tiger sign in PKAN, hyperintense streak of medial medullary lamina in MPAN, T1-weighted signal hyperintensity surrounding SN in BPAN, cerebellar atrophy in PLAN)
Parkinsonism in metabolic disorders							
Fahr's disease (SLC20A2, PDGFRB, PDGFB, XPR1, MYORG, and secondary forms)	Adulthood	AD (except for MYORG–AR)	Neuro-psychiatric features	Tremor, choreo-dystonic features	Recurrent headache	±	Symmetrical hyperdense TC signal involving predominantly basal ganglia (pontine involvement: MYORG)
Cerebrotendinous xanthomatosis (CYP27A)	Fourth to fifth decade	AR	Present	Cerebellar and pyramidal signs, polyneuropathy	Diarrhea, cataract, tendon xanthomas, osteopenia	±	Brain MRI: Cortical and cerebellar atrophy; dentate nuclei, cerebellar peduncles, and internal capsule, SN, GP, striatum T2 WM hyperintensity
Spastic paraplegia with parkinsonism							
SPG15	Second decade	AR	Present	Lower limbs spasticity ±	Retinal degeneration, dysarthria, and motor neuropathy	+	Brain MRI: Thinning corpus callosum; sign of "the ear of the lynx"

(AD: Alzheimer's disease; AR: autosomal recessive; BPAN: beta-propeller protein-associated neurodegeneration; CT: computed tomography; EOPD: early-onset Parkinson's disease; GP: globus pallidus; GRE: gradient echo; MPAN: mitochondrial membrane protein-associated neurodegeneration; MRI: magnetic resonance imaging; PD: Parkinson's disease; PKAN: pantothenate kinase-associated neurodegeneration; PLAN: PLA2G6-associated neurodegeneration; SGP: supranuclear gaze palsy; SPG15: spastic paraplegia-15; SN: substantia nigra; SWI: susceptibility weighted imaging; WM: white matter; XR: X-linked recessive) frontal-subcortical dysfunction, which directly correlates with disease duration, while language tests show no difference. Visuospatial tests worsen with disease duration and age; earlier onset correlates with poorer performance. Copper levels do not correlate with symptoms. Treatment can improve both motor and cognitive functions, though abnormalities may persist post-treatment or hepatic transplant. However, cognitive abnormalities may persist despite treatment.[14]

Neurodegeneration with Brain Iron Accumulation Spectrum

Cognitive abnormalities are prominent in various neurodegenerative disorders such as pantothenate kinase-associated neurodegeneration (PKAN), where they inversely vary with the age of onset. PLA2G6-associated neurodegeneration (PLAN) often presents with progressive cognitive decline, sometimes as the initial symptom. Adult-onset variants of mitochondrial membrane protein-associated neurodegeneration (MPAN) typically feature cognitive-behavioral syndrome and parkinsonism. Childhood-onset MPAN includes pyramidal syndrome, optic atrophy, dysarthria, and cognitive decline. A slowly progressive cognitive decline with regression of milestones is also seen in children with beta-propeller protein-associated neurodegeneration (BPAN), Fatty acid hydroxylase-associated neurodegeneration (FAHN), and COASY protein-associated neurodegeneration (CoPAN). Neuroferritinopathy shows late-cognitive decline with middle-aged onset amid chorea, parkinsonism, and orofacial dystonia. Aceruloplasminemia, marked by microcytic anemia, diabetes, and low ceruloplasmin, presents with chorea, tremor, parkinsonism, and cognitive impairment. Kufor Rakeb syndrome, part of the NBIA spectrum, includes akinetic-rigid parkinsonism, ocular movement abnormalities, pyramidal signs, facial–faucial–finger myoclonus, and variable degrees of intellectual disability.[15]

Juvenile Huntington's Disease

Typically, JHD presents before the age of 20 years. Patients present with juvenile-onset parkinsonism, associated with seizures, myoclonus, behavioral abnormalities, and prominent cognitive decline. Cognitive impairment is reported as the initial disease signs in 30–83% of JHD patients, even before the onset of motor symptoms. The cognitive profile is characterized by a subcortical form of dementia. The early signs of cognitive impairment are often associated with reduced psychomotor speed and a decline in executive functions such as attention, planning, and cognitive flexibility. Moreover, a higher incidence of developmental delay encompasses delays in cognitive, motor, language, and social development. Notably, chorea is absent in these cases. The disorder represents the most severe form of HD, caused by >60 CAG repeats in the *huntingtin* (*HTT*) gene on chromosome 4p16.3.[16]

SPECTRUM OF RAPIDLY PROGRESSIVE DEMENTIA WITH PARKINSONISM

The term "rapidly progressive dementia" (RPD) is used to characterize a cognitive disorder with rapid progression, leading to the clinical manifestation of dementia. This progression typically occurs within a relatively short timeframe, often regarded as less than either 1 or 2 years. The etiology of RPD varies widely. The ones associated with prominent parkinsonism comprise prion disorders, infective etiologies such as human immunodeficiency virus (HIV), and dural arteriovenous fistula (DAVF).[17-19]

Infectious Etiologies

Human Immunodeficiency Virus-associated Neurocognitive Disorder and HIV-encephalopathy

In a review comprising 26 patients with HIV-associated neurocognitive disorder (HAND) or HIV-associated encephalopathy (HIV-E) with Parkinsonism from 1996 to 2018, most had low CD4 counts (<200 cells/uL), with variable antiretroviral therapy (ARV) usage. Parkinsonism in HIV-E and HAND typically lacks a resting tremor, shows poor response to dopamine replacement therapy (DRT), and is linked with early mortality. Neuroimaging suggests cerebral atrophy in all cases, with some showing white matter and basal ganglia signal changes. Despite response to the highly active antiretroviral therapy (HAART), mortality is high among patients with movement disorders and HIV, particularly those with HIV-E.[20]

Whipple's Disease

Neurologic manifestations are diverse and include cognitive impairment, altered consciousness, psychiatric features, ataxia, seizures, myoclonus, supranuclear ophthalmoplegia, and sensory deficits. Pathognomonic features such as oculomasticatory and oculofacial-skeletal myorhythmia are observed in only 20% of cases, while less common manifestations encompass proximal myopathy, stroke-like episodes, progressive deafness, and EPS like parkinsonism. Cerebrospinal fluid (CSF) analysis may reveal elevated protein or pleocytosis and brain magnetic resonance imaging (MRI) may be normal or exhibit symmetric T2-weighted signal intensity in the midline involving the midbrain, hypothalamus, or mesial temporal lobes. Stereotactic brain biopsy may be considered in select cases when diagnosis remains uncertain. Treatment involves ceftriaxone for 2–4 weeks followed by maintenance therapy with trimethoprim-sulfamethoxazole one DS tablet twice daily for 1 year.[19]

Neurosyphilis

Neurosyphilis, caused by treponema pallidum, is a great imitator in medicine and an important etiology of RPD. In the late stage of neurosyphilis, patients can develop cognitive decline and neuropsychiatric symptoms such as irritability and hallucinations, speech disturbances, pupillary abnormalities, parkinsonism, myoclonus, and cerebellar ataxia. These manifestations are particularly noted in the cerebral parenchymal form of infection. Treatment with penicillin can partially improve symptoms such as parkinsonism, myoclonus, and cerebellar dysfunction while dementia significantly improved.[19]

Prion Disease

Creutzfeldt–Jakob disease (CJD) is an RPD syndrome characterized by pyramidal and extrapyramidal, with visual signs and symptoms. Approximately 90% of affected individuals develop movement disorders during the course of the disease, with myoclonus being the most common, observed in 82–100% of cases. Less commonly seen movement disorders include dystonia, choreoathetosis, tremors, and parkinsonian syndrome. Diagnosis is based on neuroimaging showing cortical ribboning or inverted hockey-stick sign, CSF biomarkers including 14-3-3 assay and characteristic electroencephalogram (EEG) abnormalities.[19]

Dural Arteriovenous Fistula

Dural arteriovenous fistulas, accounting for 10–15% of intracranial malformations, can lead to neurocognitive and motoric decline, resembling Parkinson-like symptoms, and can rapidly progress to dementia. DAVF-induced dementia includes cortical and thalamic forms. Cortical dementia involves rapid cognitive decline with focal cortical symptoms, while thalamic dementia resulting from basal ganglia/thalamic dysfunction is characterized by cognitive impairment, parkinsonism, and hypersomnolence. Treatment options, such as endovascular or surgical techniques, typically result in complete symptom resolution and MRI normalization.[17]

Autoimmune and Paraneoplastic Etiologies

Rapidly progressive PSP-like syndromes have been linked to paraneoplastic etiologies, including anti-Ma1, anti-Ma2, anti-Hu, anti-CRMP5, and anti-Ri onconeuronal antibodies. The latter is frequently correlated with breast cancer. Neoplasms associated with this syndrome include B-cell lymphoma, small cell lung carcinoma, and tonsil carcinoma. Additionally, a PSP-like syndrome may also result from an autoimmune process mediated by anti-LGI1, anti-IgLON5, and anti-DPPX antibodies. While both anti-IgLON5 disease and PSP exhibit abnormal vertical eye movements, upward gaze palsy may be predominant in anti-IgLON5 disease, while mainly downward gaze abnormalities are observed in PSP.[19]

VASCULAR ETIOLOGIES

Cerebral Small Vessel Disease

As per the International Workshop of the National Institute of Neurological Disorders and Stroke (NINDS) and the Association Internationale pour la Recherche et l'Enseignement en Neurosciences (AIREN) criteria, small vessel vascular dementia (VaD) is categorized into subcortical and cortical forms. The subcortical type is the more prevalent classic form, resulting from cerebral white matter ischemia and multiple lacunar infarcts. On the other hand, cortical small vessel disease (SVD) is primarily linked to cerebral amyloid angiopathy (CAA). Binswanger's disease, a subtype of cerebral small vessel disease (CSVD), presents with cognitive impairment and gait disturbances from small subcortical ischemic strokes and white matter hyperintensities (WMHs). Lesions in subcortical areas such as the basal ganglia lead to psychomotor slowing, memory deficits, frontal dysfunction, parkinsonism, and ataxia. Management includes controlling vascular risk factors. Memantine, an N-methyl-D-aspartate (NMDA) antagonist, potentially improves cognitive function without worsening global functioning or behavior. Antiplatelets are recommended in CSVD with or without lacunes and symptomatic atherosclerosis.[2,21]

BIOMARKERS

Cerebrospinal fluid amyloid-beta levels are typically lower in PDD compared to controls. PDD shows less amyloid-beta reduction than PD-MCI. Low amyloid-beta and A-beta 1-42/total tau predict cognitive decline in nondemented PD patients. Total alpha-synuclein remains consistent across cognitive status, but PDD is associated with more oligomeric forms. In DLB, cognitive decline correlates with CSF amyloid levels. A large proportion of DLB patients exhibit abnormal values resembling AD patterns, while PD without dementia rarely does. Elevated CSF neurofilament light chain (NFL) correlates with disease severity. CSF uric acid is reduced in PDD and DLB,

TABLE 3: CSF and imaging biomarkers of the common dementia–parkinsonism syndromes.

Disease	CSF amyloid beta	CSF tau	CSF phosphor-tau	CSF total alpha-synuclein	CSF alpha synuclein oligomers	CSF NFL	Imaging biomarkers
PDD	Low	Normal or elevated	Normal	Low	Elevated	Normal or elevated	• DAT-SPECT: Asymmetric striatal loss of DAT, more marked at the dorsal putamen, normal caudate • FDG-PET: Increased metabolic activity at basal ganglia, thalamus, decreased activity in premotor and parietal cortex
DLB	Low	Normal or elevated	Normal or elevated	Low	Elevated	Elevated	• Generalized low uptake on SPECT/PET perfusion with reduced occipital activity is evidenced as compared to AD • A more prominent hypometabolism in the anterior cingulate cortex may facilitate distinguishing DLB from PDD
PSP	Normal or low	Normal	Normal	Normal	NA	Elevated	• DAT-SPECT: Reduced putaminal uptake, putamen to caudate nucleus ratio increased, less pronounced asymmetry (not useful for differential diagnosis with PD) • FDG-PET: Asymmetric decrease in metabolic activity in basal ganglia, thalamus, and frontotemporal cortex
CBS	Normal or low	Normal or elevated	Normal	Normal	NA	Elevated	• MRI with volumetry: Atrophy of the inferior parietal cortex, the primary motor cortex, the frontal cortex and basal ganglia • FDG-PET: Asymmetric reduction in striatum, thalamus, frontal and temporoparietal cortices
MSA	Normal or low	Normal or elevated	Normal	Normal	NA	Elevated	• DAT-SPECT: Striatal uptake reduction, no significant asymmetry index (not useful for differential diagnosis with PD) • FDG-PET: Decreased metabolic activity in basal ganglia, putamen, pons, and cerebellum

(AD: Alzheimer's disease; CBS: corticobasal syndrome; CSF: cerebrospinal fluid; DLB: dementia with Lewy bodies; DAT-SPECT: dopamine transporter single-photon emission computed tomography; FDG-PET: 18-fluorodeoxyglucose positron emission tomography; MSA: multisystem atrophy; NFL: neurofilament level; PDD: Parkinson's disease with dementia; PSP: progressive supranuclear palsy)

while proteomic analysis suggests differences in proteins related to folding and neuronal signaling between demented and nondemented PD patients. In PDD, new serum and CSF biomarkers called soluble CD163 have been found to correlate with cognitive decline in PD. Additionally, retinal abnormalities measured by optical coherence tomography (OCT) show promise in predicting cognitive dysfunction, suggesting OCT's utility in PD cognitive assessment.[1] Fluid and imaging biomarkers are discussed in **Table 3**.[1,22]

MANAGEMENT ASPECTS

Management of dementia with parkinsonism requires tailored investigations and treatment of secondary causes alongside a multidisciplinary approach. Initially, potential contributors such as neuroleptic side effects and comorbidities should be addressed. While the choice of medication class in PD does not significantly impact long-term dementia rates, anticholinergic medication use is strongly linked to cognitive decline. In some regions, rivastigmine and donepezil are approved for PDD and DLB, with cholinesterase inhibitors and memantine showing potential benefits in PD-MCI, PDD, and DLB. Risk factor modification, brain-healthy lifestyle promotion, regular safety screenings, and caregiver support are essential. Deep brain stimulation targeting cholinergic pathways projecting from the nucleus basalis of Meynert has not shown clear cognitive benefits in PDD. Noninvasive brain stimulation methods have not proven effective for cognitive impairment in PD either.[1,2,7]

Recent Advances

Exploratory studies of novel treatments such as blarcamesine and neflamapimod have shown improvement in cognitive decline in PDD and DLB. Further research is underway to assess the safety and tolerability of drugs like the cortical enhancer IRL752 for cognitive enhancement. Additionally, early use of donepezil has been found to slow cognitive decline over 2 years in PD patients without dementia carrying the *apolipoprotein E* (*APOE*) ε*4* gene.[2,23]

CONCLUSION

Dementia with parkinsonism represents a broad group that ranges from inherited to acquired etiologies. The current chapter addresses the possible etiologies and provides a comprehensive understanding of the clinical manifestations of these disorders. It is important to perform a thorough clinical evaluation before ordering investigations. Clinical response relies on early diagnosis and prompt diagnosis of potentially reversible causes.

REFERENCES

1. Koros C, Stefanis L, Scarmeas N. Parkinsonism and dementia. J Neuro Sci. 2022;433:120015.
2. Goldman JG, Holden SK. Cognitive Syndromes Associated With Movement Disorders. Continuum (Minneap Minn). 2022;28(3):726-49.
3. Aarsland D, Kurz MW. The Epidemiology of Dementia Associated with Parkinson's Disease. Brain Pathol. 2010;20(3):633-9.
4. Huang J, Yuan X, Chen L, Hu B, Jiang L, Shi T, et al. Subjective cognitive decline in patients with Parkinson's disease: an updated review. Front Aging Neurosci. 2023;15:1117068.
5. Painous C, Marti MJ. Cognitive Impairment in Parkinson's Disease: What We Know so Far. Res Rev Parkinsonism. 2020;10:7-17.
6. Gonzalez-Latapi P, Bayram E, Litvan I, Marras C. Cognitive impairment in Parkinson's disease: Epidemiology, clinical profile, protective and risk factors. Behav Sci (Basel). 2021;11(5):74.
7. Zhang Q, Aldridge GM, Narayanan NS, Anderson SW, Uc EY. Approach to Cognitive Impairment in Parkinson's Disease. Neurotherapeutics. 2020;17(4):1495-510.
8. Macoir J. The Cognitive and Language Profile of Dementia with Lewy Bodies. Am J Alzheimers Dis Dement. 2022;37.
9. Höglinger GU, Respondek G, Stamelou M, Kurz C, Josephs KA, Lang AE, et al. Clinical diagnosis of progressive supranuclear palsy: The movement disorder society criteria. Mov Disord. 2017;32(6):853-64.
10. Tarazi A, Tator CH, Tartaglia MC. Chronic Traumatic Encephalopathy and Movement Disorders: Update. Curr Neurol Neurosci Rep. 2016;16(5):46.
11. Mitchell SL. Extrapyramidal features in Alzheimer's disease. Age Ageing. 1999;28(4):401-9.
12. Post B, Van Den Heuvel L, Van Prooije T, Van Ruissen X, Van De Warrenburg B, Nonnekes J. Young Onset Parkinson's Disease: A Modern and Tailored Approach. J Parkinsons Dis. 2020;10: S29-36.
13. Riboldi GM, Frattini E, Monfrini E, Frucht SJ, Di Fonzo A. A Practical Approach to Early-Onset Parkinsonism. J Parkinsons Dis. 2022;12:1-26.
14. Frota NAF, Caramelli P, Barbosa ER. Cognitive impairment in Wilson's disease. Dement Neuropsychol. 2009;3(1):16-21.
15. Hogarth P. Neurodegeneration with Brain Iron Accumulation: Diagnosis and Management. J Mov Disord. 2015;8(1):1-13.
16. Douglas I, Evans S, Rawlins MD, Smeeth L, Tabrizi SJ, Wexler NS. Juvenile Huntington's disease: a population-based study using the General Practice Research Database. BMJ Open. 2013;3(4):e002085.
17. Armocida D, Palmieri M, Paglia F, Berra LV, D'Angelo L, Frati A, et al. Rapidly progressive dementia and Parkinsonism as the first symptoms of dural arteriovenous fistula. The Sapienza University experience and comprehensive literature review concerning the clinical course of 102 patients. Clin Neurol Neurosurg. 2021;208:106835.
18. Hermann P, Zerr I. Rapidly progressive dementias—aetiologies, diagnosis and management. Nat Rev Neurol. 2022;18:363-76.
19. Geschwind MD. Rapidly Progressive Dementia. Continuum (Minneap Minn). 2016;22(2):510-37.
20. Amod F, Holla VV, Ojha R, Pandey S, Yadav R, Pal PK. A review of movement disorders in persons living with HIV. Parkinsonism Relat Disord. 2023;114:105774.
21. Van Straaten ECW, Scheltens P, Knol DL, Van Buchem MA, Van Dijk EJ, Hofman PAM, et al. Operational definitions for the NINDS-AIREN criteria for vascular dementia an interobserver study. Stroke. 2003;34(8):1907-12.
22. Peralta C, Strafella AP, van Eimeren T, Ceravolo R, Seppi K, Kaasinen V, et al. Pragmatic Approach on Neuroimaging Techniques for the Differential Diagnosis of Parkinsonisms. Mov Disord Clin Pract. 2022;9:6-19.
23. Aarsland D, Batzu L, Halliday GM, Geurtsen GJ, Ballard C, Ray Chaudhuri K, et al. Parkinson disease-associated cognitive impairment. Nat Rev Dis Primers. 2021;7(1):47.

CHAPTER

11

Clinical Approach and Management of Post-stroke Aphasia

Apoorva Pauranik, Pinki Singh

ABSTRACT

Post-stroke aphasia is a common but relatively neglected chronic disability. People with aphasia are in dire need of more attention from neurologists. Clinical assessment and management of aphasia requires a lot of time, patience, experience, and commitment from clinicians. Bedside testing of aphasia must follow a structured approach. Diagnosis and therapy should be guided by a holistic thinking, combining medical or biological model of language breakdown on one hand and a psychosocial or life participation model on the other. Classical aphasia syndromes are now considered to be of rather limited practical utility. Instead, a detailed profiling of speech and communication function is essential for planning therapeutic interventions. Speech–language therapies administered in an intensive manner by speech–language pathologists are the mainstay of management and rehabilitation. Pharmacotherapy and noninvasive brain stimulations have some complimentary role. Advances in computers, smartphones, information technology, telemedicine, and virtual reality are changing the scenario rapidly for the better. Services of caregivers, significant others (SOs), and trained volunteers must be utilized to reduce the treatment gap.

Keywords: Speech and communication, Aphasia, Rehabilitation. Speech language therapy, Neuroplasticity, Biological and psychosocial model, Assessment of aphasia, Aphasia syndromes.

INTRODUCTION

Post-stroke aphasia persists as long-term disability in about 25% of survivors (range from 21 to 38%). A community-based study from Sweden reported an incidence of 4/100,000 per year. Prevalence is around 300 per million[1] **(Table 1)**. We do not yet have a clear picture of the epidemiology of aphasia in India.

CLINICAL HISTORY TACKING

The clinical history for probable aphasia and related speech and communication disorders starts right from initial greetings and pleasantries. A significant burden of narrating the illness' story will fall upon the caregiver.

The neurologist should be "all ears" while people with aphasia (PWA) and significant others (SOs) narrate the story. We must resist the temptations to interrupt on any pretext; however, we must constantly be encouraging them.

Box 1 enumerates a list of possible symptoms which may be described or complained by PWA or SO.

WHICH TYPE OF TEST BATTERY—AD HOC OR STANDARDIZED AND VALIDATED?

A few tests have been constructed or adapted into Indian languages with all the rigor of a good test. Fewer still have been published, along with normative data and are difficult to procure as a fully commercial set.[2]

A general neurologist often uses *nonstandardized* and nonvalidated or ad hoc assessment in outpatient department (OPD) and bedside. It is a practical necessity for busy general neurologists and residents in training.

TABLE 1: Community burden of aphasia and other disorders of speech and communication.

Disease condition	Overall burden	Proportion with aphasia
Stroke	Prevalence 0.5%	25%
Head injury	Prevalence 1.2%	5–10%
Dementia	10% above the age of 60 years	Almost all have variable impairment of language functions, depending on severity
Mental retardation	5% (all) 1% (severe)	Almost all have variable impairment of language function, depending on severity
Learning disabilities (e.g., dyslexia)	5%	All have a variable handicap in reading and writing skills
Fluency and articulation disorders: Stuttering, stammering, lisping, cluttering, lalling	1%	Variable handicap in all

The methods of testing described in this chapter are *standardized* and validated but not published. Please refer to the link for appendices **(Box 2)** to access various *stimuli* and instructions about their administration and scoring as developed by the present author.[3]

A few tips may be helpful for a busy neurologist as follows:

- Always carry cards with pictures of objects, actions, scenes, printed words, and sentences in the examination bag.
- Better still, carry all the abovementioned and more variety of examples on desktop, laptop, or smartphone.
- Verbatim records of assessments of aphasia are important. Hence, keep a scoring sheet ready to enter the patient's responses to various subtests. The target answers are preprinted in one column and a parallel column is left blank to be filled verbatim immediately by the clinician.
- Make a video or an audio recording of the clinical assessment to be saved on a computer. An assistant can transcribe it later.

BOX 1 A list of possible symptoms which may be complained of by people with aphasia (PWA) and significant others (SOs).

- Not talking at all, "no speech output"—*mutism*
- "Reduced speed of talking," "speaking fewer words time," "speaking fewer utterances," "hesitating while trying to speak," "having pauses while speaking," "taking a longer time to initiate the speech act," "failing to take a turn while in conversation"—*nonfluency*
- Groping for words, "not finding the words," "getting stuck up with words"—*anomia*
- Response word differs from target word in the sound structure—*phonemic paraphasia*
- Response word differs, though the meaning is related—*semantic paraphasia*
- Uttering a word different than the one intended and which is unrelated to the target word and meaningless in the context—*semantic jargon*
- Uttering an unrecognizable string of sounds, not a word or phrase—*phonemic jargon*
- Uttering words which do not exist in the dictionary of the language (*lexicon*) known and used daily by a person with aphasia—*nonwords, neologism*
- Speech output restricted to a repetitive, meaningless, irrelevant *monosyllable* consonant–vowel pair (CV recurrent utterance)
- A correct but roundabout description—for a target word—*circumlocution*
- Uttering the same word again in response to different questions and need—*preservations*
- Speaking correctly but with distorted pronunciations which remains unchanged each time the given word or sound is uttered—*dysarthria*
- *Repeating the word* or phrase spoken by others instead of answering *(echolalia)*
- *Distorted pronunciation*, which keeps changing for a given word *(apraxia of speech)*
- *Speaking excessively*, without a sense of completion, but mostly nonunderstandable, jargon-like, talking irrelevantly *(fluent aphasia, empty speech)*
- *Not paying attention to* what others are speaking, not listening properly, not understanding whatever is being said, not following the conversation *(defective auditory comprehension)*; it may appear as if hearing acuity is reduced, but hearing is normal
- *Not being able to repeat* a *syllable* or word or phrase spoken by others, despite comprehending it well (conduction, Broca's, Wernicke aphasia)
- *Reduced interest and efficiency in reading*—PWA may be holding a newspaper in his hands, but SO are unsure if he is grasping anything. Unable to read aloud or read with distortions like phonemic and semantic paraphasia, jargon, and nonwords. It may appear as if vision is reduced, but visual acuity remains normal *(acquired alexia)*
- *Reduced memory*—maybe the memory is intact, but relatives and caregivers think so because of anomia and paraphasia
- *Total or partial failure of writing (agraphia)*—difficulties in writing with either hand—distorted handwriting. A similar range of problems in written expression as in oral verbal expressions (nonfluency, anomia, paraphasias, circumlocutions, jargon, etc.)

BOX 2 **List of appendices. These appendices are available in detail on http://neurogyan2.arth-dhwani.com/aphasia.**

- HASIT: Hindi Aphasia Screening Indore Test
- HRWIT: Hindi Reading Writing Indore Test
- LEAP-Q: Language Experience and Proficiency Questionnaire
- Handedness questionnaire
- Images for nouns
- Images for verbs
- Scenes and comic strips for picture description and narrative discourse
- Word and nonword list for repetition, reading aloud, and lexicality judgment
- Word–picture matching exercise
- Sentence–picture matching exercise
- Yes–no questions for auditory and reading comprehension
- Short story-based questions for auditory and reading comprehension
- Question for responsive naming with a single unambiguous one-word answer
- Scoring proforma
- Glossary of aphasiological terms (italicized in the main text)

Note: The link leads to a website developed by the author for public education and patient education about neurology and other subjects in Hindi. The section on aphasia hosts additional information and tools in English for neurologists and speech–language pathologists.

- If possible, train a clinical assistant in basic assessment to do the testing, recording, and later writing the notes.
- Team up with a speech–language pathologist (SLP) and clinical (neuro) psychologist long term.
- A full clinical assessment of speech and language communication in a PWA in an ideal condition is time and labor intensive and needs expertise and experience. Comprehensive *profiling* is essential for proper and complete diagnosis and therapeutic planning. SLPs are primarily suited for this task.

Hindi Aphasia Screening Indore Test (HASIT) is a *standardized* and validated *test battery*, though unpublished, modeled after Frenchy Aphasia Screening Test (FAST) from the United Kingdom (UK).[4] A more rigorous Indian *adaptation* of FAST was developed as a part of the Indian Council of Medical Research (ICMR) Toolbox for cognitive assessment across six languages and different educational levels.[5] Based on an initial briefer assessment, the neurologist or SLP must pick and choose which aspect of competence and performance he is interested in. Computers and smartphones are proving literally handy and very useful in testing aphasia because it is portable, editable, expandable, interactive, transferable, participatory, and can be individualized. Timekeeping and scoring are facilitated. Testing can be done at any time and from anywhere. Neurologists should keep themselves updated with new digital tools becoming available.[6]

BEDSIDE CLINICAL TESTING

Verbal Expression

Listen carefully to the patient and ask questions like "Tell me about your illness, your family, and the work done by you at your job." Efforts are needed to make patients speak, not merely isolated words or gestures but longer *phrases* and sentences. The patient should be asked to describe the things and actions in a picture.

Defective articulation and phonation are recognized during a conversation, reading aloud, and repetition. A list of target *syllables*, words, nonwords, and short *phrases* is needed for testing articulation. While listening to dysarthric speech, pay attention to the type of sound distortion (*phonemes*). In the case of dysarthria, the distortions will be the same each time. However, in a condition known as *apraxia of speech*, the same *stimuli* will yield slightly altered output. Dysarthria is common in nonfluent aphasias. Pure dysarthria can occur in many disorders other than aphasia.

Many measures have been used in clinical practice and research for assessment of *fluency in speech*—the number of words per minute, the total number of words, the ratio of *content words* and *grammatical or function words*, informativeness of speech, *articulatory agility*, pauses, hesitancies, *prosody, intonation*, and others.

Person with aphasia with nonfluent speech speaks in *monosyllables* or short sentences. Sometimes, only a single utterance is repetitively used in every conversation. These verbal stereotypies [consonant–vowel (CV) recurring utterances] are sometimes intoned differently to convey some meaning, as in (yes!), (yes?), and (y..y..es?).

There may be a delay in initiating a response, increased effort, apparent strain, pauses between words and sentences, and interruptions. Nonfluent speech, as in Broca aphasia, also exhibits *agrammatism* in which there is an absence or a scarcity of *function words*. The short *phrases* are composed of *content words* only, though the meaning is conveyed somehow in a manner resembling "telegraphic language" as if to economize on words.

The word-finding difficulty is also a measure of fluency. It is encountered in almost all PWA. It is manifested by repetition of determiners (a, an, or the), prepositions (this, that, which, or so), other functional or grammatical units (and or yes) and vocal and gestural mannerisms ("uh," pointing toward something), circumlocution, paraphasia, neologism, and jargon. Many PWA can fluently recite overlearned lists (automatized sequences) such as counting, alphabets, days of the week, and months of a year, while the rest of the verbal output may be very nonfluent. The same is true for singing and uttering curse words and swear words. Category Fluency Test requires the patient to think and speak names or words belonging to one specific *semantic category* within 1 minute, for example, animals, vegetables, fruits, sweets, instruments, vehicles, etc. Another fluency test is to ask the person to think and speak rapidly, words beginning with specific letters within 1 minute, e.g., F or A or S.

Fluent but empty speech in Wernicke aphasia appears effortless, with typical melody, *accent*, *prosody*, and mannerisms. However, on close observation, the content is empty and abnormal. *Phrases* and sentences are of average length or sometimes overly lengthy. The patient fails to know when to stop. They may speak excessively (logorrhea), being unaware of the abnormality. There are many paraphasias, circumlocutions, and an abundance of function or grammar words whose information load is low. The *content words*, which carry information, are scarce and are used, flouting the rules of grammar. Jargon is common.

Discourse is a linguistic unit (such as a conversation or a story) larger than a sentence. A neurologist should help SLP colleagues with discourse analysis by audio recording testing and conversation.

Auditory Comprehension

If a patient merely shows the tongue on command, nods the head this or that way, or responds to a question, this does not mean normal auditory comprehension. While giving a command, the examiner and bystanders must not help by gestures. At the sentence level, command comprehension can be complicated by involving more than one step. For example, "Fold this piece of paper and put it into your pocket," "Pick up the piece of cloth and put it into the glass and then invert the glass on the table."

Pointing test of auditory comprehension at the one-word level: The examiner speaks out the word and asks the patient to point to the corresponding picture, object, or body part. The clinician scores patients' performance in terms of correct answers, taking into account all the help or cues and time latency. Some patients may perform poorly at the single-word level (identification by pointing) but better in sentence comprehension during day-to-day life, as meanings may be discernible through the context and redundancy of words.

Yes-no questions: "Does the stone sink in water?" "Is an elephant larger than an ant?" Not uncommonly, many patients performing reasonably well in daily household communication through gestures fail miserably in these formal testing modes.

Picture-sentence matching tasks use one sentence, many picture choices, and vice versa.

Discourse level comprehension: The clinician narrates a short story and asks questions based on it.

Repetition

The examiner asks the patient to repeat words, *nonwords*, *phrases* and sentences after him. Initial *stimuli* are simple, short, and *high frequency*; later, they are long, hard to pronounce, and of *low frequency*. The errors may be sound distortions, incomplete responses, deletions, or paraphasias. Some patients may perform well on auditory comprehension tests and do well during daily life but fail miserably on repeating simple words or *phrases* (conduction aphasia). In contrast, patients with transcortical sensory and mixed aphasia repeat long, complex *phrases* mechanically or slavishly. Still, they do not follow or extract a bit of meaning from whatever they are listening to and repeating.

Naming

One begins with *naming* objects, pictures, body parts, or persons. The images used during auditory comprehension serve the purpose again, with a reversal of roles. Now, the examiner puts her finger on the object or picture and asks PWA to name it. "Responsive *naming*" involves simple questions with an unambiguous one-word answer like, "*What do we call a person who delivers a letter at home?*" Some PWA may fail or there may be a delay. Sometimes, the *response word* may be altered yet related to the target word by sound (phonemic paraphasia) or meaning (semantic paraphasia). The *response word* may be phonemic jargon (non-word) or semantic jargon (dictionary word but unconnected). Some patients may describe the word in a roundabout way (circumlocution). The clinician should give *cues* or hints. The phonemic *cue* means uttering the first one or two *phonemes* of the word or producing its rhythm. Semantic *cue* involves indicating synonyms or attributes of that word. In case of persistent failure, the examiner then offers the answer by (1) suggesting a wrong answer and asking if it is correct or not and (2) suggesting the correct answer and again looking if the patient accepts it or not.

Reading

The clinician tests the patient's ability to recognize, match, and discriminate the graphic symbols of alphabets. She asks PWA to read aloud words, *phrases*, or paragraphs, not necessarily paying attention to the meaning. Reading comprehension involves word-picture or word-object matching and carrying out some commands printed on a piece of paper (e.g., touch your hair, make a fist, etc.). A somewhat difficult task is to fill in the blanks in progressively complex sentences from a choice of detractors. The PWA reads lengthy paragraphs (unseen passages) and is asked to write answers to questions based on them. The patient can be asked to sort words and nonwords from a mixed list.

Writing

Person with aphasia with reasonably good motor dexterity of a hand should be able to reproduce his premorbid handwriting, at least in such mechanical tasks as copying from written *stimuli*, writing to dictation, and serial writing of automatized sequences (such as name, address, numbers, alphabets, weekdays, and months).

MULTILINGUALISM

We in India have an exceptional opportunity to explore the effect of the same lesions on persons who speak structurally distinct languages. Aphasia in multilingual speakers poses special challenges. It becomes imperative to assess all the languages used by PWA. The clinical profile of aphasia may vary in the two or more languages used by PWA. Language Experience and Proficiency Questionnaire (LEAP-Q) is an internationally acclaimed objective tool for assessing the efficiency and use of languages in bi- or multilingual persons.[7] A Hindi version by the present author has been acknowledged and added to the host website of LEAP-Q.

Handedness: Neurologists must use a standard and valid battery to determine right versus left-handedness degrees.[8] The present author has created a Hindi-English bilingual questionnaire for scoring handedness.

Communication in daily life: The scores obtained on formal aphasia tests (as measured on popular test batteries) and the actual communicative performance in daily life often vary. To test for the latter, we use a different set of batteries.[9]

QUALITY OF LIFE AND PSYCHOSOCIAL ISSUES

The International Classification of Functioning, Disability, and Health (ICF)—developed by the World Health Organization (WHO)—is a framework to address functioning and disability related to a health condition within the context of the individual's activities and participation in everyday life.[10]

Applying ICF to the assessment of a PWA and their family/carers leads to addressing all domains of *functioning* and disability and defines the person-centered and family-centered functional goals. The goals identified by the PWA, in partnership with the clinician and family, allow participation in meaningful activities and roles. Person-centered functional goals help in maximizing the outcomes that lead to functional improvements that are important and meaningful to the individual.[11]

It is essential to measure "quality of life (QoL)" in PWA to identify patients' problems, determine treatment priorities, manage interventions, and monitor disease periods. Indian questionnaires have been developed and validated for this purpose and should be part of the assessment protocol for aphasia.[12]

Anxiety and depression are common in PWA and interfere with therapy and rehabilitation. Simple and valid tools for assessing these mental states should also be part of testing for aphasia.

Caregivers' burden in supporting PWA may sometimes appear trivial and mutually satisfying, particularly in cultures (like in India) where family values are held high. However, in the long term, it may be unbearable. Aphasia QoL studies should include "caregiver burden" and "supportive communication strategies" used by SO and report them separately.[13,14] Clinical tales or patient stories written by patients, caregivers, and clinicians may be compiled and published.[15]

Cognitive Functions

Aphasia is not an exclusively language-related problem.[16] Other cognitive functions, such as working memory, short-term memory, recent memory, attention, executive skills, sensory perception, motor dexterity, apraxia, agnosia, and spatial orientation are simultaneously affected.[17] Aphasic deficits may be seen as impairments to working memory. It is very challenging to assess impairments in various aspects of cognition in a person whose comprehension and expression are affected.

APHASIA SYNDROMES, THEIR IRREVERENCE, AND NEWER METHODS OF ASSESSMENT

Syndromic classifications **(Flowchart 1)** have been helpful as a shorthand summary of a patient's language disorder. However, syndromes have lost their theoretical and practical relevance.[18] Newer classifications based on *neurolinguistics* and cognitive neuropsychology require modifications in methods of clinical examination. We must adopt a deficit-based approach instead of syndrome

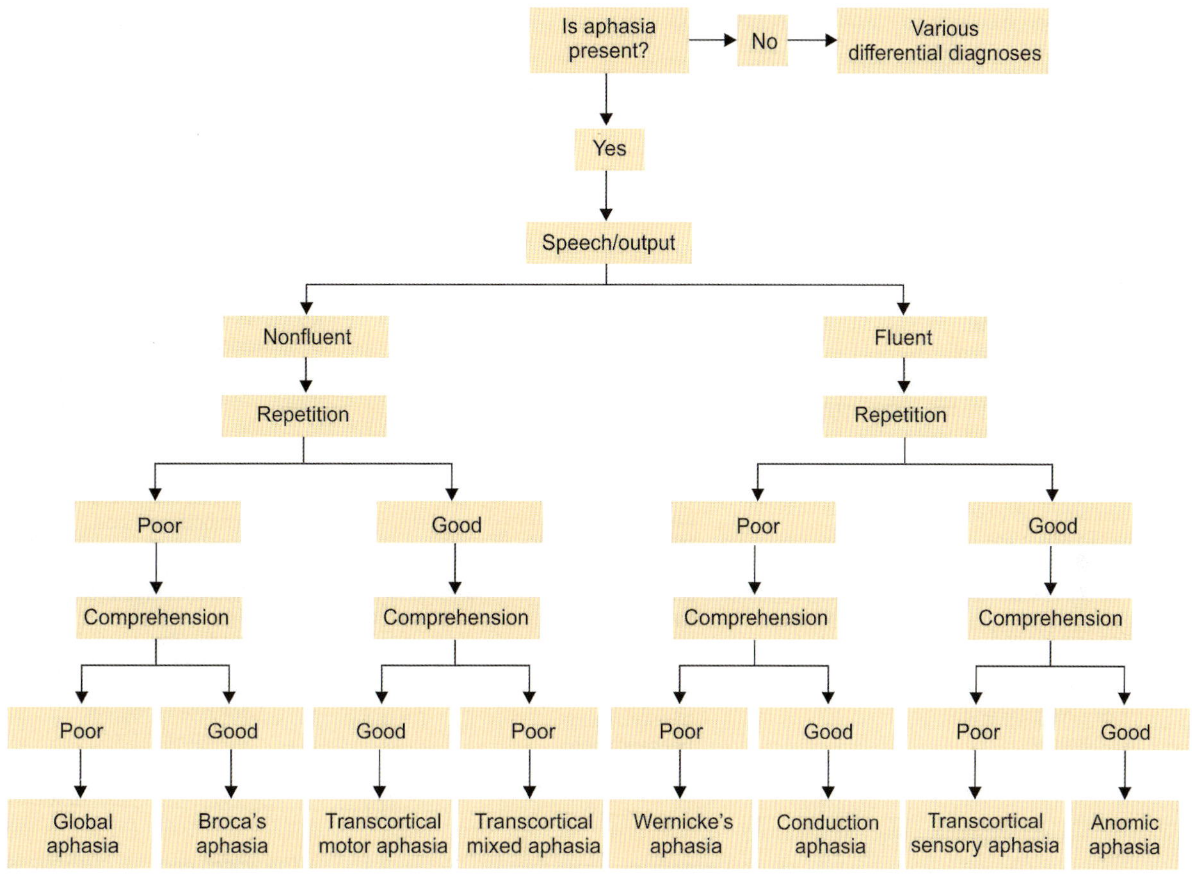

FLOWCHART 1: Algorithm: Aphasia syndrome diagnosis. Three dichotomous questions lead to the diagnosis of eight aphasia syndromes: (1) Is the speech fluent or nonfluent? (2) Is repetition good or poor? (3) Is auditory comprehension good or poor?

based. SLPs and researchers are using ingenious and experimental ways of testing the competence and performance of PWA based on the cognitive neuropsychological model of language **(Flowchart 2)**.

Aphasiologists can take a *cue* from epileptology, wherein the classification of seizures has been revised. More emphasis is on seizure semiology rather than pigeonholing subjects into a straitjacket of categories. Something like video monitoring has happened in aphasiology. Data from single patients have become the basis for cognitive neuropsychological research and therapy.[19]

DIFFERENTIAL DIAGNOSIS (TABLE 2)

It is beyond the scope of this chapter to discuss the differential diagnosis. However, it is necessary to emphasize that aphasia is a clinical diagnosis and there are no laboratory tests. The differentiation relies on a more comprehensive and repeated examination and considering the overall picture. While clinically examining a PWA, the neurologist will tailor and modify the assessment methods so as not to make errors in diagnosis.

Psychogenic syndromes (conversion or dissociative states, catatonia) can also render a person speechless for a variable period. Impaired fluency during a conversation but not during formal verbal fluency tests following a minor cerebral concussion should raise suspicion about motivation and secondary gains. The same applies if speech impairment develops many weeks or months after the event and if it keeps worsening. Another marker is the inconsistency of paraphasic errors for a particular sound. If a nearly mute person can express well in writing, it may indicate a functional disorder.

MANAGEMENT OF APHASIA

Management is a broad term encompassing many types of therapies, learning of compensatory strategies, and measures for variable degrees of rehabilitation.

The mainstay of therapy is behavioral approaches that use language-based drills. Speech-language therapy (SLT) is administered by SLPs through face-to-face interaction between a patient (PWA) and a clinician. SLP provides targeted stimulation of selected language tasks and communication skills.

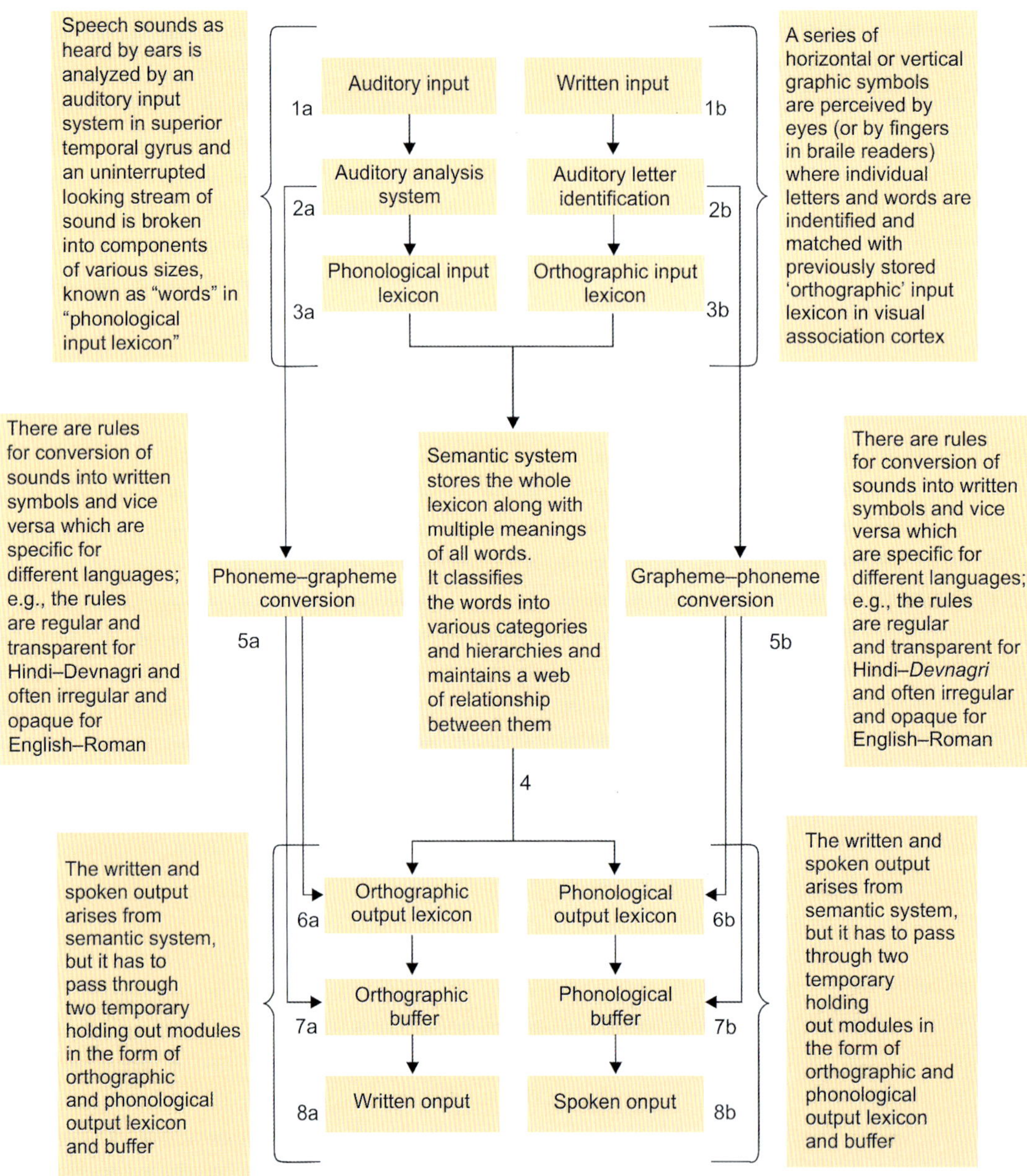

FLOWCHART 2: Cognitive neuropsychological model of language organization in the brain. A general neurologist need not memorize the model but should be aware that such frameworks lead to additional aphasia testing and profiling methods. It helps to localize the defect (not lesion on imaging) at one or more of the boxes and arrows in the model, leading to the choice of therapy.

Other means of SLT are group therapy, therapy by caregivers and trained volunteers, and computers therapy. The latter can be administered remotely also, with or without supervision of a SLP or caregiver.

Recent systemic review suggests that SLT is generally beneficial.[20] However, we do not know which treatment approach might work best for a specific patient, something akin to precision treatment.

There is an implicit assumption that SLT-assisted improvement is due to structural and functional neuroplasticity. The latter may be long lasting or short lasting. Underlying brain changes are not well understood. Neural reorganization after brain injury involves gray and white matter both. The ability of the brain to continuously adapt its structure and function based on internal and external environmental changes is the basis of neuroplasticity. The latter involves changes in neuronal morphology including glia, vascular and metabolic processes, and changes in synapse and dendrites. Ample literature is available, documenting

TABLE 2: Differential diagnosis.

Not to miss the diagnosis of aphasia when presenting a true diagnosis	
True diagnosis	*Mistaken for*
Mild aphasia	Normal variation
Receptive aphasia, mild Wernicke, pure wood deafness	Impaired hearing
Anomia	Amnesia
Alexia	Visual impairment
Jargon aphasia	Delirium psychosis
Not to make a false-positive diagnosis of aphasia when not present	
Developmental disorders of speech, learning disability	Aphasia, alexia
Developmental suppression of motor fluency, stuttering	Nonfluent aphasia
Hearing impairment, congenital deaf mutism	Receptive and global aphasia
Pure dysarthria	Nonfluent aphasia
Anarthria, mutism	Severe Broca's aphasia
Psychogenic: Mutism, hypophonia, slow speech, atypical halting	Severe Broca's or Global aphasia
Schizophrenia: Bizarre and absurd speech, flight of ideas	Jargon speech Wernicke (fluent aphasia)
Delirium, altered sensorium, muttering	Aphasia, anomia, jargon speech
Amnesia, Korsakoff syndrome	Anomia, paraphasia
Apraxia: Fails to comply with the command	Receptive aphasia

structural and functional changes in the brain parallel to aphasia recovery. Reorganization takes place in bilateral temporofrontal network, with or without therapy.[21]

Most of the recovery in speech and language function occurs in subacute stages (90 days). There is no fixed time window for recovery; it keeps improving for many more months and years spontaneously but more so with targeted intervention. Late recovery involves angiogenesis and neurogenesis. In chronic cases, it occurs due to relearning lost skills and information, retraining specific processes, and resorting to compensatory strategies, psychosocial adaptations, and environmental modifications.

THEORETICAL BASIS OF APHASIA REHABILITATION

There have been important theoretical advances in understanding the mechanism of recovery and efficacy of interventions. These advances can be described in biological as well as social models of health and illness.

Medical or Biological Model

As per biological model, the brain adapts to the imbalance between reduced resources and communication needs. Homeostatic plasticity supports the normalization of post-stroke language activity. Associative Hebbian plasticity (remember the dictum: Neurons that fire together, wire together) promotes the reconfiguration of the language network. Cognitive control processes dynamically modulate activity levels in language regions.

Postlesional neuroplasticity, or relearning, and learning in individual development as well as task learning in healthy individuals share many similarities. Creating specific learning situations repeatedly is a fundamental principle of neurorehabilitation, which aims to support neural plasticity mechanisms in stroke recovery.

Theoretical distinctions between medical approaches to therapy and rehabilitation relate not only to brain organization but often implies contrasting ideas about the nature of language processing itself.

In general, localizationist approaches focus on the structural aspects of language and its level of organization, such as phonology, lexicon, and syntax. It suggests that language is independent of other cognitive functions in terms of both processing and of neural representation.

On the other hand, the holistic approach emphasizes the unitary nature of language as a tool of communication, its relationship with other aspects of cognition, and the distributed nature of its neural substrate.

Social Model

The Social Model of health and illness, in the context of speech and communication, is exemplified by the WHO–ICF Framework[22] which focuses on real-world communication in aphasia rehabilitation. The aim of this framework is to improve every individual's ability to function in their day-to-day life. It defines language as (1) interactive, (2) multimodal, and (3) contextual.

Basically, it expands the medical model by adding treatment goal from social viewpoint and understanding the effects of physical and psychological deficits on social domains such as daily functioning, social communication, and employment capacity. Higher social goals can be achieved by leveraging compensatory strategies and interdisciplinary goal setting, even in cases where the direct restoration of some somatic functions is not possible **(Flowchart 3)**.

Aphasia intervention in acute stage is more difficult due to highly unstable clinical states and lack of awareness among team professionals and family members.

Presently, protocol related to early intervention during 2–7 days as a part of first-stage rehabilitative process has been established. This should target the preparedness

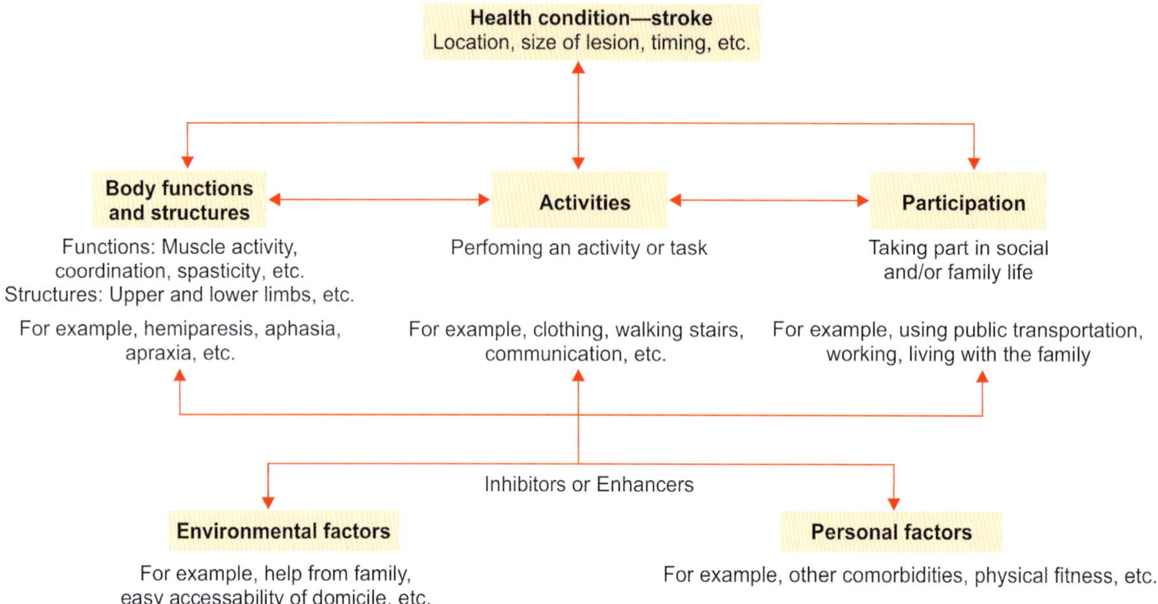

FLOWCHART 3: The International Classification of Functioning, Disability, and Health (ICF) proposed by the World Health Organization (WHO) in 2001.

of family members about upcoming issues they are going to face post discharge. Along with discussion about Supportive Communication Strategies (SCS), family members should also be guided for facilitating communication environment and to understand the different kind of burden they are going to face. This period would help to use spontaneous recovery period and neural plasticity effectively.

During the first 2–3 months, language improvement can occur in response to behavioral training and it continues in the chronic phase also.

A crucial predictor for positive language outcomes is to provide an Intensive Comprehensive Aphasia Program (ICAP) of language training lasting several hours per week (5–10) or Intensive Language Action Therapy (ILAT) of 3 hours/day for 10 days.[23]

Unfortunately, most of the PWA cannot receive the recommended amount of training estimated due to unawareness, lack of conviction, tiredness and fatigue, lack of patience for results of speech therapy, limited economic resources, lack of infrastructure, resources or services, and most sadly, the missing anguish, felt need and demand in the minds of stakeholders. As a consequence, aphasia therapies are often incomplete and inefficacious.

Additional rehabilitation techniques are desperately needed. Unconventional methods that improve overall learning (e.g., number of correct responses) or accelerate learning (e.g., vocal reaction times) have been proposed as ways to increase treatment effectiveness. There may be some role of biological interventions such as transcranial direct current stimulation (tDCS), virtual reality (VR), and pharmaceuticals.

APPROACHES TO THERAPY AND REHABILITATION

Approaches to therapy and rehabilitation may be grouped into two broad categories:

1. Impairment-based therapies which refer to one of the many "cognitive neuropsychological models of language" **(Flowchart 2)**
2. Life participation approaches emphasize overall functional communication in daily life.[24] The two approaches are not mutually exclusive or contradictory; in fact, they are complimentary to each other. A detailed description of various therapy methods is beyond the scope of this chapter.

PHARMACOTHERAPY

Many medicines have been studied in treatment of aphasia. The results have not been very impressive till now, but prospects are improving. Pharmacological augmentation of speech therapy may be more robust and reliable with stimulants, cholinesterase inhibitors, dopamine agonists, and other medications. Memantine enhanced experience-dependent neural plasticity, elicited by intensive constraint-induced aphasia therapy (CIAT).[25]

On the other hand, long-term use of a few drugs may have deleterious effect on aphasia recovery. These should be avoided or used in lower doses with caution—anxiolytics (benzodiazepines), antihypertensives (clonidine, labetalol, and prazosin), antipsychotics (haloperidol and phenothiazines), antimotility (metoclopramide), and anticonvulsant (phenobarbitone, phenytoin, and topiramate).

NONINVASIVE BRAIN STIMULATION

Noninvasive brain stimulation (NIBS) through repetitive transcranial magnetic stimulation (rTMS) and tDCS have been employed in chronic aphasia either to suppress the maladaptive and inhibitory right hemisphere activity or to stimulate compensatory left hemispheric perilesion areas. rTMS generates focal magnetic pulses, which can penetrate the skull and induce weak electrical currents that depolarize or hyperpolarize neuronal membranes. tDCS are weak and do not induce action potentials but have neuromodulatory effect. Anodal currents are excitatory and cathodal are inhibitory. tDCS is less expensive and more acceptable.

A recent meta-analysis reviewed effect of low-frequency rTMS and cathodal tDCS over the nonlesioned right hemisphere (with sham controls) and found a significant mean effect size for accuracy of naming.[26]

PSYCHOSOCIAL ISSUES

The psychosocial approach for chronic survivors as PWA looks at disability and barriers in community and outcomes such as autonomy, reintegration, empowerment, and self-help. Main aims of social approaches are: (1) To increase successful participation in authentic communication events; (2) to focus on communication at the level of conversation; (3) to provide communicative support systems within the speaker's own community; and (4) to increase communicative confidence and empower speakers with aphasia.

ROLE OF CAREGIVERS

Family members or caregivers or "significant others" bear a great burden in supporting PWA on a long-term basis. It may sometimes be considered alright and mutually satisfying, particularly in cultures (like in India) where family values are held high. However, it is also true that quite often caregiver burden may be unbearable. A few studies have documented changes in social relationship, emotional status, exhaustion, burn out, and need for support and respite for caregivers of PWA. Aphasia QOL studies should include caregivers and report separately on them.

GOAL SETTING FOR THERAPY AND REHABILITATION

Physician and SLP in collaboration with PWA and caregivers should set meaningful, relevant, specific, and challenging but achievable short-term and long-term goals for aphasia therapy and rehabilitation. Focus should be on activity and participation. The goals should be recorded, reviewed, and updated regularly.

GROUP THERAPY

Group therapy sessions can be useful in two manners: (1) Patients with nearly similar profile are offered targeted specific practice sessions and (2) heterogeneous groups are offered general purpose learning and practice opportunities (pragmatics based) to improve the overall communication skills.

Family members, caregivers, and volunteers with short-term training can act as bridge between professionals and PWA by supervising and facilitating home-based practices and exercises.

The internist and for that matter any health worker caring for a patient with aphasia should be more.

AWARENESS AND ADVOCACY

Public awareness about aphasia is crucial for any effort in the direction of its advocacy.[27] Clinicians caring for PWA should be knowledgeable about and interested in the subject. They should be convinced that speech therapy works and rehabilitation can be improved by it and other simple advices. Physicians should play some role of therapists. With increasing awareness about efficacy of physical therapy and occupation therapy for motor deficits in conditions such as hemiplegia or paraplegia, more and more physicians have developed interest and expertise in rehabilitation and restoration. They take pride in their specialization. They do not look down upon this type of work as something lowly and to be done only by physiotherapists. Similar change in the mindset is warranted with respect to aphasia.

ACCEPTANCE AND ASSISTIVE-AUGMENTATIVE DEVICES

When therapy and rehabilitation reach their limits, the clinicians become counselors about acceptance, coping, and optimum use of augmentative and assistive devices.[28] The future, however, looks bright with strides in neurobiology and better leveraging of social factors through advocacy, awareness, and life participation approach.

CONCLUSION

An expert group meeting on aphasia was organized by the present author on behalf of the Indian Academy of Neurology.[29] SLPs,clinical neuropsychologists, linguists, and imaging and computer professionals participated along with neurologists. It was realized that assessment or testing of aphasia and its management in India needs much improvement and joint efforts. There are no shortcuts. It needs time, patience, experience, and commitment from neurologists and colleagues. Practice helps. Repeated drills enhance the quality of testing in lesser time. The PWA and SOs deserve a lot more from neurologists. We must not fail them.

REFERENCES

1. Engelter ST, Gostynski M, Papa S, Frei M, Born C, Ajdacic-Gross V, et al. Epidemiology of aphasia attributable to first ischemic stroke: Incidence, severity, fluency, etiology, and thrombolysis. Stroke. 2006;37:1379-84.
2. Kaur H, Bajpai S, Pershad D, Sreenivas V, Nehra A. Development and standardization of Indian aphasia battery. J Mental Health Hum Behav. 2017;2(2):116-22.
3. Neurocognition. Aphasia (paralysis of speech). [online] Available from https://neurogyan.com/aphasia [Last accessed July, 2024].
4. Enderby P, Crow E. Frenchay Aphasia Screening Test: Validity and comparability. Disabil Rehabil. 1996;18:238-40.
5. Paplikar A, Iyer GK, Varghese F, Alladi S, Pauranik A, Mekala S, et al. A screening tool to detect stroke aphasia: Adaptation of Frenchay aphasia screening test (FAST) to the Indian context. Ann Indian Acad Neurol. 2020;23(Suppl 2):S143.
6. Privitera AJ, Ng SH, Kong AP, Weekes BS. AI and Aphasia in the Digital Age: A Critical Review. Brain Sciences. 2024;14(4):383.
7. Marian V, Blumenfeld HK, Kaushanskaya M. The Language Experience and Proficiency Questionnaire (LEAP-Q): Assessing language profiles in bilinguals and multi-linguals. J Speech Lang Hear Res. 2007;50(4):940-67.
8. Bryden MP, Steenhuis RE. Issues in the assessment of handedness. Cerebral Laterality. London: Psychology Press; 2013. pp. 35-51.
9. Stahl B, Mohr B, Dreyer FR, Lucchese G, Pulvermüller F. Communicativepragmatic assessment is sensitive and timeeffective in measuring the outcome of aphasia therapy. Front Hum Neurosci. 2017;11:223.
10. Hillari K, Byng S, Lamping DL, Smith SC. Stroke and Aphasia Quality of life Scale – 39 (SAQOL-39): Evaluation of Acceptability, Reliability and validity. Stroke. 2003;34:1994-50.
11. Hersh D, Worrall L, Howe T, Sherratt S, Davidson B. SMARTER goal setting in aphasia rehabilitation. Aphasiology. 2012;26: 220-33.
12. Mitra IH, Krishnan G. Adaptation and validation of stroke-aphasia quality of life (SAQOL-39) scale to Hindi. Ann Indian Acad Neurol. 2015;18(1):29.
13. Rombough RE, Howse EL, Bartfay WJ. Caregiver strain and caregiver burden of primary caregivers of stroke survivors with and without aphasia. Rehabil Nurs. 2006;31(5):199-209.
14. Singh P, Pauranik A. Supportive conversational strategies for persons with aphasia and their significant others. J Indian Speech Lang Hear Assoc. 2017;31:57.
15. Ackerman D. One Hundred Names for Love: A Stroke, a Marriage, and the Language of Healing. New York: Norton; 2011.
16. Fonseca J, Raposo A, Martins IP. Cognitive functioning in chronic post-stroke Aphasia. Appl Neuropsychol Adult. 2019;26(4): 355-64.
17. Weintraub S, Dikmen SS, Heaton RK, Tulsky DS, Zelazo PD, Bauer PJ, et al. Cognition assessment using the NIH Toolbox. Neurology. 2013;80:S54-64.
18. Kasselimis DS, Simos PG, Peppas C, Evdokimidis I, Potagas C. The unbridged gap between clinical diagnosis and contemporary research on Aphasia: A short discussion on the validity and clinical utility of taxonomic categories. Brain Lang. 2017;164:63-7.
19. Whitworth A, Webster J, Howard D. A Cognitive Neuro-psychological Approach to Assessment and Intervention in Aphasia: A Clinician's Guide. London: Psychology Press; 2005.
20. Burton B, Isaacs M, Brogan E, Shrubsole K, Kilkenny MF, Power E, et al. An updated systematic review of stroke clinical practice guidelines to inform aphasia management. Int J Stroke. 2023;18(9):1029-39.
21. Hickok G, Small SL (Eds). Neurobiology of Language. London: Academic Press; 2015.
22. Dantas AC, Torres GD, Corrêa CD, Pinto FC, Cera M. Categories of the International Classification of Functioning, Disability and Health in studies of people with aphasia: a scoping review. Revista CEFAC. 2022;24:e6921.
23. Singh P. Intensive Language Action Therapy for Persons with Aphasia (PWA). PhD [thesis unpublished]. Madhya Pradesh, India: Devi Ahilya University; 2017.
24. Connor LT, Ashaie S, Nicholas M. Factors contributing to life participation in people with aphasia: Current knowledge and future directions. In: Goral M, Lerman A (Eds). Advances in the Neurolinguistic Study of Multilingual and Monolingual Adults. UK: Taylor & Francis Group; 2023. pp. 156-69.
25. Berthier ML, Dávila G. Pharmacotherapy for post-stroke aphasia: what are the options? Expert Opin Pharmacother. 2023; 24(11):1221-8.
26. Kidwai J, Sharma S, Peper M, Brumberg J. Investigating NIBS for language rehabilitation in aphasia. Aphasiology. 2023; 37(8):1285-314.
27. Bennington C, Shiggins C, Isaksen J, Beesley E, Beesley K, Wallace SJ. What does it mean to be aphasia aware? An international survey of stakeholder perspectives and experiences of aphasia awareness. UK: Taylor & Francis Group; 2024. pp. 1-24.
28. Dietz A, Wallace SE, Weissling K. Revisiting the role of augmentative and alternative communication in aphasia rehabilitation. Am J Speech Lang Pathol. 2020;29(2):909-13.
29. Pauranik A, Singh P, Sahu A, Nehra A, Paplikar A, Bhat C, et al. Expert Group Meeting on Aphasia: A Report. Ann Indian Acad Neurol. 2019;22(2):137-46.

CHAPTER

12 Rapidly Progressive Dementia

Ganaraja VH, Faheem Arshad, Subasree Ramakrishnan

ABSTRACT

In recent years, the recognition of rapidly progressive dementia (RPD) has garnered increased attention within the medical community as clinicians encounter cases where cognitive decline progresses at an accelerated pace, sometimes over a matter of weeks or months. These diseases have diverse etiologies that require comprehensive diagnostic approaches. These are classified as *P*rions disease, *D*egenerative dementias, *E*ndocrinal abnormalities, *M*alignancy-related, *E*pilepsy, *N*utritional causes, *T*oxin and *M*etabolic causes, *I*nfections, *A*utoimmune diseases, and *S*troke/Vascular causes (Mnemonic *P*rogressive *DEMENTIAS*). Prion diseases were initially considered to be the prototype of RPD; however, recently, with the advent of various antibodies, the autoimmune encephalitis spectrum is increasingly being recognized as one of the potentially treatable forms of RPD. While approaching a case of RPD, it is important to have a systematic and multidisciplinary approach to ensure timely diagnosis and appropriate management. Recently, a scoring system has been developed for the early recognition of RPD, mainly to detect treatable causes of RPD. Overall, early recognition of the underlying cause can lead to timely interventions that may help slow the progression of the disease or improve symptoms.

Keywords: Progressive dementia, Autoimmune, Prion, Neuroinfections, Paraneoplastic.

INTRODUCTION

Dementia is a condition characterized by progressive cognitive decline and poses immense challenges for individuals, families, and healthcare systems worldwide.[1] While dementia often manifests as a gradual deterioration of cognitive function over time, there exists a subset of cases where the decline is alarmingly swift, leaving patients and caregivers grappling with the rapid onslaught of symptoms. This phenomenon, known as rapidly progressive dementia (RPD), presents a unique and urgent clinical conundrum, necessitating a deeper exploration of its causes, clinical manifestations, and management strategies.[1] There is no clear definition regarding the same. However, when dementia occurs in less than 1–2 years from the onset of illness, it is considered as RPD.[1] Commonly, these RPDs have symptoms duration from weeks to months for the development of dementia.[2]

Unlike the more common forms of dementia, such as Alzheimer's disease (AD), where the decline unfolds gradually, RPD presents a formidable clinical challenge due to its rapid trajectory and often ominous prognosis.[3] Prion diseases were initially considered to be the prototype of RPD; however, recently, with the advent of various antibodies, autoimmune encephalitis spectrum is increasingly being recognized as one of the potentially treatable forms of RPD and one of the common causes of RPD in Europe and North American region.[4] However, neuroinfections remain the common etiology of RPD in developing countries like India and Brazil, which is also one of the major concerns from a public health point of view.[5,6]

Owing to the heterogeneous etiology and varied presentations, it is difficult to estimate the exact incidence of RPD. In a study from China, etiological epidemiology revealed infectious, neurodegenerative, and toxic/

metabolic diseases as the three largest groups, accounting for 26.2%, 20.8%, and 16.8% of all cases, respectively.[7] In another study from Greece, neurodegenerative diseases were the most frequent causes (38%), followed by prion disease (19%) and autoimmune encephalopathy (17%).[8]

In India, in a study done in Chandigarh, it was observed that infections were the common cause (39%) among 187 patients of RPD, mainly subacute sclerosing panencephalitis (SSPE), neurosyphilis, and progressive multifocal leukoencephalopathy.[6] However, it is always challenging to make an accurate and quick diagnosis in RPD, especially when the history is too short and disease progression is very fast.

CAUSES AND PATHOPHYSIOLOGY

In general, RPDs can be categorized into:

- *Primary* as in prion diseases and other typical neurodegenerative dementias, which cause significant neuronal damage
- *Secondary*, which are due to complications of underlying illness as observed in refractory epilepsy, nutritional deficiencies, etc.[4]

There is an exhaustive list of causes for RPD. However, common causes of RPD based on the underlying pathomechanism are classified as *P*rion diseases, *D*egenerative dementias, *E*ndocrinal abnormalities, *M*alignancy related, *E*pilepsy, *N*utritional causes, *T*oxin and *M*etabolic causes, *I*nfections, *A*utoimmune diseases, *S*troke/*V*ascular causes (Mnemonic *Progressive DEMENTIAS*). These are listed in **Table 1**. Knowledge of these RPDs is essential for early and accurate diagnosis for prompt treatment.

Subtypes

Prion Diseases

Prion diseases, also known as transmissible spongiform encephalopathies (TSEs), are a group of rare and fatal neurodegenerative disorders caused by abnormally folded proteins called prions.[9] This remains a challenging area of study due to its complex pathogenesis and devastating clinical course. These diseases are characterized by the progressive accumulation of misfolded proteins in the brain, leading to neuronal damage, spongiform changes in brain tissue, and, ultimately, severe neurological dysfunction. Creutzfeldt-Jakob disease (CJD) can occur in several forms, including sporadic, genetic (familial), and acquired (variant and iatrogenic) forms. Other prion diseases in humans include Gerstmann-Sträussler-Scheinker syndrome (GSS) and fatal familial insomnia (FFI). Sporadic CJD is the most common human prion disease arising either due to somatic mutation in PRNP protein or structural change in prion protein.[9]

Prion diseases can be transmitted through contaminated food products (as seen in variant CJD, which is linked to the consumption of beef products contaminated with bovine spongiform encephalopathy or "mad cow disease"), medical procedures (iatrogenic CJD), or genetic inheritance (familial forms). Prion diseases typically present with RPD, along with a variety of neurological symptoms such as ataxia, myoclonus, visual disturbances, and behavioral changes. The course of the disease is relentlessly progressive, and patients usually succumb to the illness within months to a few years of symptom onset.[9]

TABLE 1: Etiologies of rapidly progressive dementia (Progressive DEMENTIAS).

Types		Etiology
Prions		
Degenerative		Alzheimer's disease
		Dementia with Lewy body
		Frontotemporal dementia
		Corticobasal degeneration
		Progressive supranuclear palsy
Endocrine abnormality		Hypo and hyperthyroidism
		Hyperparathyroidism
Malignancy	Primary	Gliomatosis cerebri
		Primary central nervous system (CNS) lymphoma
	Metastatic	Metastatic encephalopathy
		Carcinomatous meningitis
	Paraneoplastic neurological syndromes	Anti-Hu, Anti-Yo, Anti-CV2, etc.

Continued

Continued

Types		Etiology
Epilepsy-related		Status epilepsy
		Symptomatic epilepsy
Nutritional		Thiamine deficiency
		Vitamin B12 deficiency
Toxins and metabolic	Heavy metals toxicity	Mercury
		Aluminum
		Lead
		Arsenic
	Drug toxicity	Methotrexate
		Lithium
	Inherited metabolic disorders	Leukodystrophies
		Mitochondriopathy
		Wilson's disease
	Organ dysfunction	Hepatic encephalopathy
		Uremic encephalopathy
	Electrolyte disturbances	Hyponatremia
		Extrapontine myelinolysis
Infections	Bacterial	CNS tuberculosis
		Neurosyphilis
		Whipple's disease
	Viral	Herpes encephalitis
		Human immunodeficiency virus (HIV) dementia
		Progressive multifocal leukoencephalopathy
		Subacute sclerosing panencephalitis
	Fungal	CNS aspergillosis
	Parasitic	Neurocysticercosis
	Others	Septic encephalopathy
Autoimmune	Immune-mediated encephalitis	N-methyl-D-aspartate (NMDA), leucine-rich glioma-inactivated (LGI) antibody-mediated encephalitis, etc.
	Primary CNS demyelination	Multiple sclerosis
		Neuromyelitis optica spectrum disorder
		Acute disseminated encephalomyelitis
	Secondary CNS demyelination	CNS lupus
		Sarcoidosis
Strokes and vascular	Ischemic strokes	CNS vasculitis
		Multi infarct state
		Cerebral amyloid angiopathy
	Hemorrhagic strokes	Hypertensive hemorrhages
	Venous strokes	Venous thrombosis
	Arteriovenous (AV) malformations	Dural AV fistula
	Impaired autoregulation	Posterior reversible encephalopathy syndrome (PRES)

Note: Progressive DEMENTIAS: *P*rions, *D*rugs, *E*ndocrine abnormalities, *M*alignancy, *E*lectrolytes imbalances, *N*utritional, *T*oxins and metabolic, *I*nfections, *A*utoimmune, *S*trokes.

Various phenotypes of sporadic CJD (sCJD) have been linked at the molecular level with two distinct PrP^{Sc} protein genotypes (type 1 and type 2) and the methionine (M)/valine (V) polymorphism at *PRNP* codon 129, resulting in six main disease subtypes.[10] The commonest subtype is MM1/MV1 and is considered a classical form, and it constitutes about 65% of sCJD cases. This phenotype has very rapid disease progression and often leads to death by 4 months from symptom onset. The second common molecular subtype is VV2, which constitutes about 15–20% of sCJD cases and is characterized by early cerebellar symptoms. MV2 subtype is considered to have diverse clinical presentation, hence, definite diagnosis can be often delayed. VV1 and MM2 are uncommon subtypes with slower disease progression.[11]

Arbitrarily, it is divided into multiple stages. In early stages, often symptoms start with features of anxiety, depression, and dizziness, not impairing activities of daily living with subtle neurological signs. Later, it is characterized by impairment of higher cortical functions with impairment of activities of daily living. It further progresses with typical features of dementia and myoclonus. The late stage is characterized by reduced movement, and the terminal stage with akinetic mutism leading to death. It is also correlated with brain magnetic resonance imaging (MRI), electroencephalography (EEG), and fluid biomarkers for further characterization.[12]

The diagnosis of prion diseases is challenging and often requires a combination of clinical evaluation, neuroimaging (MRI), EEG, and cerebrospinal fluid analysis (for 14-3-3 protein and tau protein). Common findings in MRI are cortical ribboning in diffusion-weighted imaging (DWI) sequence of MRI **(Fig. 1)**. Variant CJD can show a hockey-stick sign and pulvinar sign characterized by increased signal intensity in the pulvinar thalamus and dorsomedial thalamus. Another technique for diagnosis of CJD is real-time quaking-induced conversion (RT-QuIC).[13] This technique allows the amplification and detection of PrP^{Sc} from the cerebrospinal fluid (CSF). This has high sensitivity and specificity for diagnosis of CJD and is also used as a part of clinical diagnostic criteria.[14] However, the definitive diagnosis is usually confirmed by postmortem through neuropathological examination of brain tissue. Tonsillar biopsy is also an important tool for the diagnosis of

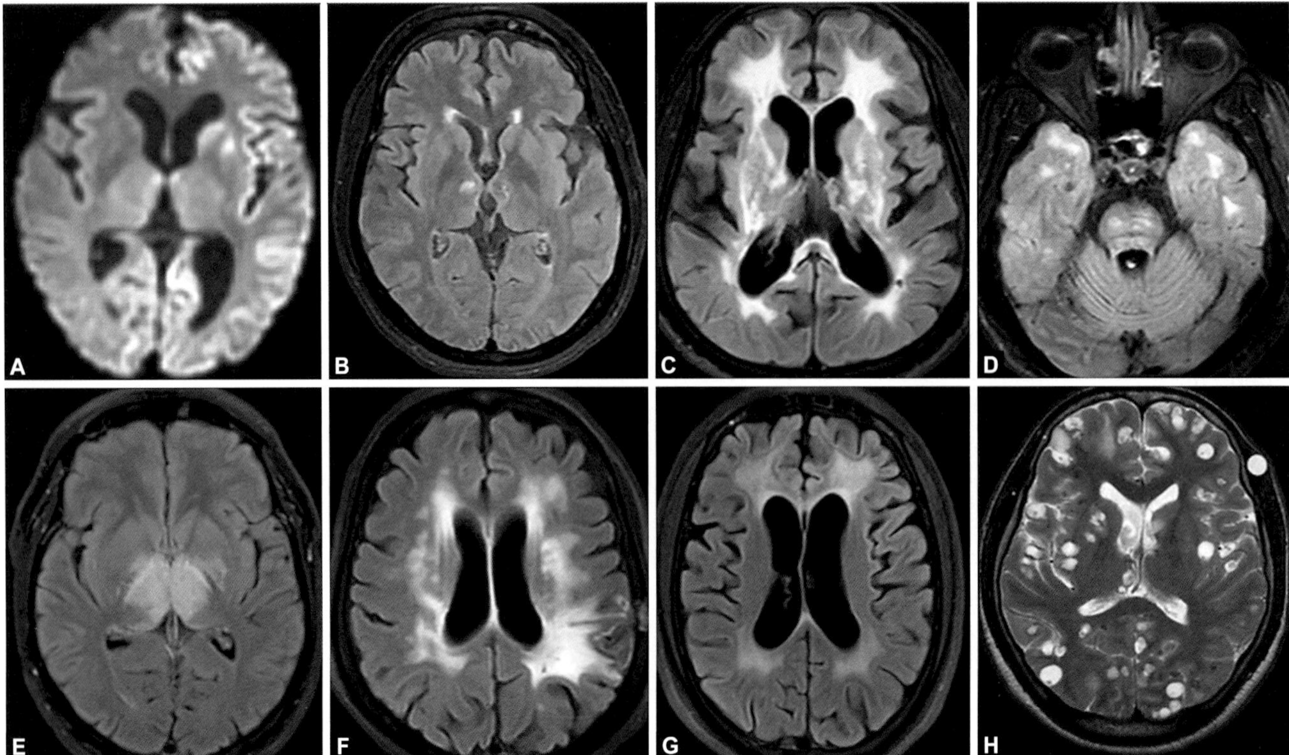

FIGS. 1A TO H: Brain MRI diffusion sequence showing gyriform diffusion brightness involving the left cerebral hemisphere and caudate and putamen in a case of CJD (A); FLAIR axial sequences showing chronic infarct with gliotic changes in bilateral thalami (B); White matter, external capsule, and anterior temporal lobe involvement in CARASIL (C and D); Hyperintensity and bilateral bulky thalamus in thalamic glioma (E); Extensive periventricular white matter changes in non-Hodgkin's lymphoma (F); Periventricular hyperintensity with diffuse cerebral atrophy in HIV encephalopathy and (G); T2 axial sequence showing multiple cystic lesions with eccentric scolex of neurocysticercosis (H).

(CJD: Creutzfeldt–Jakob disease; CARASIL: cerebral autosomal-recessive arteriopathy with subcortical infarcts and leukoencephalopathy; FLAIR: fluid-attenuated inversion recovery.; HIV: human immunodeficiency virus; MRI: magnetic resonance imaging)

variant CJD. Currently, research is focused on understanding the mechanisms of prion replication and spread, developing diagnostic tools, and exploring potential therapeutic strategies to combat these devastating diseases.

Degenerative Dementias

Degenerative dementias like AD progresses slowly, however can also progress rapidly in few cases. Rapidly progressive Alzheimer's disease (RPAD) is a rare and aggressive form of AD characterized by an unusually fast decline in cognitive function and other symptoms associated with AD.[15] It shares many pathological features with typical AD, including the accumulation of beta-amyloid plaques and tau protein tangles in the brain.[16] Though the underlying mechanisms driving the rapid progression of symptoms in RPAD are not fully understood, RPAD is shown to have higher prevalence of amyloid angiopathy.[17]

Other degenerative dementia subtypes, also found to have rapid disease progression, are due to multiple mechanisms, like in addition to underlying disease pathology in diffuse Lewy body dementia (DLBD), factors like innate immune system, genetic factors and lifestyle modifications can have an impact on disease progression and survival.[18] Corticobasal syndrome (CBS) is one of close mimicker of prion disease, as they also present with cognitive decline, pyramidal/extrapyramidal features with myoclonus. Frontotemporal dementia (FTD) with significant behavioral disturbances should also be considered in the differential diagnosis of prion disease. The presence of comorbidities such as cerebrovascular diseases, diabetes, and associated infections can accelerate cognitive decline.

Endocrine Abnormalities

Endocrine abnormalities can sometimes contribute to or be associated with progressive dementia. Hypothyroidism is one of the common endocrinal abnormalities leading to cognitive impairment. Other features include fatigue, weight gain, and depression which can progress if left untreated.[19] Diabetes mellitus, especially when poorly controlled, can lead to various complications, including cognitive impairment. Chronic high blood sugar levels can damage blood vessels and nerves, affecting brain function over time. Hypoparathyroidism, leading to low calcium levels in the blood, is also known for cognitive impairment if untreated.

Malignancy Related

The relationship between malignancy and RPD is complex and multifaceted. These tumors can be primary or metastatic. These lesions can affect cortical structures through mass effect, infiltration, altered CSF circulation, and associated edema.[20]

Primary central nervous system lymphoma (PCNSL), which is a type of non-Hodgkin lymphoma, can cause rapidly progressive cognitive decline, headaches, and neurological deficits.[21] Intravascular lymphoma is another type of central nervous system (CNS) malignancy, often presents with stroke-like and systemic symptoms and dementia features. Often tissue/brain biopsy is needed for confirmation of diagnosis.[22] Meningioma, though typically slow-growing, in some cases, can grow rapidly and compress brain tissue leading to cognitive decline and neurological symptoms.

Paraneoplastic neurological syndromes (PNS): Some cancers can trigger immune-mediated neurological disorders known as paraneoplastic syndromes. These syndromes occur when the body's immune system mistakenly attacks healthy brain tissue in response to cancer. Recently, with a newer classification of PNS, antibodies are classified as high-risk (>70% associated with cancer), intermediate-risk (30–70% associated with cancer), and lower-risk antibodies (<30% associated with cancer), based on the strength of association with cancers. Based on clinical phenotype, type of antibody detected, and presence/absence of cancers, PNS care score is used to classify PNS.[23] Overall, these PNS should be considered when there is subacute onset of ataxic, extrapyramidal syndromes with cognitive decline. If CSF shows inflammatory markers and if there is a family history of cancer, one should evaluate for PNS.[23]

Epilepsy

Epilepsy, sometimes, can be a challenging condition to manage and can have various effects on cognitive function, depending on factors such as the frequency and severity of seizures, the underlying cause of epilepsy, and the effects of medications.[24] Progressive cognitive decline in the context of refractory epilepsy can be due to several factors, like seizure activity per se, which can affect cognitive function, especially if they are frequent or severe. Prolonged or repetitive seizures can lead to neuronal damage and cognitive impairment. The underlying cause of epilepsy can also contribute to cognitive decline. In addition, some antiseizure medications can have cognitive side effects, especially at higher doses or when used in combination with other medications.[24]

Nutritional Causes

Nutritional deficiencies can contribute to progressive cognitive decline, especially when they occur over a prolonged period. Following are some key nutritional factors that can affect cognitive function:

- Thiamine deficiency is one of the common causes of cognitive decline in patients with chronic alcoholism, nutritional deficiency, and malabsorption syndromes. They present with features of subacute onset dementia with ophthalmoparesis and ataxia. Though all features may not be present, thiamine deficiency/ Wernicke encephalopathy should be considered in patients with RPD with a background of chronic alcoholism. If this is not treated early, patients can have persistent memory disturbances, which can lead to Korsakoff syndrome and may not be completely reversible.[25]
- Vitamin B12 is crucial for neurological function, and deficiency can lead to cognitive decline, memory problems, and even dementia. It is more common in older adults and vegetarians/vegans who do not supplement or consume fortified foods. Besides B12, other B vitamins like folate (B9), B6, and riboflavin (B2) are important for brain health.[26]

Toxins and Metabolic Causes

Toxins can, indeed, lead to rapidly progressive cognitive decline, depending on the type and extent of exposure. Some toxins act on the nervous system directly, while others may cause systemic effects that indirectly affect cognitive function. These etiologies should always be considered, especially in patients taking over-the-counter medicines, herbals, and energy supplements presenting with features of RPD.

Exposure to lead, often through contaminated water, paint, or certain occupations, can lead to cognitive decline, particularly in children. Exposure from mercury—both organic (e.g., methylmercury from contaminated fish) and inorganic—can lead to cognitive impairment, particularly affecting memory, attention, and language.[27] Chronic alcoholism is one of the important causes of RPD. It can be due to direct ethanol effect, associated nutritional/thiamine deficiency, or could be due to seizures secondary to alcoholism.[26]

Drug toxicity can indeed lead to cognitive decline, either through direct effects on the brain or as a side effect of systemic toxicity. Certain medications, particularly when used inappropriately or in high doses, can impair cognitive function. Some chemotherapy drugs, such as methotrexate, mood stabilizer—lithium if used in very high doses, can present with features of RPD. These effects may include difficulties with memory, attention, and processing speed.[28] Statins have been associated with cognitive side effects in some individuals, including memory loss and confusion. Drugs with anticholinergic properties, such as certain antihistamines, antidepressants, and antipsychotics, can cause cognitive impairment, especially in older adults.[28]

Mitochondriopathy, mainly MELAS (mitochondrial encephalopathy, lactic acidosis, strokes, and leukoencephalopathy), can present as RPD. These can be identified with some clues like family history, maternal inheritance, and other characteristic neurological and non-neurological clinical features. However, one may not get all clinical features of mitochondriopathy in all patients and single disease can also have varied manifestations. Organ dysfunction, like hepatic encephalopathy, also can lead to varied neuropsychiatric symptoms due to cerebral edema or due to imbalance between excitatory and inhibitory neurotransmitters

Infections

With significant geographical variability and prevalence of these infections, it is also important to identify these infectious conditions precisely, as many are treatable, and early recognition and treatment are associated with better long-term outcomes.

Japanese encephalitis and other arboviral infections-mediated encephalitis are more prevalent in the Indian subcontinent. West Nile virus is one of the most important causes of epidemic viral encephalitis in North America.[29] Recently, cognitive decline as coronavirus disease 2019 (COVID-19) infection-related delayed complications are also observed, due to delayed immune-mediated processes.[30] SSPE is an important cause of RPD in countries with low rates of measles vaccination. In India also, it is still one of the important causes of RPD. Herpes simplex virus (HSV) encephalitis is an important cause of RPD in European and North American countries.

Human immunodeficiency virus (HIV) can lead to various neurological complications including HIV-associated neurocognitive disorder (HAND). In some cases, these conditions can progress rapidly. It can also develop during HIV seroconversion and immune reconstitution.[31] In addition to direct effect of HIV, associated opportunistic infections by tuberculosis, toxoplasma, and cryptococcal infections also lead to considerable cognitive decline.[32] Neurosyphilis is also one of the important causes of cognitive decline, however, is less prevalent in recent times with availability of appropriate treatment, which prevents complications associated with primary syphilis.[33]

Whipple's disease is another condition that has a rapid course. Though it is relatively uncommon in the Indian subcontinent, one needs a high degree of suspicion to diagnose this entity. They often present with dementia, oculo-facio-skeletal myorhythmia, new psychiatric symptoms, supranuclear gaze palsy, and gastrointestinal symptoms.

Immune-mediated Etiology

Antibody-mediated encephalitis and dementia constitute a group of inflammatory brain diseases that are characterized by prominent neuropsychiatric symptoms and are associated with antibodies against neuronal cell-surface proteins, ion channels, or receptors.[34] With the increase in awareness about this new neurological entity and more availability of centers for antibody testing, recently a greater number of cases of immune-mediated RPD are being identified.

The immune encephalitis antibodies are categorized into three groups:

- *Intracellular paraneoplastic antibodies*: These are frequently associated with systemic tumors (in >90% of cases), mainly small cell lung cancers and gynecological malignancies. These patients are less responsive to immunotherapy because the antibody causes neuronal damages. These often present as PNS.
- *Cell-surface or synaptic antibodies*: These are infrequently associated with systemic tumors, e.g., N-methyl-D-aspartate (NMDA) receptor or leucine-rich glioma-inactivated 1 (LGI1) antibodies. Patients with these antibodies are more responsive to immunotherapy.
- *Antibody of unclear significance*: The classical example of encephalitis with antibodies of unclear significance is Hashimoto's encephalitis (HE), which is positive for the thyroid peroxidase antibodies, although this antibody is not directly pathogenic.

N-methyl-D-aspartate receptor-limbic encephalitis is one of the common subtypes of autoimmune encephalitis characterized by inflammation of the limbic system in the brain, primarily affecting structures involved in memory, emotion, and behavior regulation. Progressive cognitive decline is a hallmark feature of this condition, typically evolving over weeks to months.

Feature of progressive cognitive decline in this type of encephalitis is mainly memory impairment—often with loss of short-term memory. Executive dysfunction, including difficulties with planning, problem-solving, organization, and decision-making, is frequently observed. These features are often accompanied by other neurological and psychiatric symptoms, including mood changes, psychosis, seizures, and movement abnormalities.[35]

Multiple sclerosis (MS) is one of the primary demyelinating illnesses of CNS and cognitive decline is one the major and often overlooked symptoms. It is thought to be due to increased white matter lesion and gray matter damage overall leading to cortical atrophy. Nearly half of MS patients are detected to have a cognitive impairment, either symptomatic or detected during neuropsychological testing.[36] Neuromyelitis optica (NMO) is an astrocytopathy mainly affecting the spinal cord and optic nerves due to antibodies against aquaporin-4. Symptomatic cerebral syndromes are also features of NMO and can present as RPD. Acute disseminated encephalomyelitis is another immune-mediated demyelinating CNS disease that predominantly affects children, few of these symptoms are observed with myelin oligodendrocyte glycoprotein associated disease (MOGAD). Often these symptoms are triggered by a febrile illness and spontaneous presentation is also known. Seronegative autoimmune encephalitis can present as RPD, posing a diagnostic challenge due to the absence of detectable autoantibodies. It can be effectively managed with immunotherapy, particularly steroids. Early recognition and treatment are crucial for improving outcomes in these patients.

Hashimoto's encephalopathy, also known as steroid-responsive encephalopathy associated with autoimmune thyroiditis (SREAT), is a rare autoimmune disorder characterized by inflammation of the brain. It occurs in individuals with autoimmune thyroiditis (Hashimoto's thyroiditis), which is an autoimmune condition where the body's immune system attacks the thyroid gland.[37] This autoimmune form of encephalopathy can present with a wide range of symptoms, including cognitive decline, confusion, seizures, hallucinations, tremors, and stroke-like episodes. Among them, cognitive decline is a common feature of HE and can manifest as memory loss, impaired concentration, difficulty processing information, and other cognitive impairments.

Strokes/Vascular Mediated

Vascular etiologies for RPD are many, which is mainly due to reduced blood flow to the brain cells due to cerebrovascular disease, such as stroke, small vessel disease, or other conditions affecting the blood vessels in the brain. Development of cognitive impairment following a stroke, may manifest as RPD; however; the disease course is usually static in the absence of additional vascular insults.[38] Types of vascular insults are strategic strokes, multi-infarct state, dural arteriovenous fistulas (DAVFs), amyloid angiopathy, hypertensive encephalopathy, etc. Secondary causes include primary CNS vasculitis, which often presents with headache, altered cognition, focal deficits, and CSF pleocytosis.

Several factors may contribute to the rapid progression of vascular dementia: Extent of vascular damage, where there is widespread or severe vascular damage, cognitive decline may progress more rapidly; cerebral amyloid angiopathy with or without AD-related amyloid pathology; presence of microbleeds; vascular malformations; and posterior reversible encephalopathy syndromes. In addition, other factors including the frequency of ischemic events, recurrent strokes, or transient ischemic attacks (TIAs) can lead to cumulative damage to the brain and accelerate cognitive decline in vascular dementia. Multiple small strokes or infarcts can impair cognitive function and cause rapid progression of symptoms. The location of vascular lesions also plays an important factor in the clinical presentation of RPD. Lesions affecting critical areas involved in memory, executive function, or language may lead to more pronounced symptoms and faster progression, whereas lesions in thalamic regions can have features of acute mutism.

Dural arteriovenous fistula, an abnormal connection between arteries and veins within the dura mater, is recently being considered one of the important treatable causes of RPD.[39] While DAVFs can manifest in various ways depending on their location and severity, they can indeed lead to cognitive decline if they affect regions of the brain responsible for cognitive function. Rarely, mass effect by large DAVFs can exert pressure on surrounding brain tissue, leading to compression and dysfunction of nearby structures responsible for cognitive function.

DIAGNOSTIC CHALLENGES

The difficulty in RPD diagnosis is due to its rapid nature and overlapping symptoms with other conditions. Given the diverse range of potential causes of RPD, a thorough evaluation, including neurological examination, imaging studies, and laboratory tests is essential for accurate diagnosis and appropriate management. Early recognition of the underlying cause can lead to timely interventions that may help slow the progression of the disease or improve symptoms.[40] When approaching a case of RPD, it is crucial to adopt a systematic and multidisciplinary approach to ensure timely diagnosis and appropriate management.[3]

EVALUATION OF RAPIDLY PROGRESSIVE DEMENTIA

The evaluation of RPD involves the following:

- *Comprehensive history and physical examination*: Obtain a detailed medical history, including onset and progression of symptoms, past medical conditions, medications, family history of neurological disorders, and any recent infections or exposures. A crucial step in establishing the diagnosis is through proper history. Often delirium also can mimic RPD. Simple blood tests and urine analysis often helps in ruling out metabolic causes. Perform a thorough neurological examination to assess cognitive function, motor skills, reflexes, sensory function, and signs of focal neurological deficits.
- *Higher cognitive and neuropsychological assessment*: Conduct a neuropsychological evaluation to assess cognitive function, including memory, language, executive function, and visuospatial skills. Neuropsychological testing can help characterize the pattern and severity of cognitive impairment and differentiate RPD from other cognitive disorders.
- *Diagnostic imaging studies*: Perform neuroimaging studies, such as MRI or computed tomography (CT) scans of the brain, to evaluate for structural abnormalities, including atrophy, infarcts, hemorrhage, and mass lesions. Imaging findings can provide valuable clues to the underlying cause of RPD. Neuroimaging findings observed in various RPDs are shown in **Figures 1 to 3**.
- *Laboratory investigations*: Obtain routine blood tests, including complete blood count, comprehensive metabolic panel, thyroid function tests, vitamin B12 levels, and serological tests for infectious diseases (e.g., HIV and syphilis). Consider CSF analysis, including cell count, protein, glucose, and specific biomarkers (e.g., 14-3-3 protein, tau protein, and paraneoplastic/autoimmune encephalitis panel), if suspecting prion disease or autoimmune encephalitis. EEG is considered in few cases of RPD. These are shown in **Figure 4**. These investigations are prioritized based on the clinical phenotype of the case. Details are mentioned in **Table 2**.
- *Genetic testing*: Consider genetic testing for hereditary/degenerative forms of dementia, such as familial AD, FTD, or other rare genetic disorders associated with RPD.
- *Specialized testing*: Depending on the clinical presentation and suspected etiology, additional specialized testing may be warranted, such as EEG for detecting epileptiform activity and positron emission tomography (PET) imaging for amyloid or tau deposition.

Recently, a scoring system has been developed for the early recognition of RPD, mainly for detecting treatable causes and for early treatment initiation.[41] This scoring system included *S*eizures, *T*umor (disease-associated), Age <50 years, Mania, MRI features suggestive of autoimmune encephalitis, Movement abnormalities, and Pleocytosis (CSF >10 cells/mm). It is commonly described

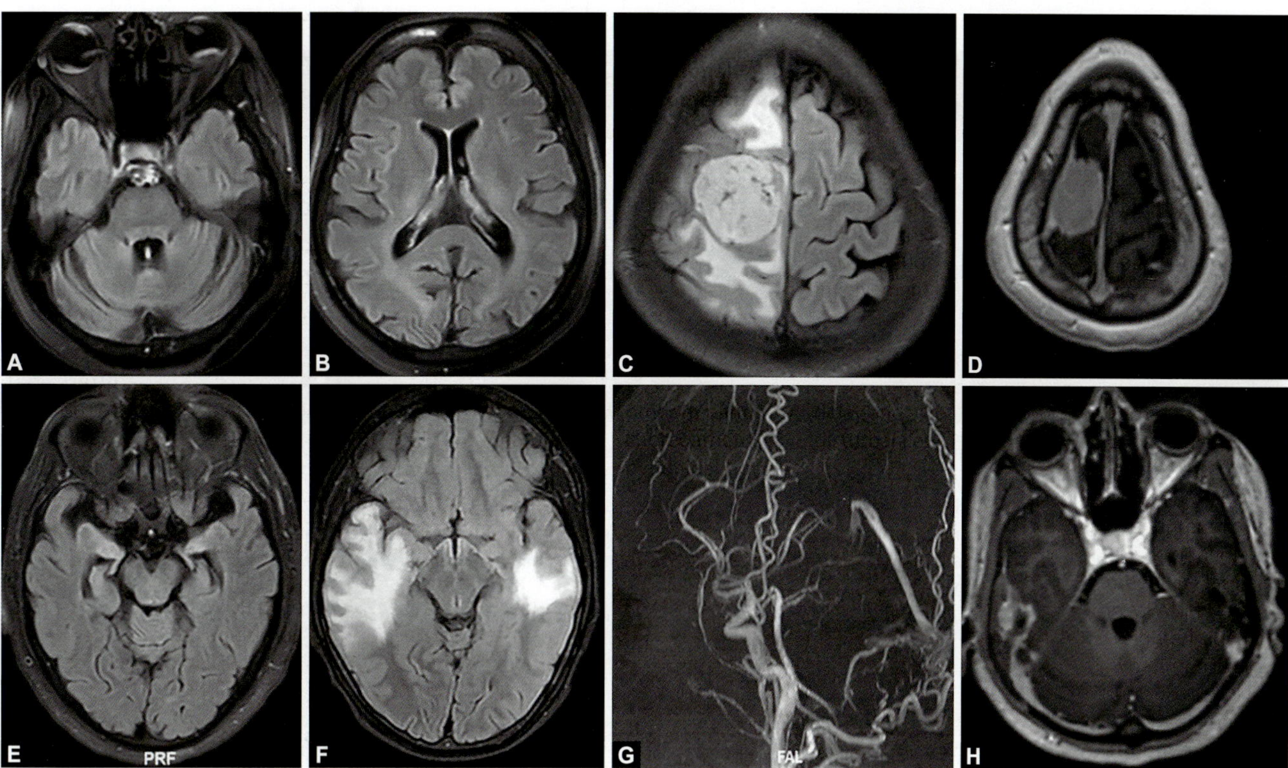

FIGS. 2A TO H: Brain MRI FLAIR axial sequences showing global cerebral and cerebellar atrophy with mild ground-glass appearance of periventricular white matter in mitochondriopathy (A and B); Well-defined extra-axial mass lesion along the parasagittal right frontoparietal convexity with perilesional edema and contrast enhancement in meningioma (C and D); Bilateral FLAIR hyperintensity and atrophic medial temporal region as a sequel of NMDA limbic encephalitis (E); FLAIR hyperintensities at bilateral peri-insula, temporal lobes in MOGAD; (F) DAVF is seen at the torcula, bilateral transverse-sigmoid sinuses with arterial feeders from bilateral middle meningeal arteries, transosseous branches of occipital arteries (G); and right mastoiditis with temporal lobe abscess in T1 axial postcontrast MRI (H).

(DAVF: dural arteriovenous fistula, FLAIR: fluid-attenuated inversion recovery; MOGAD: myelin oligodendrocyte glycoprotein associated disease; MRI: magnetic resonance imaging; NMDA: N-methyl D-aspartate)

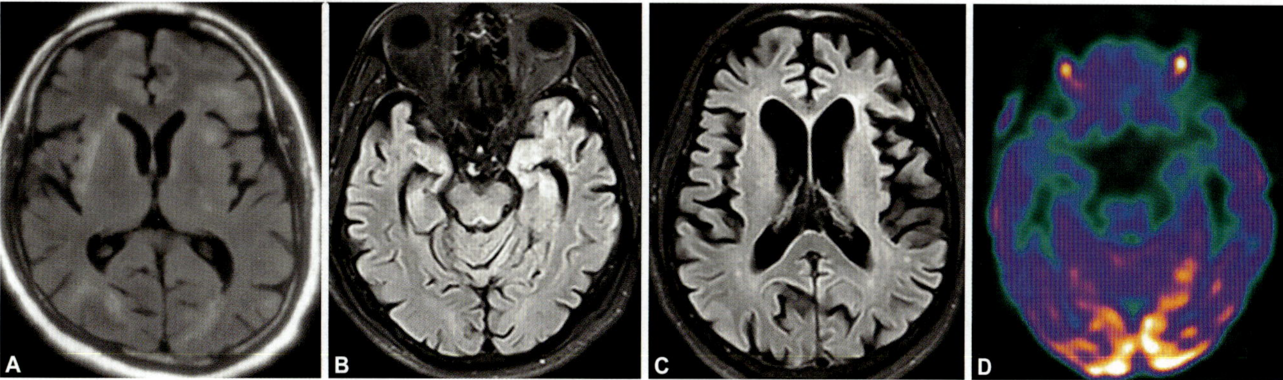

FIGS. 3A TO H: *Continued*

Continued

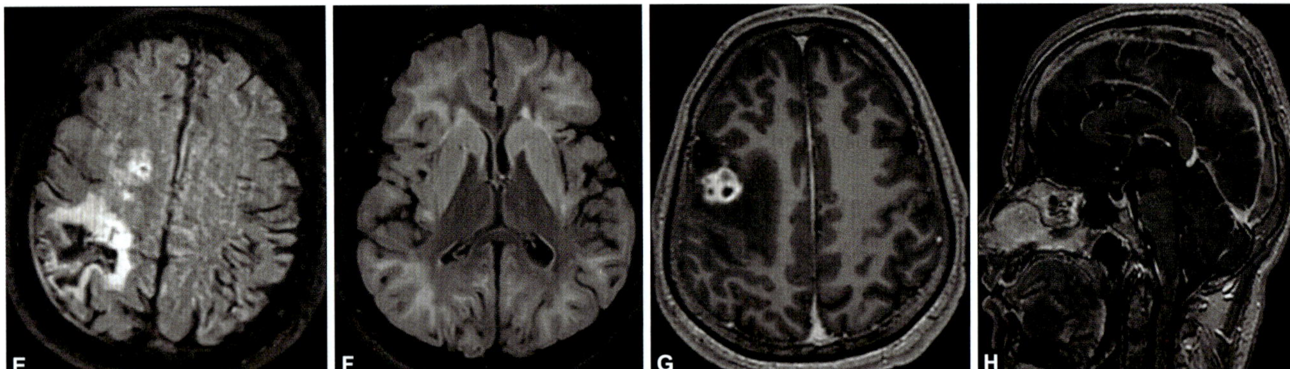

FIGS. 3A TO H: Brain FLAIR axial sequences showing multiple areas of hyperintense lesions in a case of CNS vasculitis (A); Predominant bilateral anterior temporal and frontal atrophy with reduced metabolism in PET scan in a case of frontotemporal dementia (B to D); Gliotic changes in the right parietal region due to infarct mimicking clinical features of Alzheimer's dementia (E); Bilateral symmetric predominantly subcortical white matter, bilateral striatum involvement with outer rim sign suggestive of leukodystrophy in L-2-hydroxyglutaric aciduria (F); T1 postcontrast scans suggestive of conglomerate lesions with enhancement in right frontal region in a case of CNS tuberculoma (G); and filling defect in superior sagittal sinus in cerebral venous thrombosis (H).

(CNS: central nervous system; FLAIR: fluid-attenuated inversion recovery; PET: positron emission tomography)

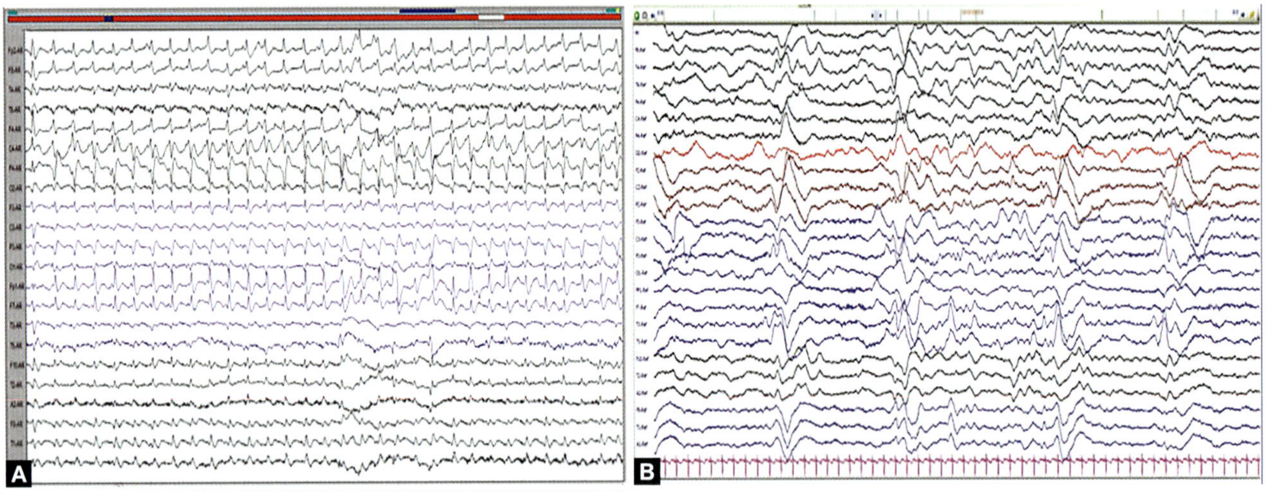

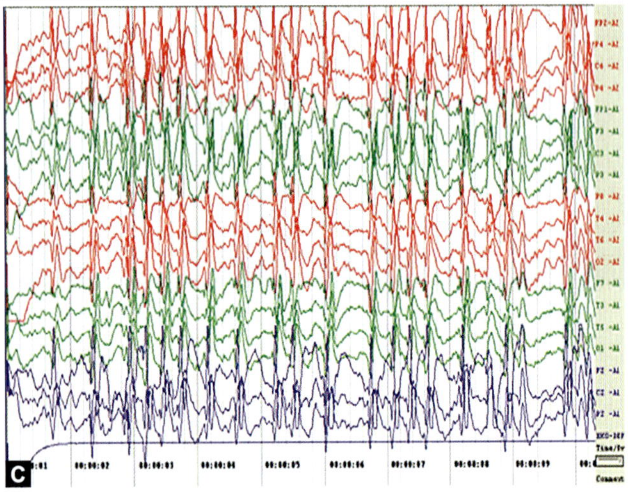

FIGS. 4A TO C: EEG. Average reference montages showing periodic short interval sharp wave complexes in CJD (A); Periodic long interval high amplitude slow wave discharges in SSPE (B); and continuous spike or spike and slow wave activity at 2–4 Hz in epileptic encephalopathy (C).

(CJD: Creutzfeldt–Jakob disease, EEG: electroencephalogram; SSPE: subacute sclerosing panencephalitis)

TABLE 2: Algorithm for the evaluation of patients with suspected rapidly progressive dementia.

First-line investigations	
Blood tests	Complete blood count, liver function test, kidney function test, serum electrolytes, ESR, CRP, Vitamin B12, homocysteine, fasting blood sugar, HbA1c, rapid plasma regain (RPR), and HIV serology
Cerebrospinal fluid (CSF) analysis	Cell type and cell count, protein, glucose, 14-3-3, and VDRL
Brain Imaging	MRI with T1, T2, FLAIR, DWI, ADC, and SWI sequences with contrast scan
Electroencephalogram (EEG)	With surface EMG electrode
Second-line investigations (based on clinical and first-line investigational observations)	
Prions disease	RT-QuIC and consider brain biopsy
Degenerative causes	PET scan brain and genetic testing
Endocrine abnormality	Anti-TG, Anti-TPO antibodies, ultrasound of thyroid gland, parathyroid hormone levels, serum calcium, and phosphorous levels
Malignancy	Tissue biopsy, tumor markers of suspected malignancy, screening of other body parts (CT chest and abdomen), mammogram, panel for paraneoplastic antibodies, and whole body PET screening
Epilepsy	Awake and sleep EEG, and autoimmune panel
Toxins and metabolic	Blood analysis for heavy metals screening and levels estimation, drug levels, copper levels, genetic testing for suspected leukodystrophies, ammonia, and lactate levels
Infections	CSF for AFB staining, India ink, cryptococcal antigen, viral PCRs and culture, tissue biopsy, and culture. Anti measles antibody titer
Autoimmune	ANA, ANCA, ACE levels, panel for autoimmune encephalitis, oligoclonal bands, and NMO and MOG antibodies
Strokes and vascular	Coagulation profile, vessel wall imaging of intra and extracranial vessels, echocardiogram, vasculitis panel, hypercoagulability testing, and genetic testing in suspected vasculopathy

(ACE: angiotensin-converting enzyme; ADC: apparent diffusion coefficient; AFB: acid-fast bacilli; ANA: antinuclear antibodies; ANCA: antineutrophil cytoplasmic antibodies; Anti-TG: antithyroglobulin antibodies; Anti-TPO: anti-treponemal antibodies; CRP: C-reactive protein; CT: computed tomography; DWI: diffusion-weighted imaging; ESR: erythrocyte sedimentation rate; EMG: electromyography; FLAIR: fluid-attenuated inversion recovery; HbA1c: glycated hemoglobin; HIV: human immunodeficiency virus; MOG: myelin oligodendrocyte glycoprotein; NMO: neuromyelitis optica; PCR: polymerase chain reaction; PET: positron emission tomography; RT-QuIC: real-time quaking-induced conversion; SWI: susceptibility-weighted imaging; VDRL: venereal disease research laboratory)

with mnemonic STAM3P. The presence of at least three or more of these features, reliably, identifies the possible etiology of treatable RPDs.

IMPACT ON PATIENTS AND FAMILIES

Beyond the clinical complexities, RPD exacts a profound emotional and psychological toll on affected individuals and their families. The sudden onset and rapid progression of symptoms often leave both patients and caregivers grappling with feelings of confusion, fear, and grief, exacerbating the already daunting challenges associated with dementia care. Furthermore, the urgency of the situation may necessitate rapid decision-making regarding treatment options and long-term care arrangements.

TREATMENT AND MANAGEMENT

Despite the formidable challenges posed by RPD, there exists a growing imperative to enhance our understanding of this condition and develop more effective strategies for its diagnosis, management, and support. There is currently no cure for prion diseases, and treatment is primarily supportive to manage symptoms and improve quality of life. However, for other degenerative dementias, supportive care counseling of the caretakers regarding illness is very important. Early recognition of other treatable dementias determines the recovery or stabilization of disease progression of these cases. The treatment principles of various RPDs are mentioned in **Table 3**.

TABLE 3: Treatment principles of various rapidly progressive dementias.

Types	Subtypes	Treatment
Prions disease		• No approved medicines available currently • Symptomatic treatment • *Depression*: SSRIs • *Agitation and psychosis*: Atypical antipsychotics • *Myoclonus*: Valproic acid and levetiracetam
Degenerative dementias	Alzheimer's disease	• Acetylcholinesterase inhibitors • N-methyl-D-aspartate receptor antagonist • Vitamin E
	Dementia with Lewy body	• Acetylcholinesterase inhibitors • Dopaminergic therapy • Avoid typical antipsychotics
	Frontotemporal dementia	• No approved therapy available • Nonpharmacological interventions • Family education • Caregiver support group
	Corticobasal degeneration	• No disease-modifying therapy available • Dopaminergic therapy for Parkinsonian features
	Progressive supranuclear palsy	• No disease-modifying therapy available • Dopaminergic therapy for Parkinsonian features • *Depression*: SSRIs
Endocrine abnormality	Hypothyroidism	• *Workup*: TSH, unbound T4, TPO antibody • Thyroid supplementation
	Hyperthyroidism	• *Workup*: TSH, unbound T4, TPO antibody • Antithyroid drugs
Malignancy	Primary/Metastasis	• Surgical removal • Chemo/radiotherapy
	Paraneoplastic neurological syndromes	• Intravenous (IV) methylprednisolone • Plasmapheresis or IV immunoglobulin • Screening for malignancy
Epilepsy		• Single/combination of antiseizure medicines • Trial of IV methylprednisolone in refractory status epilepticus
Nutritional		• Supplementation of specific nutritional deficiency • Screening for an underlying cause of nutritional deficiency
Toxins and metabolic	Heavy metals toxicity	• Chelation therapy • Preventive measures for heavy metal exposure
	Drug toxicity	• Stop the offending agent • Consider a chelation agent, if available
	Inherited metabolic disorders	• Medications for symptomatic relief • Stem cell/bone marrow transplantation in selected cases
	Hepatic encephalopathy	• Supportive care • Identify and treat precipitating factors • Treat concomitant encephalopathy
	Uremic encephalopathy	• Renal replacement therapy
	Electrolyte disturbances	• Identify the etiology • Treat underlying risk factor • Correct electrolyte disturbance

Continued

Continued

Types	Subtypes	Treatment
Infections		Select antimicrobials based on underlying organism
Autoimmune	Autoimmune encephalitis	• *Treatment of relapse*: High-dose steroids ± Plasmapheresis/IV Immunoglobulin • Maintenance therapy with immunomodulators • Screening for malignancy
	Multiple Sclerosis	• *Acute attack*: High-dose steroids • *Maintenance*: Disease modification therapy • Medicines for symptomatic relief
	NMO	*Treatment of relapse*: High-dose steroids ± Plasmapheresis/IV immunoglobulin
	MOG	Maintenance therapy with immunomodulators
	Secondary CNS demyelination	• Treatment of primary disease • Medicines for symptomatic relief
Strokes	Ischemic strokes	• *Antiplatelet agents*: Single/dual (Anticoagulation, if cardioembolic) • Treat underlying risk factors
	Hemorrhagic strokes	• Measures for controlling raised intracranial pressure • Hyperventilation • Osmotic diuresis • Treat the underlying cause
	Venous strokes	• Anticoagulation • Treat underlying risk factors
	Arteriovenous (AV) malformations	Endovascular/surgical intervention
	Impaired autoregulation	• Supportive measures • Treat underlying etiology

(MOG: myelin oligodendrocyte glycoprotein; NMO: neuromyelitis optica; SSRI: selective serotonin reuptake inhibitors; TSH: thyroid-stimulating hormone)

CONCLUSION

Rapidly progressive dementias present as one of the challenging neurological conditions. Since the list of differential diagnoses is wide, systematic approach is required for each of the patients for precise diagnosis. Common categories include prion diseases, progressive forms of degenerative dementias, endocrinal abnormalities, malignancy-related causes, epilepsy-related, nutritional, toxin-metabolic, infective causes, and stroke/vascular causes. Even after extensive evaluation, a small proportion of cases may still remain undiagnosed.

REFERENCES

1. Geschwind MD. Rapidly Progressive Dementia. Continuum (Minneap Minn). 2016;22(2 Dementia):510-37.
2. Zerr I, Hermann P. Diagnostic challenges in rapidly progressive dementia. Expert. Rev. Neurother. 2018;18(10):761-72.
3. Mahajan S, Appleby BS. Comprehensive and methodical: Diagnostic and management approaches to rapidly progressive dementia. Curr Treat Options Neurol. 2017;19(11):40.
4. Hermann P, Zerr I. Rapidly progressive dementias—aetiologies, diagnosis and management. Nat Rev Neurol. 2022;18:363-76.
5. Chandra SR, Viswanathan LG, Pai AR, Wahatule R, Alladi S. Syndromes of rapidly progressive cognitive decline-Our experience. J Neurosci Rural Pract. 2017;8:S66-71.
6. Anuja P, Venugopalan V, Darakhshan N, Awadh P, Wilson V, Manoj G, et al. Rapidly progressive dementia: An eight year (2008–2016) retrospective study. PLoS One. 2018;13(1): e0189832.
7. Liu X, Sun Y, Zhang X, Liu P. Zhang K, Yu L, et al. Prevalence and outcomes of rapidly progressive dementia: A retrospective cohort study in a neurologic unit in China. BMC Geriatr. 2023;23:142.
8. Stamatelos P, Kontokostas K, Liantinioti C, Giavasi C, Ioakeimidis M, Antonelou R, et al. Evolving causes of rapidly progressive dementia: A 5-year comparative study. Alzheimer Dis Assoc Disord. 2021;35(4):315-20.

9. Uttley L, Carroll C, Wong R, Hilton DA, Stevenson M. Creutzfeldt-Jakob disease: A systematic review of global incidence, prevalence, infectivity, and incubation. Lancet Infect Dis. 2020;20(1):e2-10.
10. Parchi P, Giese A, Capellari S, Brown P, Schulz-Schaeffer W, Windl O, et al. Classification of sporadic Creutzfeldt–Jakob disease based on molecular and phenotypic analysis of 300 subjects. Ann Neurol. 1999;46(2):224-33.
11. Meissner B, Westner IM, Kallenberg K, Krasnianski A, Bartl M, Varges D, et al. Sporadic Creutzfeldt-Jakob disease: Clinical and diagnostic characteristics of the rare VV1 type. Neurology. 2005;65:1544-50.
12. Park SY, Wang MJ, Jang JW, Park YH, Lim JS, Youn YC, et al. The clinical stages of Sporadic Creutzfeldt-Jakob disease with Met/Met genotype in Korean Patients. Eur Neurol. 2016;75(5-6): 213-22.
13. Rhoads DD, Wrona A, Foutz A, Blevins J, Glisic K, Person M, et al. Diagnosis of prion diseases by RT-QuIC results in improved surveillance. Neurology. 2020;95:e1017-26.
14. Hermann P, Laux M, Glatzel M, Matschke J, Knipper T, Goebel S, et al. Validation and utilization of amended diagnostic criteria in Creutzfeldt-Jakob disease surveillance. Neurology. 2018; 91(4):e331-8.
15. Soto ME, Andrieu S, Arbus C, Ceccaldi M, Couratier P, Dantoine T, et al. Rapid cognitive decline in Alzheimer's disease. Consensus paper. J Nutr Health Aging. 2008;12(10):703-13.
16. Liu H, Kim C, Haldiman T, Sigurdson CJ, Nyström S, Nilsson KPR, et al. Distinct conformers of amyloid beta accumulate in the neocortex of patients with rapidly progressive Alzheimer's disease. J Biol Chem. 2021;297(5):101267.
17. Seidl JN, Massman PJ. Rapidly versus slowly progressing patients with Alzheimer's disease: Differences in baseline cognition. Am J Alzheimers Dis Other Demen. 2016;31(4): 318-25.
18. Gaig C, Valldeoriola F, Gelpi E, Ezquerra M, Llufriu S, Buongiorno M, et al. Rapidly progressive diffuse Lewy body disease. Mov Disord. 2011;26(7):1316-23.
19. Yu J. Endocrine disorders and the neurologic manifestations. Ann Pediatr Endocrinol Metab. 2014;19(4):184-90.
20. van der Meulen M, Dirven L, Habets EJJ, van den Bent MJ, Taphoorn MJB, Bromberg JEC. Cognitive functioning and health-related quality of life in patients with newly diagnosed primary CNS lymphoma: A systematic review. Lancet Oncol. 2018;19(8);e407-18.
21. Kuker W, Nägele T, Korfel A, Heckl S, Thiel E, Bamberg M, et al. Primary central nervous system lymphomas (PCNSL): MRI features at presentation in 100 patients. J Neurooncol. 2005;72(2):169-77.
22. Menéndez Calderón MJ, Seguí Riesco ME, Arguelles M, Nuño Mateo J. Intravascular lymphomatosis. A report of three cases. An Med Interna. 2005;22(1):31-4.
23. Graus F, Vogrig A, Muñiz-Castrillo S, Antoine JG, Desestret V, Dubey D, et al. Updated diagnostic criteria for paraneoplastic neurologic syndromes. Neurol Neuroimmunol Neuroinflamm. 2021;8(4):e1014.
24. Mutis JA, Rodríguez JH, Nava-Mesa MO. Rapidly progressive cognitive impairment with neuropsychiatric symptoms as the initial manifestation of status epilepticus. Epilepsy Behav Case Rep. 2016;7:20-3.
25. Scalzo SJ, Bowden SC, Ambrose ML, Whelan G, Cook MJ. Wernicke–Korsakoff syndrome not related to alcohol use: A systematic review. J Neurol Neurosurg Psychiatry. 2015;86(12): 1362-8.
26. Day GS. Rapidly progressive dementia. Continuum (Minneap Minn). 2022;28(3):901-36.
27. Bolla KI, Cadet JL. Exogenous acquired metabolic disorders of the nervous system: toxins and illicit drugs. Textbook of Clinical Neurology, 3rd edition. Amsterdam, Netherlands: Elsevier Inc.; 2007. pp. 865-96.
28. von Moltke LL, Greenblatt DJ, Romach MK, Sellers EM. Cognitive toxicity of drugs used in the elderly. Dialogues Clin Neurosci. 2001;3(3):181-90.
29. Boucher A, Herrmann JL, Morand P, Buzelé R, Crabol Y, Stahl JP, et al. Epidemiology of infectious encephalitis causes in 2016. Med Mal Infect. 2017;47(3):221-35.
30. Helms J, Kremer S, Merdji H, Clere-Jehl R, Schenck M, Kummerlen C, et al. Neurologic features in severe SARS-CoV-2 infection. N Engl J Med. 2020;382(23):2268-70.
31. Wang Y, Liu M, Lu Q, Farrell M, Lappin JM, Shi J, et al. Global prevalence and burden of HIV-associated neurocognitive disorder: A meta-analysis. Neurology. 2020;95(19):e2610-21.
32. Almeida OP, Lautenschlager NT. Dementia associated with infectious diseases. Int Psychogeriatr. 2005;17(suppl 1):S65-77.
33. Ramachandran PS, Baird RW, Markey P, Singleton S, Lowe M, Currie BJ, et al. Neurosyphilis: Still prevalent and overlooked in an at risk population. PLoS One. 2020;15(10):e0238617.
34. Dalmau J, Graus F. Antibody-mediated encephalitis. N Engl J Med. 2018;378(9):840-51.
35. Heine J, Kopp UA, Klag J, Ploner CJ, Prüss H, Finke C. Long-Term Cognitive Outcome in Anti-N-Methyl-D-Aspartate Receptor Encephalitis. Ann Neurol. 2021;90(6):949-61.
36. Benedict RHB, Amato MP, DeLuca J, Geurts JJG. Cognitive impairment in multiple sclerosis: Clinical management, MRI, and therapeutic avenues. Lancet Neurol. 2020;19(10):860-71.
37. Wang J, Zhang J, Xu L, Shi Y, Wu X, Guo Q. Cognitive impairments in Hashimoto's encephalopathy: A case-control study. PLoS One. 2013;8(2):e55758.
38. Skrobot OA, O'Brien J, Black S, Chen C, DeCarli C, Erkinjuntti T, et al. The Vascular Impairment of Cognition Classification Consensus Study. Alzheimers Dement. 2017;13(6):624-33.
39. Enofe I, Thacker I, Shamim S. Dural arteriovenous fistula as a treatable dementia. Proc (Bayl Univ Med Cent). 2017;30(2): 215-7.
40. Woodruff BK Evaluation of rapidly progressive dementia. Semin Neurol. 2007;27:363-75.
41. Satyadev N, Tipton PW, Martens Y, Dunham SR, Geschwind MD, Morris JC, et al. Improving early recognition of treatment-responsive causes of rapidly progressive dementia: The $STAM_3P$ Score. Ann Neurol. 2024;95(2):237-48.

CHAPTER

13 Serum and Cerebrospinal Fluid Biomarkers in Diagnosis of Dementia

Durjoy Lahiri

ABSTRACT

Imaging and fluid biomarkers are increasingly being used in clinical practice to diagnose Alzheimer's disease. These biomarkers can detect the presence of amyloid-beta, tau and non-specific markers of neurodegeneration in the brain. CSF biomarkers are gaining access to mainstream practice due to their accuracy and cost-effectiveness. Plasma biomarkers are used for research purposes but are not yet widely used in clinical practice due to lack of established cutoffs. The future of cognitive neurology looks promising with the arrival of various biomarkers and the hope of having disease-modifying therapies in clinical practice in the near future.

Keywords: Alzheimer's, Dementia, CSF biomarkers, Serum biomarkers, Clinical practice.

INTRODUCTION

The definition of Alzheimer's disease (AD) has undergone considerable modifications in the last few years. With the advent of biomarkers for AD, the diagnosis has revolutionized to include biological or pathological status of an individual in addition to their clinical symptoms and signs. Biomarkers for AD can be classified from the vantage point of ATN scheme where A represents amyloid-beta (Aβ) which can be detected by cerebrospinal fluid (CSF) and positron emission tomography (PET) scan; T stands for tau which can be picked up in CSF and PET scan, while N designates nonspecific markers of neurodegeneration which can be interpreted from magnetic resonance imaging (MRI), fluorodeoxyglucose positron emission tomography (FDG PET), and single-photon emission computed tomography (SPECT) scans as well as CSF and plasma assays. At least one third of people having cognitive impairment resembling clinical AD can have a negative Aβ status and these cases are largely attributed to a group of clinical entities collectively called suspected non-Alzheimer pathology (SNAP) that includes hippocampal sclerosis (HS), primary age-related tauopathy (PART), and limbic-predominant age-related TDP-43 encephalopathy (LATE). CSF biomarkers are slowly gaining access to mainstream practice of cognitive neurology across the globe, mostly because of their comparable accuracy and less cost than the corresponding PET scans. Plasma biomarkers continue to be utilized widely for research purposes, mostly at the entry point for clinical trials in AD. However, they are yet to be freely used in regular clinical practice, given the lack of their established cutoffs as of now. The future landscape of cognitive neurology looks different and promising with the arrival of various biomarkers on the stage and the hope of having disease-modifying therapies in clinical practice.

DEFINITION OF ALZHEIMER'S DISEASE: CLINICAL, PATHOLOGICAL, AND PATHOBIOLOGICAL

Since its first description at the beginning of the 20th century, the definition of AD has undergone quite a few modifications over the years.[1] In 1984, when the NINCDS-ADRDA (National Institute of Neurological and Communicative Disorders and Stroke and the Alzheimer's

Disease and Related Disorders Association) criteria were published for the first time, AD was described as a clinical entity with the predominant feature being progressive memory impairment, affecting the activities of daily living.[2] This was mostly a clinical definition with an inbuilt assumption about the underlying pathophysiological process. In the following years, pathological autopsies became more frequent than earlier times, and in the late 1990s, AD came to be known as a pathological entity where Aβ plaques are demonstrated in the pathological autopsy of a person having amnestic symptoms during their lifetime.[3]

The field of cognitive neurology underwent a deep correctional phase after that period. Not only did the concept of mild cognitive impairment (MCI) become existent but several nonamnestic presentations of AD were also noted by the clinical researchers working in the field. Down the line, several biomarkers came into existence with a potential to detect underlying pathology during the lifetime of an individual with cognitive symptoms. Therefore, the diagnostic criteria were in the need of a revision in the beginning of this century. In 2011, McKhann criteria for AD reflected these recent advances in diagnosis by including biomarkers as a factor that increases diagnostic certainty in favor of AD.[4]

This led to the development of a clinicopathological definition of AD, where a clinician can make a diagnosis of AD based on the typical clinical features in an individual followed by judicious use of biomarkers to increase the diagnostic certainty. In western countries, it is a standard practice to assess biomarkers for AD in case of diagnostic dilemma or when there is a need to refer for disease-modifying therapies (more specifically antiamyloid therapies) either clinically or for trials.[5] This is slowly infiltrating into the practice of cognitive neurology here in India as well, where some hospitals and clinics do offer CSF biomarker services for AD.

TABLE 1: AT(N) classification and its interpretation in terms of predicting underlying Alzheimer's pathology in the brain.[6]

AT(N) profiles	Biomarker category	
A–T–(N)–	Normal Alzheimer's disease (AD) biomarkers	
A+T–(N)–	Alzheimer's pathologic change	Alzheimer's continuum
A+T+(N)>	AD	
A+T+(N)+	AD	
A+T–(N)+	Alzheimer's and concomitant suspected non-Alzheimer's pathologic change	
A–T+(N)–	Non-AD pathologic change	
A–T–(N)+	Non-AD pathologic change	
A–T+(N)+	Non-AD pathologic change	

BOX 1 Biomarker grouping according to the AT(N) classification.[6]

A: Aggregated Aβ or associated pathologic state
- CSF Aβ42, or Aβ42/Aβ40 ratio
- Amyloid PET

T: Aggregated tau (neurofibrillary tangles) or associated pathologic state
- CSF phosphorylated tau
- Tau PET

(N): Neurodegeneration or neuronal injury
- Anatomic MRI
- FDG PET
- CSF total tau

(Aβ: amyloid-β; CSF: cerebrospinal fluid; FDG PET: fluorodeoxyglucose positron emission tomography; MRI: magnetic resonance imaging)

AT(N) CLASSIFICATION

In modern times, AD is considered a biological disease with a continuum where the starting point is the accumulation of abnormal Aβ, which after many years, at some point in this continuum, is going to give rise to cognitive symptoms.

In 2018, Jack and colleagues proposed a new classification of AD which can be called a pathobiological classification, since it is completely based on the biomarker status of an individual regardless of clinical symptoms and signs[6] **(Table 1 and Box 1)**. This came to be known as AT(N) classification, where A stands for amyloid, T stands for tau, and N represents neurodegeneration as evidenced by brain imaging or other nonspecific biomarkers of neurodegeneration. According to this classification, someone with A+T+N+ status will be classified as having AD independent of their clinical status. People with A- status are categorized as having SNAP as a cause of their cognitive decline according to this new scheme.

There is a gray zone within the AT(N) scheme when someone has a biomarker status of A+T- which is designated as Alzheimer's spectrum.[7] Phosphorylated tau (p-tau) is a downstream neurodegenerative product that follows Aβ deposition in the brain. Therefore, logically A+ status should be accompanied by T+ status, when the degeneration is due to an Alzheimer's pathology. However, in many cases, it has been seen that A+ status is not associated with a positive p-tau status. To explain this situation, several explanations have been forwarded by the scientific community. One of the acceptable hypotheses is that this stage is AD in evolution and the p-tau status may become positive in few years down the line. The other hypothesis is that p-tau being primarily intracellular in location is not detected well enough in CSF, reflecting a falsely low value, while Aβ is more reliably detected in CSF and reflects a true-positive status.

An analogous situation occurs when A–T+ status is detected on a biomarker assay. P-tau, as explained earlier, carries a lot of significance toward AD, when accompanied by A+ status. Isolated T+ status is thought to be caused by clinical conditions such as PART which also presents in a similar way as AD except a little slower in progression.[8] This clinical entity is, however, considered distinct from AD.

Another limitation of AT(N) classification as was felt after its publication is the failure to consider the presence of copathologies which is often the case in an aging brain.[9] Single pathology is almost rarely found in the brains of individuals who are 80 years or older. Keeping this in view, the ATN scheme of classification has recently been modified in 2023 to AT(N)(X) where X accommodates copathologies, such as vascular injury and α-synuclein.[10] In the recently published revised criteria for AD diagnosis, the biomarkers are categorized based on four criteria **(Table 2)**. First, three broad mechanistic groupings are identified. Second, they are subclassified based on the proteinopathy or pathophysiologic pathway that each biomarker measures (e.g., A, T, N, etc.). Third, within the Core category, Core 1 and Core 2 biomarkers have been distinguished. Fourth, imaging and fluid analyte biomarkers are listed separately within each category.[11]

TYPES OF BIOMARKERS AVAILABLE IN ALZHEIMER'S DISEASE

Currently available biomarkers for AD can be categorized into imaging and fluid biomarkers based on the modality of testing. Notably, there has been significant recent advancement in the fluid or molecular biomarkers of AD.[12-14] **Box 1** describes the classification of biomarkers in AD according to the AT(N) system, while **Table 1** represents the interpretation of a specific AT(N) designation. In general, it is a useful scheme to understand the different categories of biomarkers used in the diagnosis of AD. A very recent document prepared by the National Institute on Aging–Alzheimer's Association (NIA-AA) workgroup on biomarkers has categorized the AD biomarkers as core biomarkers, nonspecific AD biomarkers, and non-AD copathology biomarkers (https://aaic.alz.org/diagnostic-criteria.asp). This modernized scheme is presented in **Table 2**.

Imaging Biomarkers

Magnetic Resonance Imaging

Magnetic resonance imaging is a commonly used imaging biomarker for AD. One of the most well-known MRI markers for AD is medial temporal lobe atrophy (MTLA),[15] which can be quantified by using the Scheltens' Scale or MTLA score.[16] This score ranges from 0 to 3 depending on the magnitude of atrophy seen within the medial

TABLE 2: Biomarkers are categorized in this table based on four criteria.

Biomarker category	CSF or plasma analytes	Imaging
Core biomarkers		
Core 1		
A (Aβ proteinopathy) Aβ42	Aβ42	Amyloid PET
T1 (phosphorylated and secreted AD tau)	p-tau217, p-tau181, p-tau231	
Core 2		
T2 (AD tau proteinopathy)	pT205, MTBR-243, nonphosphorylated tau fragments	Tau PET
Biomarkers of nonspecific processes involved in AD pathophysiology		
N (injury, dysfunction, or degeneration of neuropil)	NfL	Anatomic MR or CT, FDG PET
I (inflammation) Astrocytic activation	GFAP	
Biomarkers of non-AD copathology		
V vascular brain injury		Anatomic infarction, WMH
S α-synuclein	αSyn-SAA*	

*Means only informative in CSF.

(αSyn-SAA: alpha-synuclein seed amplification assay; Aβ: amyloid beta; AD: Alzheimer's disease; CT: computed tomography; FDG PET: fluorodeoxyglucose positron emission tomography; GFAP: glial fibrillary acidic protein; MR: magnetic resonance; NfL: neurofilament light chain; p-tau: phosphorylated tau; WMH: white matter hyperintensity)

Source: Alzheimer's Association. Criteria for Diagnosis and Staging of Alzheimer's Disease. [online] Available from https://aaic.alz.org/diagnostic-criteria.asp [Last accessed July, 2024].

temporal lobes (MTL) on the coronal sections of the MRI brain, focusing on hippocampal volume. Some other MRI biomarkers of AD are parietal atrophy score (Koedam score) and global cortical atrophy score. AD pathology is typically associated with global atrophy of the brain volume alongside more shrinkage of the MTL. However, several variations have been observed in practice, such as minimal atrophy, hippocampal predominant, and hippocampal sparing.[17]

Single-photon Emission Computed Tomography

Single-photon emission computed tomography is a special form of computed tomography (CT) scan technique that can reveal brain perfusion in different areas. One of the classic patterns seen in AD is bilateral parietal hypoperfusion. This modality is also not specific for AD. In addition, the sensitivity of SPECT in early AD particularly is not very high. One of the factors that can cause variability in perfusion scans is starting a symptomatic medication for AD such as donepezil which can reportedly increase brain perfusion.[18]

Fluorodeoxyglucose Positron Emission Tomography Scan

Positron emission tomography is used to assess the metabolism in different areas of brain by injecting the individual with FDG. Typical pattern seen in AD is bilateral parietal hypometabolism. This pattern is more sensitive and specific than a SPECT scan.

Amyloid and Tau Positron Emission Tomography Scans

Amyloid and tau PET scans are highly specific and sensitive PET scans that can detect the deposition of Aβ and p-tau in the brain, which are the signature pathologic changes seen in AD.[19] The main drawback is that they are not easily available in most of the countries. In the United States of America (USA), they are available for clinical use, while in Canada and Europe, they are primarily accessible for research purposes. Another flip side is the extremely high expenses of conducting such scans.

Fluid Biomarkers in Alzheimer's Disease

Fluid biomarkers in AD can be primarily of two types: CSF and blood (plasma).[20]

Cerebrospinal Fluid Biomarkers

Amyloid-β42

It is understood that in AD, the central pathology starts from the deposition of abnormal amyloid in different brain areas.[21] Corollary to that notion, there is inadequate secretion of Aβ in the body fluids, mostly CSF, which can be utilized to detect the presence of Aβ pathology within the brain parenchyma.[22]

Amyloid-β42 levels start going down in the CSF at least 10–15 years before the onset of cognitive symptoms and therefore gives a clinician an opportunity to detect the amyloidopathy way before an individual starts having memory or other cognitive complains.[23] Several laboratories have different cutoff values for determining Alzheimer's pathology in the brain. The most used cutoff value is 1,030 ng/L. Below this level, an individual is considered to have Aβ42 positivity. Aβ42 values in CSF are however subject to individual variations and therefore, some cases can be false positive or false negative. The concordance of CSF amyloid with PET amyloid is close to 90% indicating a good agreement between the two modalities.[22,24]

While most of the laboratories commonly measure Aβ42 in the CSF, the measurement of Aβ40 is also available for research purposes. The role of Aβ40 is to predominantly differentiate between AD and cerebral amyloid angiopathy (CAA). Both AD and CAA are amyloid deposition disorders where AD is characterized by deposition of Aβ42 specifically, while a global decline of amyloid values (both Aβ42 and Aβ40) has been observed in CAA, indicating a more widespread β-amyloidopathy.[25]

As per prevalent understanding, Aβ plaque deposition in the brain along with formation of neurofibrillary tangles is considered central to the pathogenesis of AD. Several researchers have documented evidence that tends to challenge the primacy of the Aβ hypothesis in AD pathophysiology. Probably the most striking evidence in this context is that neither all cognitively normal brains are devoid of Aβ plaques nor does its removal lead to resolution of cognitive symptoms with certainty. Furthermore, the recent failure of some large-scale clinical trials in demonstrating clinical cognitive improvement by targeting Aβ in the brain has pulled the Aβ cascade hypothesis under scrutiny.[26]

At least one third of individuals with cognitive impairment resembling AD can have negative amyloid status in the CSF (or PET).[27-29] These people are known as Alzheimer phenotype or Alzheimer syndrome. Several explanations have been put forward to explain this clinic-biologic dissociation. One of these hypotheses pertain to the fact that there are several non-Alzheimer pathologies that can take place leading to cognitive impairment. These conditions are collectively known as SNAP, which include HS, PART, and LATE.[30]

Phosphorylated-tau

Phosphorylated-tau is another analyte that is commonly assayed in the CSF for AD biomarkers. P-tau is considered a downstream marker of neurodegeneration in AD that follows Aβ deposition. It is understood that while the extracellular plaques, pathognomonic of AD, are composed of Aβ, the intracellular neurofibrillary tangles, another hallmark of AD, consist of p-tau.[23]

Phosphorylated-tau is assayed alongside Aβ42 in the CSF and higher than cutoff values are considered abnormal unlike the lower values for Aβ. The normal range of values of p-tau in CSF are 18–27 ng/L. CSF p-tau is a good reflection of tau deposition in the brain as it has good concordance with tau PET scans. However, there are individual variations in tau clearance from the system which can influence the p-tau levels in the body fluid, giving a false interpretation of the underlying pathology. In some cases, p-tau is more densely situated in the neuronal synapses and therefore is not adequately secreted in the body fluids. This can also lead to a false, low estimation, confusing the clinical picture.

Overall, the ratio of Aβ and p-tau is more important than their individual values. A low Aβ in the face of a rising p-tau value can give the clinician indication of an underlying Alzheimer's pathology going on. The normal ratio of p-tau/Aβ42 is <0.024 and values greater than that are indicative of AD pathology. This ratio takes out of the equation, to a great extent, any individual variation in clearance of these molecules from the system. In clinical situations, therefore, this specific ratio is viewed with higher importance than the individual levels of these two analytes.

Total Tau

Total tau (T-tau) is an assay that is often included in the CSF biomarker panel for AD. T-tau is a nonspecific marker of neurodegeneration. This molecule is found to be raised in different neurodegenerative conditions, besides AD, such as frontotemporal dementia (FTD) and Creutzfeldt–Jakob disease (CJD). It does not have a predictive value for AD as its specificity is lower than Aβ and p-tau.

Plasma Biomarkers

Plasma biomarkers are being increasingly used in the field of AD mostly for research purposes. This method has the potential to come to regular clinical practice in memory clinics worldwide, since this is easier to access than a lumbar puncture and less expensive. However, there are a few drawbacks that need to be borne in mind while interpreting the results of plasma biomarker assays in AD. While some plasma assays have shown excellent accuracy in the diagnosis of AD (keeping PET and CSF as reference standards), others have not been that successful. In general, none of the plasma assays has so far received regulatory approval for use in mainstream clinical practice.[31]

The specificities are discussed in the following sections in relation to the specific molecules.

Amyloid-β42

Plasma Aβ42 is measured to evaluate the presence of AD pathology in the brain with the same idea that this molecule will be secreted less in the body fluids, in this case plasma, with an ongoing AD pathology. The sensitivity of plasma Aβ42 is variable, ranging from 60 to 90%, dependent on the technique used and the laboratory involved.[32] One of the factors that is commonly implicated is our lack of understanding of the CSF–blood dynamics in terms of Aβ movements across these two compartments.

Plasma Aβ40 is also assayed sometimes in laboratories to generate a ratio of Aβ42/40 which presumably has a better sensitivity toward diagnosing AD pathology than their individual absolute values. This ratio falls below the normal range in case of AD pathology as compared to CAA where there is a global Aβ decline in the body fluids.

Phosphorylated-tau

Plasma p-tau levels reflect the progression of AD pathology as this marker is specific for neurodegeneration in AD.[33] It has been seen that p-tau181 is a reliable predictor of Aβ pathology, even more than that of Aβ itself. Another molecule that has drawn quite a lot of attention recently in this context is p-tau217 which has reflected high sensitivity and specificity for AD.[34] A combination of these biomarkers is more useful sometimes for biological interpretation than their isolated values.

Neurofilament Light Chain

Neurofilament light chain (NfL) is a nonspecific marker on neurodegeneration measured in the plasma and has the potential to be clinically used in cognitive clinics around the world.

Glial Fibrillary Acidic Protein

Glial fibrillary acidic protein (GFAP) is another nonspecific marker of neurodegeneration that is being increasingly used in modern practice to assess the presence of brain inflammation in AD. Several recent research studies have used this molecule to argue that people living with AD have more magnitude of neuroinflammation ongoing as compared to their non-AD counterparts, indicating that AD is fundamentally a neuroinflammatory disorder, at least partially.

TDP-43

TDP-43 is an interesting recent development in the field of plasma biomarkers. TDP-43 is a molecule that is physiologically found in plasma. Therefore, greatly sensitive assays are required to detect the presence of very small pathological TDP-43 in the blood. This technique is called single molecular assay (SIMOA), which is extremely sensitive and can detect the presence of pathological TDP-43 in the plasma.[35]

Autopsy studies demonstrated that almost 50% of people living with AD have concurrent TDP-43 pathology ongoing in their brains. Presence of dual pathologies may indicate a rapid progression or more severe cognitive deficit. More importantly, as mentioned earlier, some people with AD like cognitive impairment do not show Aβ deposition in their brains and they may harbor a non-AD pathology, such as LATE which cannot be easily diagnosed by antemortem investigations. Plasma assay of TDP-43 can open new avenues for diagnosis of LATE when Aβ assays turn out negative.

In brief, plasma biomarkers are at the point where they are coming into clinical use in a very limited capacity in very specific settings and this is only happening in the United States and few select European countries. Priority biomarkers are Aβ, NfL, and GFAP, with p-tau181 and -217 coming out as major front runners. It is also important to note that these biomarkers are meant to detect pathology and not at the point of screening for disease since parameters for using them to detect cognitive decline have not been established. This is also often framed as a good reason to use biomarkers for clinical trials to determine if someone has the pathology the drug targets. In the screening process of many clinical trials, plasma biomarkers are being employed as a variable to decide on PET amyloid screening in a specific case, since the latter is more expensive and time-consuming.

Box 2 presents in a nutshell the key points about CSF and plasma biomarkers in AD.

TEMPORAL RELATION OF BIOMARKERS IN ALZHEIMER'S DISEASE

The temporal relation of biomarkers among each other is a subject of deep interest both to clinicians and researchers working in the field of AD. It has been noted that biomarker abnormalities start in the system at least 10–15 years before the onset of memory or other cognitive symptoms. The first biomarker to become abnormal in this context is Aβ42 which can be picked up in the CSF analysis and later the PET scan that is able to demonstrate the presence Aβ plaques in the brain. Strikingly, imaging abnormalities such as MRI and FDG-PET scans also start becoming abnormal before the onset of clinical phase in AD. It has been hypothesized that people with higher

BOX 2 Utilities and drawbacks of different AD biomarkers in a nutshell.

Aβ42:
- Early biological diagnosis, mostly in high-risk group
- Insight into pathogenesis of AD
- CSF assays are concordant with PET amyloid in 90% cases
- Important for inclusion in clinical trials of antiamyloid agents
- Ratio of p-tau/Aβ42 is more meaningful than their individual values
- Plasma Aβ42 is not as accurate as CSF assays
- Not much is known about the diurnal or individual variations and blood–CSF dynamics of this molecule

P-tau:
- Downstream marker of neurodegeneration in the Aβ cascade
- Specific for AD pathogenesis
- Often interpreted as a ratio with Aβ42
- Important in clinical trials of antiamyloid agents
- Plasma tests for p-tau181 and p-tau217 are accurate and more specific than plasma Aβ42 for AD pathology
- The dynamics between CSF and blood are not well understood
- May not reflect the p-tau deposition in the brain accurately sometimes
- Individual variations are not well understood and can lead to discrepant results

T-tau:
- Nonspecific marker of neurodegeneration
- Often measured in CSF in association with other biomarkers of AD

NfL:
- Nonspecific marker of neurodegeneration
- Measured in plasma samples

GFAP:
- Nonspecific marker of neurodegeneration measured in plasma
- Associated with neuroinflammation
- Studies argue that AD has a component of neuroinflammation

TDP-43:
- Measured in plasma by using SIMOA technique which is extremely sensitive
- Sometimes found associated with AD pathology in the brain
- Can give important clues when there is a suspected non-AD pathology

Aβ40:
- Measured in plasma as an indicator of amyloidopathy in the brain
- Interpreted with Aβ42 as a ratio to discriminate AD (specific decline in Aβ42) and CAA (global Aβ decline)

(Aβ: amyloid beta; AD: Alzheimer's disease; CAA: cerebral amyloid angiopathy; CSF: cerebrospinal fluid; GFAP: glial fibrillary acidic protein; NfL: neurofilament light chain; PET: positron emission tomography)

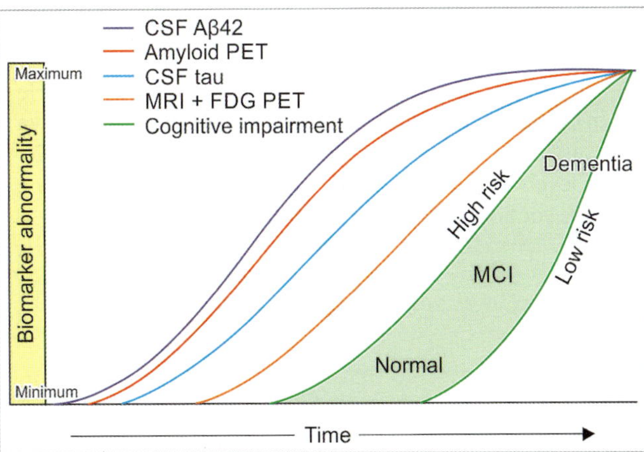

FIG. 1: The hypothetical model showing temporal progression of different biomarkers in AD. It is demonstrated that the cognitive symptoms fall behind the biomarker abnormalities by 10–15 years. This model is one of the most popular and well established one for understanding the temporal relation of biomarkers in the pathogenesis of AD.[23]

(Aβ: amyloid beta; AD: Alzheimer's disease; CSF: cerebrospinal fluid; FDG PET: fluorodeoxyglucose positron emission tomography; MCI: mild cognitive impairment; MRI: magnetic resonance imaging)

risk factors will likely have a more rapid progression in AD symptoms as compared to low-risk individuals. Protective genetic profile, higher cognitive reserve, and lesser comorbidities constitute a low risk profile for the development of AD.[6,23] This concept has been depicted in **Figure 1**.

The clinical implications for understanding the temporal relation among the AD biomarkers are multifold. First, it gives us an opportunity to diagnose the onset of AD pathology in the brain years before symptom onset or neuroimaging changes, more so in people with risk factors. Second, it gives us an insight about the pathogenetic process ongoing in AD and what to expect biologically at different stages of the disease. Third, current disease-modifying treatments in AD have a narrow therapeutic window. They are applicable to individuals with MCI or early dementia but mostly not beyond that. By the judicious use of biomarker assays, one can widen the therapeutic window of these disease-modifying agents by making an early biological diagnosis.

FLUID BIOMARKERS IN NON-ALZHEIMER'S DISEASE DEMENTIAS

Biomarkers for non-AD dementias is not as well established as AD in clinical practice so far. While there are some imaging modalities that have good predictive values for a particular form of dementia, fluid biomarkers are yet to come to mainstream clinical practice.

Frontotemporal Dementia

Biomarkers can help distinguish FTD from AD and sometimes in detection of presymptomatic individuals with a positive family history of FTD.[36] CSF t-tau is often used as a marker for nonspecific neurodegeneration. Similarly, plasma NfL value would indicate a neurodegenerative process. In several studies, plasma GFAP, a measure of astrogliosis, has been found raised in people with FTD, mostly GRN mutation carriers. Plasma TDP-43 has been found raised in people living with semantic dementia, a form of FTD. No specific fluid biomarker for FTD is available in clinical practice till date.

Dementia with Lewy Bodies

Based on clinical features and neuroimaging, dementia with Lewy bodies (DLB) is often considered in the twilight zone between AD and Parkinson's disease (PD). Aβ42 in body fluids is found diminished in both AD and DLB, while an oxidized form of Aβ40 is raised in CSF in people living with DLB. A promising biomarker for DLB is α-synuclein which is decreased in the body fluids in DLB.[37] It has however, yet to come to mainstream clinical practice. Understandably, nonspecific neurodegenerative markers are also to be found elevated in the body fluids.

Creutzfeldt–Jakob Disease

Cerebrospinal fluid t-tau is often found elevated in CJD that represents a neurodegenerative process. 14-3-3 is a protein that is commonly measured in the context of CJD but again is nonspecific. Real-time quaking-induced conversion (RT-QuIC) is a reliable method to detect the presence of prion protein in CSF and it has good sensitivity as well as specificity.

CASE VIGNETTES

In the current section, the author is going to describe a few typical real-life case scenarios that we often face in the memory/cognitive clinics worldwide. A summary of the case is presented in the beginning followed by the diagnostic question that led to the prescription of a CSF biomarker assay. In the end, the biological interpretation of the assay along with its clinical implication have been noted. Readers are requested to consult **Table 2** of this chapter to formulate the ATN classification in each of these cases.

CASE 1

Mr H, a 61-year-old highly educated man, presented with subjective complain of episodic memory impairment for 3 years. He did not have a family history of AD. There were no comorbidities either. Cognitive screening tests, including Montreal Cognitive Assessment (MoCA), were within normal limits. Clinically, he would be classified as having subjective cognitive impairment (SCI). MRI scan was largely unremarkable except mild cortical atrophy. Serum levels of vitamin B12 and thyroid-stimulating hormone (TSH) are within normal limits. However, his subjective memory complains continued to persist in the follow-up visit.

Diagnostic question: Is the SCI caused by Alzheimer's pathology?

The CSF test for biomarkers was as follows:

- Aβ42: 514 ng/L (>1,030 ng/L)
- P-tau: 18.62 ng/L (<28 ng/L)
- T-tau: 184.4 ng/L (<301 ng/L)
- P-tau/Aβ42: 0.0361 (<0.024)

According to the biomarker results, he is positive for Aβ pathology in the brain, suggestive of Alzheimer spectrum pathology, while his tau status is negative. He is at a higher risk of developing Alzheimer's dementia in the future given his positive biomarker status.

CASE 2

Mrs C, a 59-year-old lady, presented with anxiety, depression, and irritability for 2 years. This has affected her job as a nurse as she sometimes is forgetful too. Her father had a diagnosis of dementia at a later age. Cognitive test, MoCA, revealed a borderline score of 25/30 (cutoff 26/30). MRI brain showed mild ischemic vascular changes in the periventricular regions.

Diagnostic question: Could the anxiety and stress be an early manifestation of AD neuropathology in this case?

The CSF test for biomarkers was as follows:

- Aβ42: <150 ng/L (>1,030 ng/L)
- P-tau: 33.56 ng/L (<28 ng/L)
- P-tau/Aβ42: 0.224 (<0.024)

According to the biomarker results, she is positive for Aβ pathology in the brain. Her mild cognitive decline is likely associated with AD pathology. It has been noted that people with cognitive impairment and a positive Aβ status are more prone to developing neuropsychiatric symptoms than their Aβ negative counterparts.

CASE 3

Mrs B, a 64-year-old female, presented with rapid significant cognitive decline and walking difficulty for last 1 year. There were a few instances of urinary urgency and incontinence as well. MRI revealed supratentorial ventriculomegaly and acute callosal angles with gyral crowding and enlarged subarachnoid spaces, suggestive of normal pressure hydrocephalus (NPH).

Diagnostic question: Is there an additional amyloid pathology in the brain accounting for the out-of-proportion magnitude of cognitive impairment?

The CSF test for biomarkers was as follows:

- Aβ42: 1,063 ng/L (>1,030 ng/L)
- P-tau: 9.75 ng/L (<28 ng/L)
- P-tau/Aβ42: 0.009 (<0.024)

According to the biomarker results, she is negative for Aβ pathology in the brain. Therefore, this lady seems to have a non-AD pathology ongoing. It needs to be borne in mind that in NPH, due to hyperdynamic CSF flow, the biomarkers in the CSF may be diluted and reflect a falsely low estimation of p-tau. However, the Aβ value is on the higher side in this case, indicating only a minor role of CSF dilution in this specific individual's brain.

CONCLUSION

The definition of AD has undergone quite a few modifications in the last couple of decades. Currently, the diagnosis of AD is still majorly clinical and supported by relevant biomarker status. However, the research definition considers only the biomarker status of an individual to determine the presence of AD pathology. CSF biomarkers are slowly coming into clinical practice with some centers in India regularly performing these assays. This can not only help a clinician make a diagnosis of AD with higher certainty but also is essential when considering an individual's eligibility for disease-modifying clinical trials. Plasma biomarkers, although being used widely for research purposes, have some drawbacks in terms of accuracy. That said, p-tau181 and p-tau217 have shown excellent accuracy in predicting Aβ pathology. Modern cognitive neurology is taking its first few steps toward disease modification by bringing biomarkers into the scope of mainstream clinical practice. It has, however, a long way to go as the old Chinese proverb says, *"Journey of a thousand miles begins with a step."*

ACKNOWLEDGMENTS

I am sincerely thankful to my mentors Dr Howard Chertkow and Dr Stefano Cappa for their teachings and insights on biomarkers in dementia. My sincere gratitude to Dr Clifford R Jack for allowing me to freely use his illustrations for academic purposes. I would also thank each member of the clinical trials unit at the Rotman Research Institute, Toronto, for supporting me throughout my journey in cognitive neurology. A special note of thanks to Jennifer Cooper (University of British Columbia) for her valuable inputs in the plasma biomarker section. Above all, without the unwavering support of innumerable patients and their families, my journey in dementia biomarkers and clinical trials would never have started.

REFERENCES

1. Knopman DS, Petersen RC, Jack CR. A brief history of "Alzheimer disease": Multiple meanings separated by a common name. Neurology. 2019;92(22):1053-9.
2. McKhann G, Drachman D, Folstein M, Katzman R, Price D, Stadlan EM. Clinical diagnosis of Alzheimer's disease: Report of the NINCDS-ADRDA Work Group under the auspices of Department of Health and Human Services Task Force on Alzheimer's Disease. Neurology. 1984;34(7):939-44.
3. Bennett DA, Schneider JA, Buchman AS, Mendes De Leon C, Bienias JL, Wilson RS. The Rush Memory and Aging Project: Study Design and Baseline Characteristics of the Study Cohort. Neuroepidemiology. 2005;25(4):163-75.
4. McKhann GM, Knopman DS, Chertkow H, Hyman BT, Jack CR, Kawas CH, et al. The diagnosis of dementia due to Alzheimer's disease: Recommendations from the National Institute on Aging-Alzheimer's Association workgroups on diagnostic guidelines for Alzheimer's disease. Alzheimers Dement. 2011;7(3):263-9.
5. Cummings JL. Biomarkers in Alzheimer's disease drug development. Alzheimer Dement. 2011;7(3):e13-44.
6. Jack CR, Bennett DA, Blennow K, Carrillo MC, Dunn B, Haeberlein SB, et al. NIA-AA Research Framework: Toward a biological definition of Alzheimer's disease. Alzheimers Dement. 2018; 14(4):535-62.
7. Clark CM, Xie S, Chittams J, Ewbank D, Peskind E, Galasko D, et al. Cerebrospinal Fluid Tau and β-Amyloid: How Well Do These Biomarkers Reflect Autopsy-Confirmed Dementia Diagnoses? Arch Neurol. 2003;60(12):1696.
8. Crary JF, Trojanowski JQ, Schneider JA, Abisambra JF, Abner EL, Alafuzoff I, et al. Primary age-related tauopathy (PART): a common pathology associated with human aging. Acta Neuropathol. 2014;128(6):755-66.
9. Bennett DA, Schneider JA, Buchman AS, Barnes LL, Boyle PA, Wilson RS. Overview and Findings from the Rush Memory and Aging Project. Curr Alzheimer Res. 2012;9(6):646-63.
10. Hampel H, Cummings J, Blennow K, Gao P, Jack CR Jr, Vergallo A. Developing the ATX(N) classification for use across the Alzheimer disease continuum. Nat Rev Neurol. 2021;17(9): 580-9.
11. Jack CR, Andrews JS, Beach TG, Buracchio T, Dunn B, Graf A, et al. Revised criteria for diagnosis and staging of Alzheimer's disease: Alzheimer's Association Workgroup. Alzheimer's Dement. 2024;1-27.
12. Lashley T, Schott JM, Weston P, Murray CE, Wellington H, Keshavan A, et al. Molecular biomarkers of Alzheimer's disease: progress and prospects. Dis Model Mech. 2018;11(5): dmm031781.
13. Rabbito A, Dulewicz M, Kulczyńska-Przybik A, Mroczko B. Biochemical Markers in Alzheimer's Disease. Int J Mol Sci. 2020;21(6):1989.
14. Sharma N, Singh AN. Exploring Biomarkers for Alzheimer's Disease. J Clin Diagn Res. 2016;10(7):KE01-6.
15. Jeong HE, Shin DH, Lee DC. Medial Temporal Atrophy Alone is Insufficient to Predict Underlying Alzheimer's Disease Pathology. Korean J Fam Med. 2020;41(5):352-8.
16. Wahlund LO. Visual rating and volumetry of the medial temporal lobe on magnetic resonance imaging in dementia: a comparative study. J Neurol Neurosurg Psychiatry. 2000; 69(5):630-5.
17. Ferreira D, Nordberg A, Westman E. Biological subtypes of Alzheimer disease: A systematic review and meta-analysis. Neurology. 2020;94(10):436-48.
18. Tepmongkol S, Hemrungrojn S, Dupont P, Tunvirachaisakul C, Aniwattanapong D, Likitjareon Y, et al. Early prediction of donepezil cognitive response in Alzheimer's disease by brain perfusion single photon emission tomography. Brain Imaging Behav. 2019;13(6):1665-73.
19. Suppiah S, Didier MA, Vinjamuri S. The Who, When, Why, and How of PET Amyloid Imaging in Management of Alzheimer's

Disease—Review of Literature and Interesting Images. Diagnostics. 2019;9(2):65.

20. Zetterberg H. Applying fluid biomarkers to Alzheimer's disease. Am J Physiol Cell Physiol. 2017;313(1):C3-10.
21. Hampel H, Hardy J, Blennow K, Chen C, Perry G, Kim SH, et al. The Amyloid-β Pathway in Alzheimer's Disease. Mol Psychiatry. 2021;26(10):5481-503.
22. Hansson O, Seibyl J, Stomrud E, Zetterberg H, Trojanowski JQ, Bittner T, et al. CSF biomarkers of Alzheimer's disease concord with amyloid-β PET and predict clinical progression: A study of fully automated immunoassays in BioFINDER and ADNI cohorts. Alzheimers Dement. 2018;14(11):1470-81.
23. Jack CR, Knopman DS, Jagust WJ, Petersen RC, Weiner MW, Aisen PS, et al. Tracking pathophysiological processes in Alzheimer's disease: an updated hypothetical model of dynamic biomarkers. Lancet Neurol. 2013;12(2):207-16.
24. Fagan AM, Mintun MA, Mach RH, Lee S, Dence CS, Shah AR, et al. Inverse relation between in vivo amyloid imaging load and cerebrospinal fluid Aβ 42 in humans. Ann Neurol. 2006; 59(3):512-9.
25. De Kort AM, Kuiperij HB, Jäkel L, Kersten I, Rasing I, Van Etten ES, et al. Plasma amyloid beta 42 is a biomarker for patients with hereditary, but not sporadic, cerebral amyloid angiopathy. Alzheimers Res Ther. 2023;15(1):102.
26. Bateman RJ, Cummings J, Schobel S, Salloway S, Vellas B, Boada M, et al. Gantenerumab: an anti-amyloid monoclonal antibody with potential disease-modifying effects in early Alzheimer's disease. Alzheimers Res Ther. 2022;14(1):178.
27. Lahiri D, Roncero CT, Lima BS, Verhoeff NPLG, Freedman M, Al-Shamaa S, et al. A comparative study of Amyloid positive and negative individuals with "Alzheimer Syndrome." Alzheimers Dement. 2023;19(S14):e075037.
28. Landau SM, Horng A, Fero A, Jagust WJ; For the Alzheimer's Disease Neuroimaging Initiative. Amyloid negativity in patients with clinically diagnosed Alzheimer disease and MCI. Neurology. 2016;86(15):1377-85.
29. Rabinovici GD, Gatsonis C, Apgar C, Chaudhary K, Gareen I, Hanna L, et al. Association of Amyloid Positron Emission Tomography With Subsequent Change in Clinical Management Among Medicare Beneficiaries With Mild Cognitive Impairment or Dementia. JAMA. 2019;321(13):1286.
30. Nelson PT, Dickson DW, Trojanowski JQ, Jack CR, Boyle PA, Arfanakis K, et al. Limbic-predominant age-related TDP-43 encephalopathy (LATE): consensus working group report. Brain. 2019;142(6):1503-27.
31. Hansson O, Blennow K, Zetterberg H, Dage J. Blood biomarkers for Alzheimer's disease in clinical practice and trials. Nat Aging. 2023;3(5):506-19.
32. Brand AL, Lawler PE, Bollinger JG, Li Y, Schindler SE, Li M, et al. The performance of plasma amyloid beta measurements in identifying amyloid plaques in Alzheimer's disease: a literature review. Alzheimers Res Ther. 2022;14(1):195.
33. Zabala-Findlay A, Penny LK, Lofthouse RA, Porter AJ, Palliyil S, Harrington CR, et al. Utility of Blood-Based Tau Biomarkers for Mild Cognitive Impairment and Alzheimer's Disease: Systematic Review and Meta-Analysis. Cells. 2023;12(8):1184.
34. Thijssen EH, La Joie R, Strom A, Fonseca C, Iaccarino L, Wolf A, et al. Plasma phosphorylated tau 217 and phosphorylated tau 181 as biomarkers in Alzheimer's disease and frontotemporal lobar degeneration: a retrospective diagnostic performance study. Lancet Neurol. 2021;20(9):739-52.
35. Álvarez-Sánchez L, Peña-Bautista C, Ferré-González L, Balaguer A, Baquero M, Casanova-Estruch B, et al. Assessment of Plasma and Cerebrospinal Fluid Biomarkers in Different Stages of Alzheimer's Disease and Frontotemporal Dementia. Int J Mol Sci. 2023;24(2):1226.
36. Ntymenou S, Tsantzali I, Kalamatianos T, Voumvourakis KI, Kapaki E, Tsivgoulis G, et al. Blood Biomarkers in Frontotemporal Dementia: Review and Meta-Analysis. Brain Sci. 2021;11(2):244.
37. Schade S, Mollenhauer B. Biomarkers in biological fluids for dementia with Lewy bodies. Alzheimers Res Ther. 2014; 6(5-8):72.

CHAPTER

14

Neurogenetics of Dementia

Mohammed Faruq, Himanshi Kapoor

ABSTRACT

Dementia, an umbrella term encompassing various neurodegenerative disorders, heralds a daunting challenge in global healthcare. It leads to a progressive decline in cognition, emotional regulation, and behavioral patterns, significantly compromising individuals' functional ability. As longevity and life expectancy rise globally, the aging population burgeons, with a consequential surge in individuals aged 60 years and above. The World Alzheimer's Report 2015 forecasts a staggering rise in dementia prevalence, from approximately 55 million in 2020 to a projected 132 million by 2050, equating to a substantial increase of 25 million cases per decade. Alarmingly, low- and middle-income countries (LMICs) bear the brunt, accounting for 60% of current cases, and expected to escalate to approximately 70% by 2050. Within this context, it is disconcerting that an estimated 90% of individuals with dementia in India remain undiagnosed, underscoring pervasive healthcare disparities. In this context, understanding the genetic underpinnings of dementia holds paramount significance for diagnosis, prognosis, and targeted therapeutic interventions. As genetic research advances, personalized approaches to dementia management hold promise for mitigating the burgeoning global dementia burden. Therefore, the prime focus of this chapter is to encase the genetic factors associated with different dementia types and their prospective role in pathophysiology, diagnosis, and therapeutics.

Keywords: Genetic predisposition, Alzheimer's disease, Lewy body dementia, Frontotemporal dementia, Vascular dementia, Genome-wide association studies (GWAS), Next-generation sequencing (NGS).

INTRODUCTION

Dementia, a spectrum of neurodegenerative disorders, presents with clinical heterogeneity, overlapping symptoms, and poor prognosis. It severely affects cognition, behavior, and physical functioning in the diseased. Currently, over 55 million are affected due to dementia and aging is an important risk factor for the entire spectrum.[1,2] Thus, with rising longevity and life expectancy, it is bound to rise steeply. As per a global estimate, there will be an expected increase in people living with dementia to 132 million in 2050, a 25 million increase each decade.[3] Interestingly, the share of dementia burden from low- and middle-income countries (LMICs) is 60% and will be more by 2050 (~70%), yet given the inequality in access to healthcare in LMICs, it is estimated that 90% of Indian people living with dementia are not diagnosed.[3]

With the available clinical, paraclinical, and molecular tools, the dementia spectrum can be classified as Alzheimer's disease (AD), frontotemporal dementia (FTD), dementia with Lewy bodies (DLB), and vascular dementia (VaD). Despite advances in classification techniques, a considerable portion of cases within each subtype remain etiologically ambiguous. Although many dementia cases emerge to be sporadic, the involvement of genetic component and its modifications are instrumental for disease development and progression. Genetic factors exert significant influence, with both high-impact and modest-low-impact variations implicated in early and late-onset cases of dementia, respectively.[1,2] Understanding the neurogenetic basis of dementia is crucial for developing advanced therapeutics, prognostication, and for setting ease of diagnosis in a democratic way. In addition, superlative genetic tools like the next-generation sequencing (NGS), can pave the way for multipronged approach to tackling the disease, facilitating early picking of disease signatures and its etiology, and target-based drug development.

GENETIC DETERMINATION OF DIFFERENT DEMENTIA TYPES

Alzheimer's Disease

Alzheimer's disease represents the most prevalent dementia form, accounting for 60–80% of the diagnosed cases.[3] It presents as a typical proteinopathy, occurring due to extracellular accumulation of amyloid-beta (Aβ) plaques. Parallelly, the AD brain also exhibits the formation of hyperphosphorylated tau protein neurofibrillary tangles intracellularly. A majority of AD cases are known to be sporadic (late onset), whilst a few follow a distinct pattern of inheritance (familial-early onset). Etiologically, the causative reasons for AD can only be ascertained in a meaningful way in rare instances when the disease occurs in Mendelian fashion, while the majority of AD population remains unknown for its cause.[4,5] With the identification of amyloid precursor protein (*APP*) gene defects in familial AD (1990), and the subsequent presenilin 1 (*PSEN1*) and presenilin 2 (*PSEN2*) in monogenic AD, a contemplating theory of amyloid pathology was established.[6-8] Later, apolipoprotein E (*APOE4*) was identified as the main risk factor for late-onset (sporadic) AD.[9]

Amyloid-beta is the small (37–43 residue long) abnormal breakdown product of 2 consecutive cleavages of APP. As per the amyloid cascade hypothesis, the Aβ peptide accumulation, particularly Aβ42, leads to plaque formation, neuroinflammation, synaptic dysfunction, and neuronal death. Mutations in *APP*, *PSEN1*, and *PSEN2* exacerbate this process by increasing the production and aggregation of Aβ42.[4-9]

Genetic Factors Known in Association with Alzheimer's Disease

Early-onset Alzheimer's Disease (EOAD)

This accounts for less than 5% of AD cases and typically manifests before the age of 60. It shows a strongly associated genetic component. The likelihood of observing a genetic defect in known genes of AD is as high as ~80% in the multiple generations of an affected family. While young-onset AD without family history will manifest known gene defects in rare instances, together three of the genes, *APP*, *PSEN1*, and *PSEN2* explain 86% of cases with multigenerational history of AD[7-10] **(Fig. 1)**.

Amyloid precursor protein (APP):

- *Gene location and expression:* The *APP* gene is located on chromosome 21, which is why individuals with Down syndrome (trisomy 21) often develop AD pathology early. APP is ubiquitously expressed with high levels in neuronal tissues. Mutations in *APP* explain 15% cases of Mendelian AD.[7,11]
- *Structure of APP:* APP is a type I transmembrane protein comprising several domains: Extracellular E1 and E2 domains, a single transmembrane domain, and an intracellular C-terminal domain. The extracellular region includes the Kunitz protease inhibitor (KPI) domain in some isoforms.[7,11]
- *Processing pathways of APP*:
    - *Non-amyloidogenic pathway:* Alpha-secretase cleavage occurs within the Aβ domain, preventing Aβ peptide formation. This pathway produces soluble APP-alpha (sAPPα), and a non-toxic C-terminal fragment (CTF83).[7-9,11]

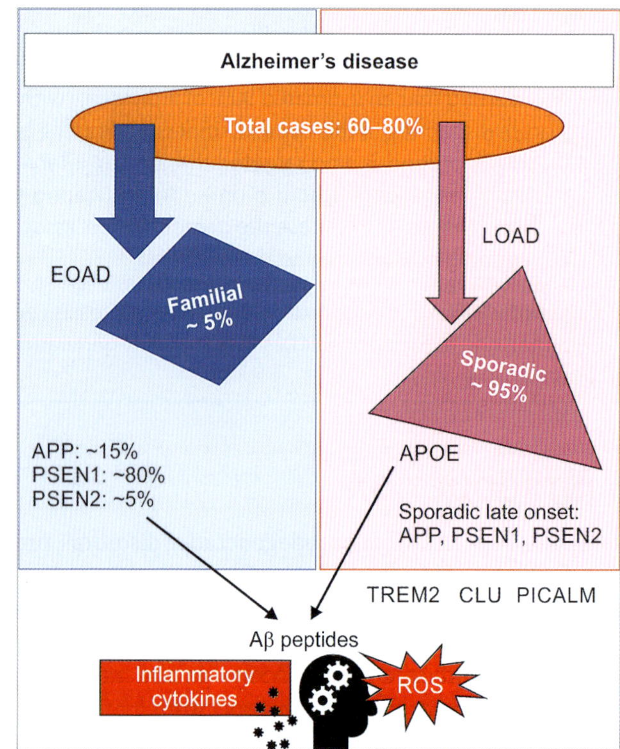

FIG. 1: Genetic determinants of early as well as late-onset Alzheimer's disease.

(Aβ: amyloid beta; APP: amyloid precursor protein; APOE: apolipoprotein E; CLU: clusterin; EOAD: early-onset Alzheimer's disease; LOAD: late-onset Alzheimer's disease; PICAKM: phosphatidylinositol binding clathrin-assembly protein; PSEN: presenilin; ROS: reactive oxygen species; TREM2: triggering receptor expressed on myeloid cells 2)

  - *Amyloidogenic pathway*: Beta-secretase cleavage occurs in APP at the N-terminus of the Aβ sequence, generating soluble APP-beta (sAPPβ) and a membrane-bound C-terminal fragment (CTF99 or C99).[7-9,11]
    - Gamma-secretase cleavage further cleaves C99 within the membrane, producing Aβ peptides, including Aβ40 and Aβ42, the latter being more prone to aggregation.[7-9,11]
- *APP mutations and their impact*: There are the following types of mutations **(Table 1)**:
  - *Point Mutations:* Single nucleotide changes leading to amino acid substitutions **(Table 1)**.
  - *Duplications:* Extra copies of the *APP* gene are made leading to increased expression and subsequent Aβ production **(Table 1)**.[9,10,12-21]
- Consequences of mutations in APP:
  - *Enhanced Aβ production*: Mutations like the Swedish mutation increase the substrate availability for γ-secretase, thereby raising overall Aβ levels.
  - *Altered Aβ42/Aβ40 ratio*: Mutations like the London mutation, which are near the γ-secretase cleavage site, preferentially increase Aβ42 production, which is more fibrillogenic and pathogenic.
  - *Increased Aβ aggregation*: Mutations within the Aβ sequence itself, such as the Arctic and Dutch mutations, promote the aggregation of Aβ peptides into oligomers and fibrils, contributing to plaque formation.
  - *Neurotoxicity and synaptic dysfunction*: The aggregation of Aβ peptides into oligomers and plaques

TABLE 1: Notable amyloid precursor protein (APP) mutations in Alzheimer's disease (AD).

APP mutation	Location	Impact	Clinical significance
Swedish mutation (KM670/671NL)	β-secretase cleavage site	Increases β-secretase cleavage, resulting in elevated production of both amyloid-beta 40 (Aβ40) and Aβ42 peptides	Associated with early-onset AD with rapid progression
Arctic mutation (E693G)	Within the amyloid-beta (Aβ) sequence	Promotes the formation of protofibrils, enhancing Aβ aggregation	Causes early-onset AD with severe amyloid pathology
London mutation (V717I)	γ-secretase cleavage site	Alters γ-secretase cleavage, increasing the Aβ42/Aβ40 ratio	Leads to early-onset AD with predominant amyloid plaque formation
Flemish mutation (A692G)	Within the Aβ sequence	Increases Aβ production and enhances aggregation propensity	Associated with cerebral amyloid angiopathy (CAA) and AD
Dutch mutation (E693Q)	Within the Aβ sequence	Enhances aggregation and CAA	Predominantly associated with hereditary cerebral hemorrhage with amyloidosis (HCHWA)
Iowa mutation (D694N)	Within the Aβ sequence	Increases Aβ aggregation and toxicity.	Leads to both AD and CAA, often with severe vascular amyloid deposition
Austrian mutation (T714I)	Near the γ-secretase cleavage site	Increases the Aβ42/Aβ40 ratio	Causes early-onset AD with pronounced amyloid pathology
Indiana mutation (V717F)	Similar to the London mutation, within the transmembrane domain	This mutation shifts the γ-secretase cleavage towards the production of Aβ42, enhancing its aggregation potential	Associated with early-onset AD, characterized by a rapid progression of cognitive decline
Iberian mutation (I716F)	Leads to an increased production of Aβ42 by altering γ-secretase cleavage	Leads to increased production of Aβ42 by altering γ-secretase cleavage	Causes early-onset AD with severe amyloid pathology
Italian mutation (E693K)	Within the Aβ domain	Increases the propensity of Aβ peptides to form toxic aggregates and enhances their neurotoxicity	Associated with early-onset AD and CAA
Tottori mutation (D678N)	Near the β-secretase cleavage site	Increases the production of Aβ42, enhancing its aggregation	Leads to early-onset AD and the formation of amyloid plaques.
Belgian mutation (E693Q)	Within the Aβ domain	Promotes aggregation and fibril formation of Aβ peptides	Causes early-onset AD and CAA

lead to synaptic dysfunction, neuroinflammation, and neuronal death.

- *Impact on cerebral vasculature:* Some APP mutations, like the Flemish mutation, also lead to cerebral amyloid angiopathy (CAA), characterized by the deposition of Aβ in the walls of cerebral blood vessels. This can cause vascular damage and microhemorrhages, and contribute to the overall pathogenesis of AD.[9,10,12-21]

Presenilin 1 and presenilin 2: *PSEN1* and *PSEN2* genes are known to be highly homologous. While missense mutations in *PSEN1* gene are one of the most frequent (60% cases of familial AD) causes of autosomal dominant AD, the PSEN2 mutations, on the contrary, are least frequent/rare. More than 185 mutations on *PSEN1* gene and 14 mutations on *PSEN2* gene account for inherited AD. Mutations in *PSEN1* gene cause the most severe AD forms, exhibiting complete penetrance. *PSEN1* gene mutation also leads to an early onset of the disease, at around 25 years of age. These mutations alter the γ-secretase activity, affecting both the site and efficiency of APP cleavage in Aβ fragments. These mutations lead to an elevated Aβ1–42/Aβ1–40 ratio, which may be because of an enhanced Aβ1–42 production or lower production of Aβ1–40, or a combination of both.[5-9]

- *Structure and function of presenilin:* PSEN1 and PSEN2 are integral membrane proteins and the catalytic core of the γ-secretase complex. This complex is responsible for the final cleavage of APP within its transmembrane domain to produce Aβ peptides. PSEN1 is more widely expressed and has a more prominent role in γ-secretase activity compared to PSEN2.[5-9]
- *Mutations in PSEN1 and PSEN2:* As discussed above, *PSEN1* mutations are the most common cause of familial AD, whereas the *PSEN2* mutations are less common but both result in a similar function—increase in Aβ42 production. Examples of PSEN1 and PSEN2 mutations include:
  - PSEN1 mutations—M146L, L286V, and E280A are well-documented mutations linked to early-onset AD. These mutations typically lead to a higher Aβ42/Aβ40 ratio.
  - PSEN2 mutations—N141I and M239V are examples, although less frequent, they also contribute to increased Aβ42 production and early-onset AD.[5-9]
- *Mechanisms of pathogenesis*:
  - *Amyloid cascade hypothesis:* This is the central theory in AD pathogenesis, according to which the accumulation of Aβ peptides (particularly Aβ42) leads to plaque formation, neuroinflammation, synaptic dysfunction, and neuronal death. Mutations in APP, PSEN1, and PSEN2 exacerbate this process by increasing the production and aggregation of Aβ42.
  - *Neuroinflammation and oxidative stress*: Aβ aggregates trigger microglial activation, leading to chronic neuroinflammation and the release of cytokines and reactive oxygen species (ROS), further damaging neurons.
  - *Synaptic dysfunction*: Aβ oligomers disrupt synaptic function by altering neurotransmitter release, receptor function, and synaptic plasticity, contributing to cognitive decline.[5-14]

Late-onset Alzheimer's Disease (LOAD)

It mostly presents with the disease after 65 years of age and is influenced by both genetic and environmental factors. Apoliporotein E (*APOE*) gene is the most significant genetic risk factor in LOAD.

APOE allele and AD: APOE is found on chromosome 19 and encodes for a polymorphic glycoprotein expressed in brain, liver, monocytes, and macrophages. The *APOE* ε4 (Arg112-Arg158) allele increases risk in familial and sporadic EOAD and LOAD, but it is not sufficient to cause disease whereas ε2 (Cys112-Cys158) allele is associated with protection against LOAD. In general population, *APOE* ε3 (Cys112-Arg158) is more prevalent. Thus, in general population, the frequency of *APOE3/APOE3* genotype is more common, while the risk of AD with genotype *APOE2/APOE2, APOE2/APOE3,* and *APOE4/APOE4* is 0.5-, 3-, and 8-fold. It is important to mention that nearly 50% cases of AD do not show APOE risk allele. The presence of the ε4 allele of the *APOE* gene significantly increases the risk of developing AD. APOE is a major component of high-density lipoproteins (HDL)-like particles in the brain and acts as a ligand in the brain for the transfer of cholesterol and lipids. APOE expression is observed in astrocytes and microglia. APOE isoforms have structural differences and have differential binding to low-density lipoproteins (LDL) receptors, APOE ε2 has the least binding affinity to them. APOE glycoproteins after lipidation, get extruded from the astrocytes to interact with the amyloid protein produced from the neuronal cells. APOE colocalizes with amyloid aggregates and facilitates its clearance. APOE ε4 is less effective at clearing Aβ from the brain compared to the more common ε3 allele followed by ε2, and thus aggregation propensity of amyloid is most seen in APOE ε4. Conversely, Aβ independent pathways are also involved in APOE-mediated AD pathogenesis as they can cause direct neuroinflammation, affect cerebral vascular integrity, metabolism, synaptic plasticity, and transcription.[5-9]

Common Genetic Markers for Sporadic Late-onset Alzheimer's Disease

As high-impact rare variations in *APP, PSEN1,* and *PSEN2* explain Mendelian forms of early-onset familial AD, on the other hand, common variants have been implicated with sporadic late-onset AD as elucidated by genome-wide association studies (GWAS). Genome-wide analysis leverage onto studying association with genetic markers in two phenotypically distinct groups using several thousand single nucleotide polymorphisms (SNPs). So far, studies conducted have identified close to 100 SNPs as GWAS signals in multiple genes ($n = 80$) **(Table 2)**.[4-6,20,21]

Along with *APOE*, numerous other genetic loci have been implicated in AD through GWAS. Majorly, these are involved in immunity, cholesterol metabolism, amyloid, protein ubiquitination, endocytosis, Tau and vascular components. Of the 80 GWAS-implicated AD risk loci, 49 are replicated by more than 1 study. These include genes involved in immune response [e.g., triggering receptor expressed on myeloid cells 2 (TREM2)], lipid metabolism [e.g., clusterin (CLU)], endocytosis [e.g., phosphatidylinositol binding clathrin-assembly protein (PICALM)], and other cellular processes. The cumulative effect of these variants, each contributing a small risk, can be substantial **(Table 2; Box 1 and Fig. 1)**.[2,4-6,20,21]

- *TREM 2:* Variants in TREM2, involved in microglial activation and response to injury, significantly increase AD risk. TREM2 mutations impair microglial function,

TABLE 2: Genome-wide association studies (GWAS) implicated loci.

Genes with >two studies supporting association	Genes with at least two studies supporting association	Novel associations		
SORL1	*NCK2*	*AGRN*	*PILRA*	*ZFP3*
SLC24A4	*MME*	*SORT1*	*NYAP1*	*MYO15A*
CR1	*TNIP1*	*ADAMTS4*	*CNTNAP2*	*GRN*
BIN1	*TREML2*	*ADAM17*	*CTSB*	*FAM171A2*
INPP5D	*TMEM106B*	*PRKD3*	*OPLAH*	*WNT3*
CD2AP	*SPDYE3*	*WDR12*	*SHARPIN*	*ABI3*
EPHA1	*ZCWPW1*	*HESX1*	*ABCA1*	*ALPK2*
CLU	*ECHDC3*	*IDUA*	*TSPAN14*	*CNN2*
FERMT2	*ANK3*	*RHOH*	*BLNK*	*KLF16*
ABCA7	*MS4A6A*	*ANKH*	*PLEKHA1*	*MEIOSIN*
CASS4	*EED*	*COX7C*	*PSMC3*	*MAMSTR*
HLA-DQA1	*TMEM121*	*MEF2C*	*CELF1*	*SIGLEC11*
MS4A4A	*SPPL2A*	*HAVCR2*	*TPCN1*	*LILRB2*
PICALM	*MINDY2*	*RASGEF1C*	*SNX1*	*LILRA5*
CLNK	*BCKDK*	*HLA-DRB1*	*CTSH*	*RBCK1*
UNC5CL	*IL34*	*OARD1*	*IQCK*	*CSTF1*
TREM2	*ZNF652*	*HS3ST5*	*DOC2A*	*SLC2A4RG*
PTK2B	*TSPOAP1*	*UMAD1*	*KAT8*	
USP6NL	*CYB561*	*ICA1*	*WWOX*	
SPI1	*ACE*	*JAZF1*	*MAF*	
ADAM10	*NECTIN2*	*GPR141*	*FOXF1*	
APH1B	*APP*	*EPDR1*	*PRDM7*	
PLCG2	*ADAMTS1*	*SEC61G*	*WDR81*	
SCIMP				
APOE				
CD33				

BOX 1 Gene ontology terms for genome-wide association studies (GWAS) signals.

- Regulation of amyloid-beta formation (GO:1902003)
- Negative regulation of amyloid precursor protein catabolic process (GO:1902992)
- Positive regulation of MAPK cascade (GO:0043410)
- Macrophage activation (GO:0042116)
- Negative regulation of macromolecule metabolic process (GO:0010605)
- Regulation of gene expression (GO:0010468)
- Negative regulation of amyloid-beta formation (GO:1902430)
- Negative regulation of neuron death (GO:1901215)
- Microglial cell activation (GO:0001774)
- Positive regulation of supramolecular fiber organization (GO:1902905)

(MAPK: mitogen-activated protein kinase)

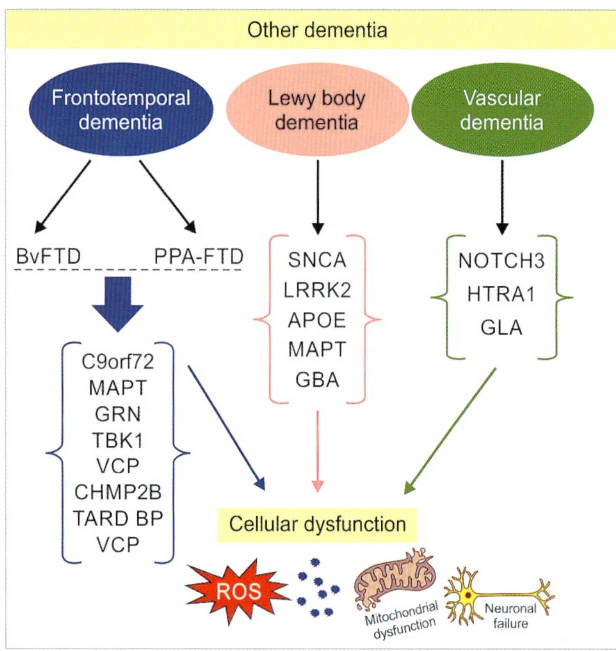

FIG. 2: Genetic determinants of other different dementia types.

leading to reduced clearance of Aβ and increased neuroinflammation.[2, 4-6,20,21]

- *CLU:* Involved in lipid transport and clearance of cellular debris, it is another gene implicated in AD. Variants in CLU may affect its protective role against Aβ aggregation.[2, 4-6,20,21]
- *PICALM:* It plays a role in clathrin-mediated endocytosis, essential for Aβ clearance. Variants in PICALM are thought to influence endocytic trafficking and Aβ metabolism.[2-6,20,21]

Role of Next-generation Sequencing in AD Genetics

Next-generation sequencing, being high throughput, has supported efficient AD diagnosis and prognosis. It is helpful in screening potential AD pathogenic variants as well as identifying the gain or loss of function in genes, if any. The technological advancements in NGS are now capable of detecting the presence of tandem deletion and duplications in the targeted disease-causing genes or any novel gene leading to the disease. With the advent of NGS, the genetic network of AD and associated genes has been explored extensively. This is instrumental for clinicians to trace the cause and progression of AD at molecular levels. Both hypothesis-free (whole-genome and whole-exome) and hypothesis-driven (targeted-exome) approaches for NGS will iron out the disease genetics further and help in designing novel and precision-based therapeutics.[22] *SORL1, TREM2, ABCA7, ABCA1, ATP8B4,* and *ADAM10* loci have been implicated through whole exome/whole genome studies. One study reported rare variants related to synaptic dysfunction, *FNBP1L, SEL1L, LINC00298, PRKCH, C15ORF41, C2CD3, KIF2A, APC, LHX9, NALCN, CTNNA2, SYTL3,* and *CLSTN2.*[23]

Frontotemporal Dementia

Frontotemporal dementia is a heterogeneous disorder characterized by degeneration of the frontal and temporal lobes, leading to changes in personality, behavior, and language **(Fig. 2)**.[24,25]

Clinical Variants of Frontotemporal Dementia

Frontotemporal dementia encompasses several clinical syndromes, primarily affecting personality, behavior, and language. The two main variants are:

- *Behavioral variant FTD (BvFTD):* Characterized by prominent changes in personality and social behavior, it involves degeneration of the frontal lobes.[24,25]
- *Primary progressive aphasia (PPA):* This variant primarily affects language abilities and is associated with atrophy in the temporal lobes. Further, PPA can be categorized into nonfluent/agrammatic, logopenic, and semantic variants.[24,25]

Nearly 30% of FTD is familial and genetic causes are identified in an autosomal dominant fashion. FTD with genetic causality is more common among bvFTD than PPA-FTD.[24,25]

Genetic Variants

Chromosome 9 open reading frame 72 (C9orf72) related FTD: C9orf72 is the most common genetic cause of FTD and amyotrophic lateral sclerosis (ALS). A hexanucleotide repeat expansion (GGGGCC) within the noncoding region of the gene is the primary mutation. Normal individuals typically have fewer than 30 repeats, while pathogenic expansions can range from 100 to 1,000. Clinically, patients with c9orf72 mutation have FTD-ALS presentation and cognitive dysfunction is global.[25-32]

- *Pathogenesis*: The exact mechanism by which the C9orf72 repeat expansion causes FTD is not fully understood, but several hypotheses have been proposed:
- *RNA toxicity*: The expanded repeats may form abnormal RNA structures, that may sequester RNA-binding proteins, disrupting normal cellular function.
- *Dipeptide repeat proteins*: Repeat-associated non-AUG (RAN) translation of the expanded RNA can produce toxic dipeptide repeat proteins.
- *Haploinsufficiency*: Reduced levels of C9orf72 protein may impair its normal function in endosomal trafficking and autophagy.

Microtubule-associated protein tau (MAPT) related FTD: Mutations in MAPT, encoding the tau protein, are a major cause of familial FTD (5–10%). Tau is essential for microtubule stabilization in neurons. Patients with MAPT defects are more affected by memory function.[25-32]

- *Pathogenesis*: Mutations in MAPT lead to the production of abnormal tau proteins that aggregate into neurofibrillary tangles, a hallmark of several neurodegenerative diseases, including FTD and AD.
- *Splicing mutations*: Some MAPT mutations affect the splicing of exon 10, altering the ratio of 3-repeat (3R) and 4-repeat (4R) tau isoforms, which can promote tau aggregation.
- *Missense mutations*: Other mutations alter the amino acid sequence of tau, reducing its ability to bind microtubules and promoting aggregation.
- *Clinical features*: MAPT mutations typically present with bvFTD, but can also lead to PPA, characterized by language deficits. The age of onset and clinical progression can vary widely among individuals.

Progranulin (GRN) related FTD: GRN mutations lead to haploinsufficiency of progranulin, a protein involved in neuronal survival and inflammation regulation. Reduced progranulin levels lead to increased neuroinflammation and neuronal loss, contributing to FTD pathology. GRN mutations are another significant cause of familial FTD. GRN encodes progranulin, a protein involved in cell growth, inflammation, and tissue repair. Clinically, PPA-FTD is associated with *GRN* gene defect. GRN mutations are associated with worsening attention function.[25-32]

- *Pathogenesis*: Mutations in GRN, often nonsense or frameshift, lead to progranulin haploinsufficiency. Reduced progranulin levels result in neuroinflammation and neuronal death.
- *Progranulin deficiency*: Insufficient progranulin disrupts lysosomal function and enhances neuroinflammatory responses, contributing to neurodegeneration.
- *Clinical features*: GRN mutation carriers typically present with bvFTD, but can also exhibit PPA. GRN mutations are associated with a wide range of symptoms, including Parkinsonism and corticobasal syndrome.

Additional Genetic Factors

Other genes, such as *TBK1, VCP, CHMP2B, TARDBP*, and *FUS*, have also been implicated in FTD, although they are less common. Each gene contributes to the complex genetic landscape of FTD, highlighting the disorder's heterogeneity.[25-32]

TAR DNA-binding protein 43 (TARDBP): Mutations in TARDBP (encoding TDP-43) lead to its mislocalization and aggregation. TDP-43 pathology is a hallmark of several FTD subtypes.[30]

Valosin-containing protein (VCP): Mutations in VCP (involved in protein homeostasis) cause inclusion body myopathy with early-onset Paget disease and FTD (IBMPFD). VCP mutations result in impaired protein degradation and accumulation of ubiquitinated proteins.[31]

Lewy Body Dementia

Lewy body dementia and Parkinson's disease dementia (PDD) are neurodegenerative disorders characterized by the presence of Lewy bodies—abnormal aggregates of the protein alpha-synuclein in neurons. Although they share clinical and pathological features, these conditions have distinct genetic predispositions[32-36] **(Fig. 2)**.

Genetic Predisposition to Lewy Body Dementia

- *Alpha-synuclein gene (SNCA): SNCA* (encodes alpha-synuclein) gene mutations are rare but significant. These include point mutations (e.g., A53T and E46K) and gene multiplications (duplications and triplications), leading to increased production or altered conformation of alpha-synuclein, promoting its aggregation into Lewy bodies.[33-37]
- *Glucocerebrosidase gene (GBA)*: Mutations in the *GBA* gene, which encodes the lysosomal enzyme glucocerebrosidase, are the most common genetic risk factor for LBD. These mutations reduce enzyme activity, leading to the accumulation of substrates that promote alpha-synuclein aggregation.[33-37]
- *Leucine-rich repeat kinase 2 (LRRK2)*: Mutations in the *LRRK2* gene are more commonly associated with Parkinson's disease but have also been found in some

cases of LBD. The LRRK2 protein is involved in various cellular processes, including neuronal survival and inflammation.[38,39]

- *APOE*: The APOE ε4 allele, known for its association with AD, also increases the risk of LBD. Its role in Lewy body pathology may involve lipid metabolism and Aβ deposition.[40]

Genetic Predisposition to Parkinson's Disease Dementia

- *SNCA gene*: Similar to LBD, mutations and multiplications of the *SNCA* gene increase the risk of developing PDD by enhancing alpha-synuclein levels or altering protein structure, promoting aggregation.[33-37]
- *GBA gene*: *GBA* mutations disrupt lysosomal function, leading to increased alpha-synuclein aggregation, and are a significant genetic risk factor for PDD.[33-37]
- *MAPT*: Certain haplotypes of the *MAPT* gene, which encodes the tau protein, are associated with an increased risk of developing PDD. Tau pathology often coexists with alpha-synuclein pathology, exacerbating neurodegeneration.[33-37]
- *LRRK2 Gene*: *LRRK2* mutations confer an increased risk for PDD. LRRK2 is thought to affect various cellular processes, including autophagy and mitochondrial function.[38,39]

Impact of SNCA Mutations on Lewy Body Pathology

Alpha-synuclein is abundant in the brain and implicated in synaptic function. Its abnormal aggregation is a hallmark of both LBD and PDD.[33]

Pathogenic mechanisms of *SNCA* mutations:

- *Increased expression:* Gene duplications and triplications result in increased alpha-synuclein expression, overwhelming cellular degradation pathways and leading to aggregation.[33,41]
- *Structural alterations:* Point mutations (e.g., A53T, E46K, and A30P) alter the structure of alpha-synuclein, making it more prone to misfolding and aggregation.[32,40]
- *Propagation:* Misfolded alpha-synuclein can act as a template, inducing normal alpha-synuclein to adopt a pathological conformation, spreading Lewy pathology throughout the brain.[33-41]

Effects on cellular function:

- *Synaptic dysfunction:* Alpha-synuclein aggregates disrupt synaptic vesicle trafficking, impairing neurotransmitter release and synaptic function.[33,41]
- *Mitochondrial dysfunction:* Aggregated alpha-synuclein impairs mitochondrial function, leading to energy deficits and increased oxidative stress.[33,41]
- *Autophagy and proteasome dysfunction:* Alpha-synuclein aggregates overwhelm cellular degradation pathways, including autophagy and the ubiquitin-proteasome system, leading to further protein accumulation and cell death.[33,41]

Vascular Dementia

Vascular dementia results from cerebrovascular pathology, including strokes and small vessel disease, leading to cognitive impairment. The genetic underpinnings of VaD are diverse and often overlap with those of cardiovascular diseases. Vascular dementia encompasses several subtypes, including multi-infarct dementia, strategic single-infarct dementia, subcortical ischemic vascular disease, and mixed dementia (VaD with AD pathology). These subtypes reflect the diverse cerebrovascular pathologies leading to cognitive impairment[2,42,43] **(Fig. 2)**.

Key Genetic Factors in Vascular Dementia

NOTCH3: Mutations in the *NOTCH3* gene cause cerebral autosomal dominant arteriopathy with subcortical infarcts and leukoencephalopathy (CADASIL), a hereditary form of small vessel disease leading to VaD.[42,43]

HTRA1: Mutations in the *HTRA1* gene are associated with cerebral autosomal recessive arteriopathy with subcortical infarcts and leukoencephalopathy (CARASIL), another genetic form of small vessel disease.[42,43]

Other Genetic Loci Implicated in Monogenic Form of Vascular Dementia

Alpha galactosidase enzyme A (GLA) (Fabry disease): In patients with Fabry disease (X-linked recessive disease), multiorgan accumulation of glycosphingolipid (globotriaosilceramide) may lead to small or large vessel disease, ischemic attack, renal disease, and cardiomyopathy.[42,43]

Retinal vasculopathy with cerebral leukodystrophy (RVCL): This is an autosomal dominant disorder, caused by frameshift mutations in three prime repair exonuclease 1 (*TREX1*), with manifestation typically occurring in fourth to fifth decade of life and has small vessel affection.[42,43]

COL4A1-A2 gene-related arteriopathy: In this disorder, autosomal dominant arteriopathies affecting small vessels occur and cause intracranial hemorrhage.[42,43.]

THERAPEUTIC IMPLICATIONS OF NEUROGENETICS IN DEMENTIA

The profound understanding of neurogenetics in dementia brings forth significant implications for targeted therapeutic approaches. By unraveling the genetic foundations of various dementia types, avenues for personalized medicine, gene-targeted therapies, and novel drug development strategies are paved. This section navigates through the current and future therapeutic landscape in dementia, spotlighting personalized medicine's potential, advancements in gene-targeted therapies and clinical trials, and the associated challenges and prospects in drug development.

Personalized Medicine Approaches

Genetic Profiling and Risk Assessment

Genetic profiling analyzes individual genetic variants to gauge dementia risk, allowing for proactive monitoring and early intervention strategies discussed as follows:

- *Personalized therapeutic strategies:* Tailored treatments based on genetic mutations include targeted therapeutics and biomarker-based treatments.
- *Early-onset AD:* This requires proactive cognitive assessments and participation in clinical trials for γ-secretase inhibitors in families with PSEN1 mutations.
- *FTD with GRN mutation:* This requires participation in clinical trials for gene therapy to increase progranulin levels.

Gene-targeted Therapies and Clinical Trials

Types of gene-targeted therapies: Dementia holds a huge burden on the individuals as well the nations. Although, its genetic predisposition and molecular underpinnings have been explored extensively but are poorly understood. The current therapeutic strategies available to tackle different forms of dementia are diffuse in mechanism and efficiency. Gene-targeted therapies for dementia are the need of hour as they are precise and promising, as seen in other diseases with strong genetic involvement. The following are some of the prospects of gene therapies in dementia:

- *Gene editing:* CRISPR-Cas9 technology for correcting pathogenic mutations, such as those in the *APP* gene
- *Gene therapy:* Introduction of functional copies of genes, like GRN, using viral vectors
- *Antisense oligonucleotides (ASOs):* Targeting MAPT mRNA to reduce abnormal tau protein production

Clinical trials and their outcomes:

- *Aducanumab in AD:* Mixed results regarding cognitive benefits highlight the need for further research.
- *Tau-targeted therapies in FTD:* Promising results in slowing disease progression through ASOs and small molecules
- *Progranulin replacement therapy:* Early-phase trials demonstrating safety and feasibility

Challenges and Prospects in Drug Development

Challenges in Drug Development

Complexity of disease mechanisms: Dementia is a multifactorial disease with varying pathogenesis. Overall, it is essential that the specific causative pathway be identified in order to administer effective therapeutics. Diagnosis of dementia itself is difficult, both due to obscure clinical presentations and detailed investigations required. This complexity in presentation and pathophysiological mechanisms renders difficulty in designing therapeutic interventions.

Blood-brain barrier (BBB): It is a semipermeable barrier which gatekeeps between the blood and the brain interstitium to protect the brain from systemic insults. While this is essential physiologically, it significantly hampers drug delivery to the brain through the accessible oral or peripheral intravenous routes. It is significantly challenging to overcome the hinderance of the BBB to drug delivery. One of the methods for this involves the use of alternative delivery routes such as the intrathecal, which are significantly invasive and prone to complications. Alternatively, emerging concepts to increase delivery across the BBB are being developed, which increase paracellular transport across the layer as well as evade the efflux mechanisms to pump molecules out of the interstitium. Some of these methods involve focused ultrasound-based delivery mechanisms, inducing transient inflammatory reaction, and use of nanoparticle packaging or even biomimicking like strategies.[44,45]

Clinical trial design: Dementia is a debilitating disease that presents with long trajectories and variable cognitive decline, which sometimes is very slow. Clinical trials for this require long study durations, which leads to attrition and multiple hurdles. Moreover, due to the varied pathophysiology, dementia tends to be a heterogenous disorder that requires reasonably accurate subgroup analysis in order to derive clinical insights from these trials.

Prospects in Drug Development

Combination therapies: Considering dementia is a group of disorders with varying pathophysiologies, it may be important to target multiple pathways simultaneously to improve efficacy.

Biomarker-driven approaches: To enhance the application of precision medicine in dementia therapeutics, it is important to guide therapy based on biomarkers to identify the major mechanisms to target in the disease. Biomarkers also enable precise tracking of disease progression and treatment response, to allow clinical decision-making regarding aggressiveness of therapy.

Artificial intelligence (AI) and big data: Accelerating drug discovery through data analytics and machine learning may help to introduce novel therapeutics in dementia. Data analysis may also allow for identification of dementia sub-phenotypes and endotypes based on accessible, parsimonious biomarker panels.

FUTURE DIRECTIONS

The future directions involve the following.

- *Regenerative medicine:* Stem cell therapies hold promise for replacing lost neurons and restoring neural function.
- *Epigenetic therapies:* These involve modulating epigenetic modifications to restore normal gene function.
- *Patient-centric trials:* These include incorporating patient perspectives and real-world evidence into clinical trials.

In conclusion, the therapeutic implications of neurogenetics in dementia are transformative. Personalized medicine approaches promise tailored treatments, while gene-targeted therapies and ongoing clinical trials offer hope for disease modification. Addressing challenges in drug development requires innovative strategies and collaboration across disciplines. As our understanding of the genetic basis of dementia advances, the goal of effective, personalized treatments draws closer.

CONCLUSION

The neurogenetics of dementia is a rapidly advancing field, providing critical insights into the mechanisms underlying these complex disorders. While significant progress has been made in identifying genetic risk factors and understanding their pathogenic roles, continued research is essential. Collaborative efforts in genetic research, coupled with advances in technology and therapeutics, will pave the way for improved diagnosis, treatment, and prevention of dementia. By translating genetic discoveries into clinical practice, we can offer hope to patients and families affected by these devastating conditions.

REFERENCES

1. Arvanitakis Z, Shah RC, Bennett DA. Diagnosis and management of dementia: Review. JAMA. 2019;322(16):1589-99.
2. Hinz FI, Geschwind DH. Molecular genetics of neurodegenerative dementias. Cold Spring Harb Perspect Biol. 2017;9(4):a023705.
3. Alzheimer's Disease International. (2015). World Alzheimer Report 2015. [online] Available from https://www.alzint.org/resource/world-alzheimer-report-2015/ [Last accessed July, 2024].
4. Neuner SM, Tcw J, Goate AM. Genetic architecture of Alzheimer's disease. Neurobiol Dis. 2020;143:104976.
5. Latimer CS, Lucot KL, Keene CD, Cholerton B, Montine TJ. Genetic insights into Alzheimer's disease. Annu Rev Pathol. 2021;16:351-76.
6. Bateman RJ, Xiong C, Benzinger TL, Fagan AM, Goate A, Fox NC, et al. Clinical and biomarker changes in dominantly inherited Alzheimer's disease. N Engl J Med. 2012;367(9):795-804.
7. Nilsberth C, Westlind-Danielsson A, Eckman CB, Condron MM, Axelman K, Forsell C, et al. The "Arctic" APP mutation (E693G) causes Alzheimer's disease by enhanced Abeta protofibril formation. Nat Neurosci. 2001;4(9):887-93.
8. Hendriks L, van Duijn CM, Cras P, Cruts M, Van Hul W, van Harskamp F, et al. Presenile dementia and cerebral haemorrhage linked to a mutation at codon 692 of the beta-amyloid precursor protein gene. Nat Genet. 1992;1(3):218-21.
9. Quan M, Cao S, Wang Q, Wang S, Jia J. Genetic phenotypes of Alzheimer's disease: Mechanisms and potential therapy. Phenomics. 2023;3(4):333-49.
10. Goate A, Chartier-Harlin MC, Mullan M, Brown J, Crawford F, Fidani L, et al. Segregation of a missense mutation in the amyloid precursor protein gene with familial Alzheimer's disease. Nature. 1991;349(6311):704-6.
11. Hardy J, Selkoe DJ. The amyloid hypothesis of Alzheimer's disease: Progress and problems on the road to therapeutics. Science. 2002;297(5580):353-6.
12. Prasher VP, Farrer MJ, Kessling AM, Fisher EM, West RJ, Barber PC, et al. Molecular mapping of Alzheimer-type dementia in Down's syndrome. Ann Neurol. 1998;43(3):380-3.
13. Levy E, Carman MD, Fernandez-Madrid IJ, Power MD, Lieberburg I, van Duinen SG, et al. Mutation of the Alzheimer's disease amyloid gene in hereditary cerebral hemorrhage, Dutch type. Science. 1990;248(4959):1124-6.
14. Grabowski TJ, Cho HS, Vonsattel JP, Rebeck GW, Greenberg SM. Novel amyloid precursor protein mutation in an Iowa family with dementia and severe cerebral amyloid angiopathy. Ann Neurol. 2001;49(6):697-705.
15. Murrell J, Ghetti B, Cochran E, Macias-Islas MA, Medina L, Varpetian A, et al. The A431E mutation in *PSEN1* causing Familial Alzheimer's Disease originating in Jalisco State, Mexico: an additional fifteen families. Neurogenetics. 2006;7(4):277-9.
16. Lanoiselée HM, Nicolas G, Wallon D, Rovelet-Lecrux A, Lacour M, Rousseau S, et al. APP, PSEN1, and PSEN2 mutations in early-onset Alzheimer disease: A genetic screening study of familial and sporadic cases. PLoS Med. 2017;14(3):e1002270.
17. Kamino K, Orr HT, Payami H, Wijsman EM, Alonso ME, Pulst SM, et al. Linkage and mutational analysis of familial Alzheimer disease kindreds for the APP gene region. Am J Hum Genet. 1992;51(5):998-1014.
18. Tomiyama T, Nagata T, Shimada H, Teraoka R, Fukushima A, Kanemitsu H, et al. A new amyloid beta variant favoring oligomerization in Alzheimer's-type dementia. Ann Neurol. 2008;63(3):377-87.

19. Sellal F, Wallon D, Martinez-Almoyna L, Marelli C, Dhar A, Oesterlé H, et al. APP mutations in cerebral amyloid angiopathy with or without cortical calcifications: Report of three families and a literature review. J Alzheimers Dis. 2017;56(1):37-46.
20. Lambert JC, Ibrahim-Verbaas CA, Harold D, Naj AC, Sims R, Bellenguez C, et al. Meta-analysis of 74,046 individuals identifies 11 new susceptibility loci for Alzheimer's disease. Nat Genet. 2013;45(12):1452-8.
21. Andrews SJ, Renton AE, Fulton-Howard B, Podlesny-Drabiniok A, Marcora E, Goate AM. The complex genetic architecture of Alzheimer's disease: Novel insights and future directions. EBioMedicine. 2023;90:104511.
22. Hardy J, Selkoe DJ. The amyloid hypothesis of Alzheimer's disease: Progress and problems on the road to therapeutics. Science. 2002;297(5580):353-6.
23. Chandy T. Intervention of next-generation sequencing in diagnosis of Alzheimer's disease: Challenges and future prospects. Dement Neuropsychol. 2023;17:e20220025.
24. Prokopenko D, Morgan SL, Mullin K, Hofmann O, Chapman B, Kirchner R; Alzheimer's Disease Neuroimaging Initiative (ADNI); et al. Whole-genome sequencing reveals new Alzheimer's disease-associated rare variants in loci related to synaptic function and neuronal development. Alzheimers Dement. 2021;17(9):1509-27.
25. Bang J, Spina S, Miller BL. Frontotemporal dementia. Lancet. 2015;386(10004):1672-82.
26. Seelaar H, Rohrer JD, Pijnenburg YA, Fox NC, van Swieten JC. Clinical, genetic and pathological heterogeneity of frontotemporal dementia: A review. J Neurol Neurosurg Psychiatry. 2011;82(5):476-86.
27. DeJesus-Hernandez M, Mackenzie IR, Boeve BF, Boxer AL, Baker M, Rutherford NJ, et al. Expanded GGGGCC hexanucleotide repeat in noncoding region of C9ORF72 causes chromosome 9p-linked FTD and ALS. Neuron. 2011;72(2):245-56.
28. Rohrer JD, Warren JD. Phenotypic signatures of genetic frontotemporal dementia. Curr Opin Neurol. 2011;24(6):542-9.
29. Hutton M, Lendon CL, Rizzu P, Baker M, Froelich S, Houlden H, et al. Association of missense and 5'-splice-site mutations in tau with the inherited dementia FTDP-17. Nature. 1998;393(6686):702-5.
30. Baker M, Mackenzie IR, Pickering-Brown SM, Gass J, Rademakers R, Lindholm C, et al. Mutations in progranulin cause tau-negative frontotemporal dementia linked to chromosome 17. Nature. 2006;442(7105):916-9.
31. Mackenzie IR, Rademakers R, Neumann M. TDP-43 and FUS in amyotrophic lateral sclerosis and frontotemporal dementia. Lancet Neurol. 2010;9(10):995-1007.
32. Watts GD, Wymer J, Kovach MJ, Mehta SG, Mumm S, Darvish D, et al. Inclusion body myopathy associated with Paget disease of bone and frontotemporal dementia is caused by mutant valosin-containing protein. Nat Genet. 2004;36(4):377-81.
33. Koriath CAM, Kenny J, Ryan NS, Rohrer JD, Schott JM, Houlden H, et al. Genetic testing in dementia—utility and clinical strategies. Nat Rev Neurol. 2021;17(1):23-36.
34. Singleton AB, Farrer M, Johnson J, Singleton A, Hague S, Kachergus J, et al. Alpha-synuclein locus triplication causes Parkinson's disease. Science. 2003;302(5646):841.
35. Zarranz JJ, Alegre J, Gómez-Esteban JC, Lezcano E, Ros R, Ampuero I, et al. The new mutation, E46K, of alpha-synuclein causes Parkinson and Lewy body dementia. Ann Neurol. 2004;55(2):164-73.
36. Sidransky E, Nalls MA, Aasly JO, Aharon-Peretz J, Annesi G, Barbosa ER, et al. Multicenter analysis of glucocerebrosidase mutations in Parkinson's disease. N Engl J Med. 2009;361(17):1651-61.
37. Schapira AH, Chiasserini D, Beccari T, Parnetti L. Glucocerebrosidase in Parkinson's disease: Insights into pathogenesis and prospects for treatment. Mov Disord. 2016;31(6):830-5.
38. Paisán-Ruíz C, Jain S, Evans EW, Gilks WP, Simón J, van der Brug M, et al. Cloning of the gene containing mutations that cause PARK8-linked Parkinson's disease. Neuron. 2004;44(4):595-600.
39. Healy DG, Falchi M, O'Sullivan SS, Bonifati V, Durr A, Bressman S, et al. Phenotype, genotype, and worldwide genetic penetrance of LRRK2-associated Parkinson's disease: A case-control study. Lancet Neurol. 2008;7(7):583-90.
40. McKeith IG, Boeve BF, Dickson DW, Halliday G, Taylor JP, Weintraub D, et al. Diagnosis and management of dementia with Lewy bodies: Fourth consensus report of the DLB Consortium. Neurology. 2017;89(1):88-100.
41. Liao F, Yoon H, Kim J. Apolipoprotein E metabolism and functions in brain and its role in Alzheimer's disease. Curr Opin Lipidol. 2017;28(1):60-7.
42. Greaves CV, Rohrer JD. An update on genetic frontotemporal dementia. J Neurol. 2019;266(8):2075-86.
43. Ikram MA, Bersano A, Manso-Calderón R, Jia JP, Schmidt H, Middleton L, et al. Genetics of vascular dementia—review from the ICVD working group. BMC Med. 2017;15(1):48.
44. Paulson HL, Igo I. Genetics of dementia. Semin Neurol. 2011;31(5):449-60.
45. Hersh DS, Wadajkar AS, Roberts N, Perez JG, Connolly NP, Frenkel V, et al. Evolving drug delivery strategies to overcome the blood brain barrier. Curr Pharm Des. 2016;22(9):1177-93.

CHAPTER

15

Language Assessment and Speech Therapy in Primary Progressive Aphasia

Avanthi Paplikar, Aparna Venugopal, Sneha Rozelena Anthony

ABSTRACT

Primary progressive aphasia (PPA) is classified based on distinct speech and language characteristics. A comprehensive assessment of speech and language abilities by a trained speech–language pathologist is essential for diagnosis and planning individualized therapeutic goals for PPA. PPA assessment by a speech–language pathologist should focus on multiple domains such as speech motor production, comprehension, naming, conceptual knowledge, syntax, repetition, reading, and spelling. Therapeutic targets can be planned based on the extent of impairment in each of these domains. Using an impairment-based therapeutic approach, compensatory strategies, and group education of individuals with PPA and their caregivers, quality of life of patients will be improved. Successful delivery of services by speech–language pathologists is only possible through creating awareness among related health professionals about the importance of timely referrals for speech–language assessment and intervention.

Keywords: Neurodegenerative disorders, Primary progressive aphasia, Frontotemporal dementia, Speech and language assessment, Speech and language therapy.

INTRODUCTION

Primary progressive aphasias (PPAs) are a heterogeneous group of clinical disorders resulting from relatively focal neurodegeneration of frontal and temporal areas of the brain responsible for speech and language. It features communication difficulties affecting daily functionality, without any primary cognitive/behavioral impairments. Since communication difficulties are most prominent symptoms at the onset and initial stages of PPA, comprehensive evaluation by a speech-language pathologist (SLP) is an integral part of the diagnostic and rehabilitative process. This aids in identification, differential diagnosis of PPA phenotypes, setting up therapy goals, prediction, and monitoring cognitive-linguistic changes over time.

There are three clinical phenotypes of PPA: Semantic (svPPA), nonfluent/agrammatic (nfvPPA), and logopenic (lvPPA) based on distinct speech and language impairments and specific neural networks involved. The criteria for three clinical variants are developed by an international group of PPA investigators.[1] The diagnostic labeling based on the core features is represented in **Flowchart 1**.

SPEECH AND LANGUAGE ASSESSMENT OF PRIMARY PROGRESSIVE APHASIA

A comprehensive understanding of the onset and progression of language disturbances in PPA is possible through detailed case history and speech-language assessments. A clinician should record sociodemographic details, language background, relevant family history, medical/psychiatric illness, sensory impairment, and nonlinguistic symptoms (motor, cognitive, and behavioral). Further assessment of PPA by SLP should focus on multiple domains: Speech motor functioning, single word and sentence comprehension, naming,

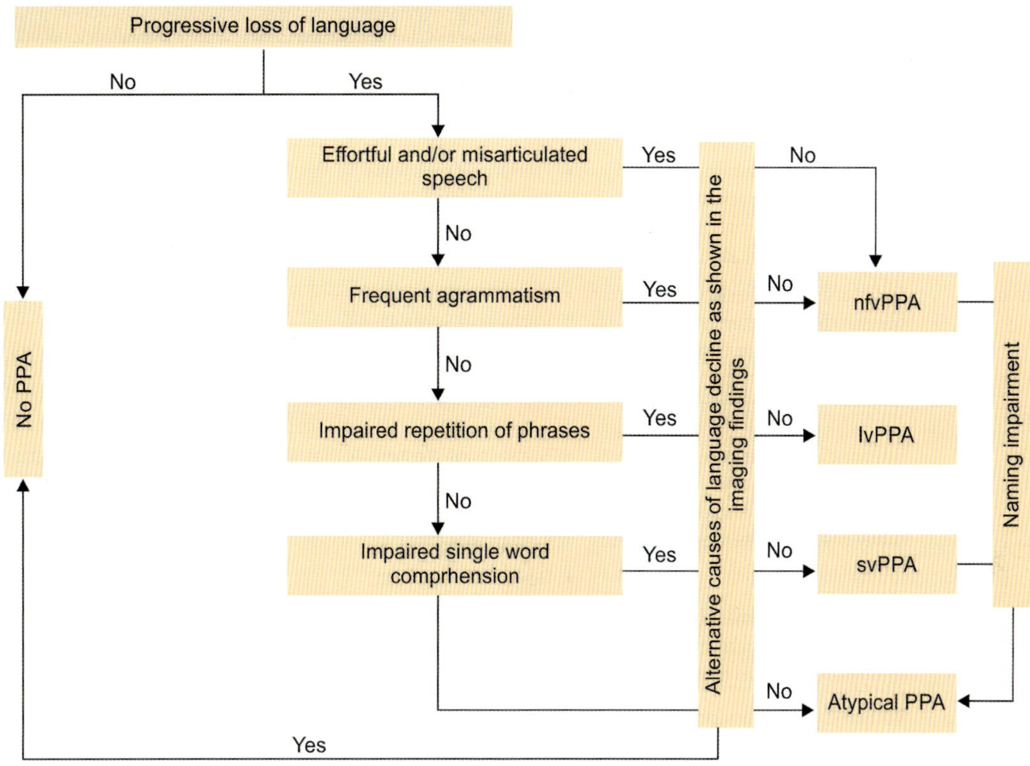

FLOWCHART 1: The diagnostic tree diagram of PPA variants based on the key features.

(lvPPA: logopenic variant of primary progressive aphasia; nfvPPA: nonfluent/agrammatic variant primary progressive aphasia; PPA: primary progressive aphasia; SvPPA: semantic variant primary progressive aphasia)

conceptual knowledge, syntax, repetition, reading, and spelling that are impaired in PPA. Most of the common test batteries developed for poststroke aphasia are sometimes used in conjunction with case history and interviews for accurate diagnosis of PPA.

Assessment of Global Language Function

Overall linguistic abilities and severity of communication impairment at baseline and during PPA progression are profiled using test batteries like the Western Aphasia Battery (WAB)[2] and the Boston Diagnostic Aphasia Examination (BDAE).[3] In India, the adapted version of WAB,[4] All India Institute of Medical Sciences (AIIMS) Diagnostic Test of Aphasia,[5] and the Indian Aphasia Battery[6] are the most commonly used language tests. These test batteries may lack the sensitivity to detect early speech and linguistic changes in PPA.[7] Hence, specific tests have been developed to diagnose and monitor PPA progression.

Differential Diagnosis and Severity Rating of Primary Progressive Aphasia

Mini Linguistic Status Examination (MLSE)[8] is a novel screening tool for the differential diagnosis of classical variants of PPA. Sydney Language Battery[9] and Repeat and Point test[10] are also quick and simple tests for PPA classification. Progressive Aphasia Severity Scale (PASS)[11] assesses the severity of impairments based on structured interview of informants and individuals with PPA. The Progressive Aphasia Language Scale (PALS)[12] is another quick and simple bedside measure for PPA grading.

Assessment of Specific Language Domains in Primary Progressive Aphasia

It is essential to administer tests for assessment of specific language domains and differential diagnosis of PPA variants **(Table 1)**. Naming tests are used to assess the degree of naming impairment which is highest in svPPA followed by lvPPA and nfvPPA. Semantic association and word-to-picture matching tasks suggest impairment in object/person knowledge and single-word comprehension, which is prominently seen in svPPA. Tests of syntax such as Northwestern assessment of verbs and sentences, and Northwestern anagram test reveal poor performance on receptive and expression of syntactical structures in nfvPPA.[13] Phonological memory deficits in lvPPA can cause difficulties in formulating complex and low-probability sentence structures in lvPPA. Word and sentence repetition assessments imply

TABLE 1: Tasks and tests for speech and language evaluation to identify primary progressive aphasia (PPA).[1]

Speech and language subdomains	Tasks	Specific tests in a global context	Impaired in
Speech production			
Motor speech mechanism	Speech motor examination, spontaneous speech, diado-chokinetic movements, and repetition of multisyllabic utterances	• Frenchay Dysarthria Assessment[29] • Apraxia Battery of Adults[14]	Nonfluent/agrammatic variant
Syntax/grammar	Spontaneous speech, connected speech tasks, sentence generation, and sentence completion task	• Northwestern Assessment of Verbs and Sentences[30] • Northwestern Anagram Test[13]	Nonfluent/agrammatic variant
Comprehension			
Sentence comprehension	Responding to yes/no questions, following single- and multiple-step commands, and matching orally presented sentences with pictures	• Subtests of Western Aphasia Battery[2] • Boston Diagnostic Aphasia Examination[3] • Revised Token Test[31]	• Nonfluent/agrammatic variant with presence of difficulty in grammatically complex sentences • Logopenic variant with difficulty in long and less frequent sentences
Single-word comprehension	Word-to-picture matching, word-to-synonym matching, and word-to-definition matching	• Pyramids and Palm Tree[32] • Peabody Picture Vocabulary Test[33]	Semantic variant
Confrontation naming	Verb and noun naming task	• Boston Naming Test[34] • Northwestern Naming Battery[13]	• Semantic variant > logopenic variant • Semantic errors in semantic variant • Phonemic errors in logopenic variant
Repetition	Repetition of words and phrases of increasing length and complexity and repetition of nonwords	• Subtests of Western Aphasia Battery[2] • Boston Diagnostic Aphasia Examination[3]	Logopenic variant with the presence of phonemic paraphasia
Conceptual knowledge (objects/persons)	Picture–picture matching based on given semantic relations, gesture–object matching, auditory stimuli–picture matching, semantic associations task, and odd-one out	• Pyramids and Palm Tree test[32] • Peabody Picture Vocabulary Test[33]	Semantic variant
Reading, writing/ spelling	Reading of regular, irregular, nonwords, spoken word–written word matching matching, writing to dictation	Arizona Battery of Reading and Spelling[35]	• Semantic variant with the presence of surface dyslexia (regularize irregular words) • Logopenic variant with presence of phonological errors

difficulty in repeating complex and low-probability words and sentences, nonwords, and semantically anomalous sentences due to the phonological working memory deficits for lvPPA. Meanwhile, repetition errors in nfvPPA are attributed to motor speech impairment like dysarthria and apraxia.

Motor speech evaluation involves the examination of speech subsystem, which includes diadochokinetic rate, repetition of multisyllabic utterances of increasing length and complexity, and articulatory groping.[14] Surface dyslexia/dysgraphia, difficulty reading nonwords and irregular words associated with lvPPA can be detected using reading and spelling tests. Although the connected speech analysis demands expertise and effort, picture description using a WAB-picnic scene or cookie theft picture of BDAE can classify PPA by revealing multi-faceted elements like speech fluency, rate, mean utterance length, grammar, word retrieval, and motor speech impairment.

The currently available test batteries are time-consuming and are not ecologically valid for PPA. Hence, clinicians often carry out informal assessments using simple tasks to determine clinical subtype of PPA **(Table 1)**. In the Indian context, there are limited tools for speech and language assessment specifically in PPA. Tests developed for the English-speaking population cannot be used in the Indian context due to the linguistic and cultural differences. Linguistically and culturally relevant tools in the Indian context for assessing semantic impairment are Indian Semantic Battery (ISMB)[15] the Indian Council of Medical Research-Picture Naming Test (ICMR-PNT)[16] The "Autorickshaw task" a nonverbal association task of ISMB is sensitive to detect semantic impairment among PPAs.

The extent of impairment in daily functionality, quality of life, and participation limitation in PPA can be assessed using specific scales and questionnaires.[17] Ecologically validated neuropsychological tests can detect nonlinguistic cognitive impairments developing at later stages of PPA along with linguistic assessments to supplement differential diagnosis of PPA.

SPEECH THERAPY FOR PRIMARY PROGRESSIVE APHASIA

The communication difficulties in PPA range from trouble expressing basic needs and preferences to engaging in complex interactions that involve the communication of financial and legal decisions. Through comprehensive assessment and individualized treatment plans that target specific impairments, SLPs enable individuals with PPA to communicate independently in all levels of social situations. Evidence from research, practice, and preferences of a fully informed patient is used for deciding the intervention plans. According to literature, speech and language interventions for PPA can be divided into: Impairment-based approaches, compensatory-based approaches, and group education and support.

Impairment-based Approach

Lexical Retrieval Treatment

Lexical retrieval treatment is the most extensively researched impairment-based approach that reduces word-finding difficulty and slows down further decline of personally relevant and meaningful words. This involves a cueing heirarchy based on "lexical retrieval cascade treatment." It has proven to be beneficial for individuals with svPPA and lvPPA. Furthermore, this intervention method facilitates word retrieval and encourages self-cueing by recruiting spare semantic, phonological, and orthographic knowledge.[18] The intervention starts with semantic self-cueing, followed by orthographic, phonemic, and repetition. Semantic cues were found to be useful in svPPA whereas phonological cues were better for nfvPPA. Semantic elaboration improved the naming for lvPPA, and the effect was maintained for 6 months post-therapy. The benefit also extended to untreated items, syntactic generation tasks, and discourse measures.[19] The selection of personally relevant stimuli and retraining daily vocabulary are vital for the success of this approach.

Repetition Treatment

Repetition and/or reading in the presence of a picture (RRIPP) is another word retrieval treatment.[20] It is a look, listen, and repeat strategy to improve oral naming for trained items with or without generalization and maintenance of gains.

Constraint-induced Aphasia Therapy

Constraint-induced aphasia therapy (CIAT) is a method widely used in treating persons with poststroke aphasia. The following principles underpin this approach: Massed practice, shaping, and constraint of compensatory communication (nonverbal) strategies. Intensive CIAT in groups with computer-based home programs was found to significantly improve noun and verb retrieval as well as grammatical structure in nfvPPA.[21]

Spaced Retrieval

Spaced retrieval therapy helps individuals with dementia in recalling a variety of information over longer periods of time. Spaced retrieval, combined with semantic therapy, improves naming and generation of semantic attributes. Treatment effects last for 5 weeks following termination of therapy with or without generalization.[22]

Cueing Hierarchy

A cue serves as a signal that guides the production of the correct response. Several cues that benefit individuals with anomia are functional cues, semantic cues, categorical cues, and phonemic cues. lvPPA had more advantage on naming than svPPA using the cueing technique.[23] Moreover, only lvPPA exhibited generalization of treatment across untreated items. These results indicate that cueing hierarchy promotes access to the phonological lexicon, in turn improving naming skills in PPA. The cueing hierarchy used is as follows:

- Spontaneous naming of the pictured object
- Written naming of the pictured object, followed by oral reading of written name
- Search for the written name of the stimulus, followed by oral reading of the written name
- Read the written name after it is identified by the clinician
- Repeat the name of the stimulus

Transcranial Magnetic Stimulation and Transcranial Direct Current Stimulation

Transcranial magnetic stimulation (TMS) is a noninvasive procedure that normalizes neural activity in cortical areas of metabolic dysfunction. High-frequency TMS directly strengthens neural connections in the damaged cortical area. In recent studies, researchers have utilized TMS to enhance verb production and oral and written language in individuals with PPA.[24] Further, transcortical direct current stimulation (tDCS) was proven to strengthen the effects of lexical retrieval treatment when used along with speech-language therapy.[25] There is a need for future studies to evaluate the effectiveness of tDCS and TMS as the current evidence is limited.

Script Training

Script training is a technique that involves repeated practice of phrases and sentences in the form of a monologue or a dialogue to improve fluency and speech production. It can be used to treat apraxia, nonfluent speech, and agramatism by repeating syntactically accurate utterances in nfvPPA. Video-implemented script training for aphasia (VISTA) was found to have both immediate and long-term effects in nfvPPA.[26] Treatment involved repeated rehearsal of the script with the clinician and intensive home practice using speech entrainment (imitation of audiovisual speech model in real-time). Post-treatment results showed a considerable improvement in accuracy, intelligibility of scripted words for the trained topic, and an overall reduction in grammatical errors. The treatment effect was maintained for a duration of 1 year.

Treating Apraxia of Speech

Gradual decline in speech motor planning (apraxia of speech) is one of the most prominent symptoms of nfvPPA. Motor speech deficits are mild in the early stage of the disease and persist for several years.[27] Early intervention may help to slow down the progression of speech motor deficits. Henry et al investigated the effectiveness of structured oral reading as a therapy approach for improving the production of multisyllabic words in an individual with nfvPPA. Initially, the individual was made to read aloud until an incorrect production of a word. The word was then underlined in the text and divided into its constituent syllables. Further, the individual was instructed to say the word syllable-by-syllable until each syllable was produced correctly. The whole word was then repeated in a syllabified manner. Finally, once the word was mastered in isolation, the participant was asked to read from the beginning of the text and attempt to produce the word again. Treatment sessions lasted for 1 hour each week for 12 weeks. Results demonstrated a reduction in speech errors during the reading of text that was maintained for 1 year post-treatment.

Multimodal Strategy

Multimodal language stimulation improves everyday communication skills in PPA.[28] This approach focuses on developing comprehension and expression skills by engaging in activities such as picture naming, picture description, comprehension of complex commands, and enhancing conversational skills. Communication strategies are incorporated through conversation tasks that involve speaking, writing, drawing, or gesturing. Moreover, individuals are given opportunities to develop effective strategies for overcoming communication barriers. This approach mitigates the gradual decline of language abilities in individuals with PPA.

Computer-based Interventions

MossTalk Words is an evidence-based computer-assisted program specifically designed for treating individuals with aphasia. This program constitutes separate modules for auditory comprehension, word retrieval, and reading comprehension. Clinician-guided therapy using MossTalk Words will benefit nfvPPA and svPPA to relearn lost words and increase the quality of life.[19]

Compensatory-based Approach

Speech therapists are now prioritizing communication skills training and the use of augmentative and alternative communication to manage individuals with PPA. These approaches emphasize developing functional communication and everyday conversation skills between individuals with PPA and their family members. It begins by evaluating communication facilitators (gestures accompanied by verbal communication) and barriers (abrupt topic shifting and interrupted utterances). Conversation tasks with the use of facilitative behaviors by communication partners will have add-on advantage in individuals with PPA in terms of overall communication. Additionally, the use of assistive augmentative communication devices like smartphones and communication books can support conversations with trained partners and other activities of daily living. Use of communication books will foster interactions between people with PPA and communication partners.

Group Education and Support

Group education and support programs provide valuable opportunities to practice effective communication strategies for the individual with PPA and their communication partners. Individuals with PPA and their families feel more confident and valued when attending group sessions. These group sessions also play a role in educating both individuals with PPA and family members about the progression of symptoms and support groups that assist in addressing future challenges.

CONCLUSION

It is widely recognized that speech-language assessment and communication intervention for individuals with PPA are vital and successful. The needs of individuals with PPA and their families change with time and therefore require long-term support. In all stages of the progression, individuals with PPA and their families benefit from SLP support in the form of impairment-based and compensatory-based interventions, and education. Targeting improving linguistic abilities and facilitating communication interactions can greatly enhance overall communication, independence, and quality of life over an extended period of time. However, PPA remains one of the most underserved populations in terms of language disorders. As a solution, it is essential to create awareness among healthcare providers about the scope in practice of SLPs and the benefits of communication therapy. Besides that, increasing SLP's knowledge and confidence in assessing and managing PPA will lead to superior quality service.

REFERENCES

1. Gorno-Tempini ML, Hillis AE, Weintraub S, Kertesz A, Mendez M, Cappa SF, et al. Classification of primary progressive aphasia and its variants. Neurology. 2011;76(11):1006-14.
2. Kertesz A. Western aphasia battery-revised (WAB-R). United States: Pearson Clinical; 2006.
3. Goodglass H, Kaplan E, Weintraub S. BDAE: The Boston diagnostic aphasia examination. Philadelphia: Lippincott Williams & Wilkins; 2001.
4. Chengappa SK, Kumar R. Language in India. (2008). Normative & Clinical Data on the Kannada Version of Western Aphasia Battery (WAB-K). [online] Available from http://www.languageinindia.com/june2008/normativechengappa.pdf [Last accessed July, 2024].
5. Bhatnagar SC. AIIMS diagnostic test of aphasia. nd Unpublished test and manuscript.
6. Nehra A, Pershad D, Sreenivas V. Indian Aphasia battery: Tool for specific diagnosis of language disorder post stroke. J Neurol Sci. 2013;333:e165.
7. Henry ML, Grasso SM. Assessment of individuals with primary progressive aphasia. Semin Speech Lang. 2018;39(3):231-41.
8. Patel N, Peterson KA, Ingram RU, Storey I, Cappa SF, Catricala E, et al. A 'Mini Linguistic State Examination' to classify primary progressive aphasia. Brain Commun. 2022;4(2):fcab299.
9. Savage S, Hsieh S, Leslie F, Foxe D, Piguet O, Hodges JR. Distinguishing subtypes in primary progressive aphasia: Application of the Sydney language battery. Dement Geriatr Cogn Disord. 2013;35(3-4):208-18.
10. Hodges JR, Martinos M, Woollams AM, Patterson K, Adlam ALR. Repeat and point: Differentiating semantic dementia from progressive non-fluent aphasia. Cortex. 2008;44(9):1265-70.
11. Sapolsky D, Domoto-Reilly K, Dickerson BC. Use of the Progressive Aphasia Severity Scale (PASS) in monitoring speech and language status in PPA. Aphasiology. 2014;28(8-9):993-1003.
12. Leyton CE, Villemagne VL, Savage S, Pike KE, Ballard KJ, Piguet O, et al. Subtypes of progressive aphasia: Application of the international consensus criteria and validation using β-amyloid imaging. Brain. 2011;134(Pt 10):3030-43.
13. Weintraub S, Mesulam MM, Wieneke C, Rademaker A, Rogalski EJ, Thompson CK. The Northwestern anagram test: Measuring sentence production in primary progressive aphasia. Am J Alzheimers Dis Other Demen. 2009;24(5):408-16.
14. Dabul B. ABA-2: Apraxia battery for adults. Austin, TX: Pro-ed; 2000.
15. Paplikar A, Vandana VP, Mekala S, Darshini KJ, Arshad F, Iyer GK, et al. Semantic memory impairment in dementia: A cross-cultural adaptation study. Neurol Sci. 2022;43(1):265-73.
16. Paplikar A, Varghese F, Alladi S, Vandana VP, Darshini KJ, Iyer GK, et al. Picture-naming test for a linguistically diverse population with cognitive impairment and dementia. Int J Lang Commun Disord. 2022;57(4):881-94.
17. de Carvalho IA, Mansur LL. Validation of ASHA FACS–functional assessment of communication skills for Alzheimer disease population. Alzheimer Dis Assoc Disord. 2008;22(4):375-81.
18. Grasso SM, Shuster KM, Henry ML. Comparing the effects of clinician and caregiver-administered lexical retrieval training for progressive anomia. Neuropsychol Rehabil. 2019;29(6):866-95.
19. Jokel R, Graham NL, Rochon E, Leonard C. Word retrieval therapies in primary progressive aphasia. Aphasiology. 2014;28(8-9):1038-68.
20. Croot K, Taylor C, Abel S, Jones K, Krein L, Hameister I, et al. Measuring gains in connected speech following treatment for word retrieval: A study with two participants with primary progressive aphasia. Aphasiology. 2015;29(11):1265-88.
21. Hameister I, Nickels L, Abel S, Croot K. "Do you have mowing the lawn?"–improvements in word retrieval and grammar following constraint-induced language therapy in primary progressive aphasia. Aphasiology. 2017;31(3):308-31.
22. Bier N, Macoir J, Gagnon L, Van der Linden M, Louveaux S, Desrosiers J. Known, lost, and recovered: Efficacy of formal-semantic therapy and spaced retrieval method in a case of semantic dementia. Aphasiology. 2009;23(2):210-35.
23. Newhart M, Davis C, Kannan V, Heidler-Gary J, Cloutman LL, Hillis AE. Therapy for naming deficits in two variants of primary progressive aphasia. Aphasiology. 2009;23(7-8):823-34.
24. Trebbastoni A, Raccah R, De Lena C, Zangen A, Inghilleri M. Repetitive deep transcranial magnetic stimulation improves verbal fluency and written language in a patient with primary progressive aphasia-logopenic variant (LPPA). Brain Stimul. 2013;6(4):545-53.
25. Tippett DC, Hillis AE, Tsapkini K. Treatment of primary progressive aphasia. Curr Treat Options Neurol. 2015;17(8):362.
26. Henry ML, Hubbard HI, Grasso SM, Mandelli ML, Wilson SM, Sathishkumar MT, et al. Retraining speech production and

fluency in non-fluent/agrammatic primary progressive aphasia. Brain. 2018;141(6):1799-814.
27. Henry ML, Rising K, DeMarco AT, Miller BL, Gorno-Tempini ML, Beeson PM. Examining the value of lexical retrieval treatment in primary progressive aphasia: Two positive cases. Brain Lang. 2013;127(2):145-56.
28. Farrajota L, Maruta C, Maroco J, Martins IP, Guerreiro M, De Mendonça A. Speech therapy in primary progressive aphasia: A pilot study. Dement Geriatr Cogn Dis Extra. 2012;2(1):321-31.
29. Enderby PM, Palmer R. Frenchay Dysarthria Assessment: FDA-2, Vol. 2. Texas: Pro-Ed; 2008.
30. Thompson CK. Northwestern Assessment of Verbs and Sentences (NAVS). Evanston, IL: Northwestern University; 2012.
31. McNeil MR, Prescott TE. Revised Token Test. Baltimore, MD: University Park Press; 1978.
32. Breining BL, Lala T, Martínez Cuitiño M, Manes F, Peristeri E, Tsapkini K, et al. A brief assessment of object semantics in primary progressive aphasia. Aphasiology. 2015;29(4):488-505.
33. Dunn DM. Peabody Picture Vocabulary Test (5th ed.). Bloomington: MN: NCS Pearson; 2019.
34. Kaplan E, Goodglass H, Weintraub S. Boston naming test. Austin: Pro-Ed; 2001.
35. Beeson PM, Rising K, Kim ES, Rapcsak SZ. A treatment sequence for phonological alexia/agraphia. J Speech Lang Hear Res. 2010;53(2):450-68.

CHAPTER

16

Role of Modifiable Lifestyle Factors in Neurodegenerative Dementias

Anu Gupta, Manjari Tripathi

ABSTRACT

The elderly population, including those living with dementia, is increasing globally. Evidence supports the role of 12 potentially modifiable risk factors for degenerative dementias.

Forty percent of dementia cases could be prevented globally by targeting these risk factors. The potential for prevention is higher in low-income and middle-income countries, including India, where dementia is underrecognized and low education and vascular risk factors are highly prevalent. In this chapter, we summarize the available evidence for each of these modifiable factors, interventions based on them, and the guidelines for primary prevention of dementia using multidomain measures. The future of memory clinics envisages the development of personalized risk profiling and implementing risk reduction interventions in addition to diagnosing and treating late-stage disease.

Keywords: Risk factors, Elderly population, Degenerative dementias, India.

INTRODUCTION

Dementia is a global concern with increasing prevalence worldwide. Nearly, 416 million people are estimated to be on the Alzheimer's disease (AD) continuum globally (22% of all persons aged 50 years and above), which includes 315 million people with preclinical AD, 69 million at the prodromal stage, and 32 million with dementia due to AD.[1] In India, the prevalence of dementia is estimated to be 7.4%.[2] Progressive disability, caregiver burnout,[3] financial distress (the annual cost of care per patient with mild-to-moderate and severe major neurocognitive disorder was ₹78,288 and ₹167,808, respectively, as per a study done in 2021[4]), and lack of widespread availability of cost-effective and specific disease-modifying therapies are a clarion call to institute preventive measures for this entity.

Etiologically, AD accounts for 60%, whereas vascular dementia accounts for approximately 30% of the dementias in developing countries.[5] The latest Lancet Commission report of 2020 has summarized 12 modifiable risk factors (less education, hypertension, diabetes, obesity, physical inactivity, smoking, alcohol consumption, depression, low social contact, hearing impairment, air pollution, and traumatic brain injury) using population attributable fractions (PAFs) that affect nearly 40% of dementias worldwide.[6] Studies from India estimate a slightly higher PAF (41.2%) than Western countries with greater weightage for less childhood education, smoking, hypertension, obesity, and diabetes.[7] Also, some risk and protective factors may be unique to the Indian setting such as hyperhomocysteinemia, pickles in diet, and living in joint families.[8] These modifiable factors can be potential targets for prevention and even mild improvement in them at the individual level can lead to considerable impact at the population level.

In this chapter, we will discuss these modifiable risk factors in terms of their contribution to pathophysiology and the available evidence base for their role in prevention of neurodegenerative dementia, the seventh leading cause of mortality globally in all ages.[9]

VASCULAR RISKS

Hypertension

Hypertension has the highest PAF for dementia among the vascular risk factors,[10] but the effect appears to differ with age. Midlife hypertension is associated with cognitive impairment later in life, while hypertension in late life is reported to have either a null or inverse association with neurocognitive outcomes.[11] The most important etiopathogenic mechanism underlying high blood pressure (BP) and impaired cognition is cerebral small vessel disease. The factors contributing to the same include oxidative stress, endothelial dysfunction, inflammation, increased blood brain barrier permeability, arterial stiffness and tortuosity, altered physiological parameters such as nocturnal dipping of BP, and changes in renin angiotensin system. These alterations predispose the brain to chronic vascular damage, strokes, reduced amyloid clearance, and brain atrophy.[12]

In a meta-analysis based on individual patient data from 34,519 community-dwelling older adults (17 longitudinal cohort studies), untreated hypertension was associated with greater propensity for dementia compared to treated hypertension, and this association was not modified by age, baseline BP, gender, or race.[13] This is in contradiction to a previous individual patient data meta-analysis[14] and some other studies[15] which have either reported a negative linear association of systolic BP with dementia risk (low point being 185 mm Hg and effect modified by age) or found a U shape between late-life BP and dementia risk (lowest-risk BP variable across studies).

While population-based studies of people aged >60 years have mostly found higher BPs to be associated with lower dementia risk, clinical trial results based on antihypertensive usage are the opposite. A recent systematic review and meta-analysis of 14 randomized controlled trials (RCTs) reported that BP lowering with antihypertensive agents significantly reduced the incidence of dementia or cognitive impairment compared to controls.[11] Another meta-analysis in 2022 (individual patient data of 28,008 participants of randomized clinical trials) found an adjusted odds ratio of 0.87, favoring treatment of hypertension for dementia risk reduction.[16] Age moderated this association, with less benefit seen in participants aged 80 years or older. No difference was seen between outcomes of male and female participants.

Considering the contradictory results, it is important to understand that BP in late life is a highly variable biomarker and one has to consider several factors while treating hypertension in elderly like white coat effect, interclinician measurement differences, diurnal variation, poorer autoregulation, atherosclerosis (systolic BP becomes less reflective of central BP), and reverse causality (association of lower BP in late life may be due to loss of central vascular control due to dementia itself). On the other hand, it is prudent to target systolic BP of <130 mm Hg in midlife to reduce the risk of late-life dementia.

Diabetes

Epidemiological studies have established an increased risk of dementia and mild cognitive impairment among individuals with type 2 diabetes (T2D), particularly in older individuals.[17] In a systematic review and meta-analysis (122 studies, 9,359,005 individuals, 49.9% women, and mean age 40.4–87.8 years), diabetes vested a 1.25- to 1.91-fold excess risk for cognitive disorders (cognitive impairment and dementia). Subjects with prediabetes also had higher risk for dementia.[18] In another pooled meta-analysis (14 cohort studies, 2.3 million individuals with T2D across, including 102,174 with dementia), diabetes was associated with an increased risk of any dementia [Relative risk (RR) 1.6; 95% confidence interval (CI) 1.5–1.8 for women and 1.6, 1.4–1.8 for men].[19] The risk of dementia increased with the duration and severity of diabetes. Also, younger age at diabetes onset is more strongly associated with incidence of dementia.[20] Diabetes-associated microvascular and macrovascular disease, comorbid hypertension, dyslipidemia, and depression are other potential risk factors for cognitive dysfunction in diabetes. The diabetes-associated RRs for vascular dementia have been reported to be 2.34 (95% CI 1.86–2.94) in women and 1.73 (95% CI 1.61–1.85) in men, and for nonvascular dementia, the RRs are 1.53 (95% CI 1.35–1.73) in women and 1.49 (95% CI 1.31–1.69) in men.[19] Although pathology-based studies do not report an increase in AD pathology in people with diabetes, still 40% of individuals with T2D have intermediate-to-severe AD pathology in their brain at the time of death. Cerebral insulin resistance and advanced glycation end products are the possible links between diabetes and AD pathology.[17]

The effect of diabetes treatment on dementia outcomes remains unclear, with different studies reporting different results. As far as intensity of blood glucose control is concerned, it is generally agreed that intensive control does not decrease the risk of dementia. A Cochrane review of RCTs reported that intensive diabetes control showed no impact on cognitive decline (RR 1.0; 95% CI 0.9–1.1) or dementia (1.3, 0.9–1.9) compared to standard diabetes control over 5-year follow-up ($n = 11{,}140$).[21] On the other hand, severe hypoglycemic episodes are clearly associated with a nearly twofold increased risk of incident dementia.[22]

The effect of different diabetic medications on cognitive outcomes is also unclear. One meta-analysis (cohort studies of T2D) reported that metformin use was associated with lower prevalence of cognitive impairment cross-sectionally and reduced incidence of dementia longitudinally.[23] Another meta-analysis (27 cohort/case-control studies, n = 3,046,661) did not corroborate this protective effect of metformin for incident dementia in the Eastern population.[24] Potential protective effects have been reported with thiazolidinedione exposure (RR 0.71; 95% CI 0.55–0.93),[22] with a recent meta-analysis reporting 47% of reduced risk of dementia with the use of pioglitazone.[18]

Finally, guidelines propose that intensive blood glucose control has a less favorable risk–benefit ratio in older individuals with diabetes, particularly for those having cognitive impairment, so glycemic targets should be higher.[25] On the other hand, vascular risk factor management and lifestyle modifications have the highest impact if these are started in midlife and maintained throughout.

Obesity

Midlife obesity [body mass index (BMI) ≥ 30 kg/m^2] is known to increase the risk of late-life dementia. A review of 19 longitudinal studies, including 589,649 people aged between 35 and 65 years, reported 30% increased risk of dementia over a 42-year follow-up.[26] Another meta-analysis revealed that midlife underweight, obesity, and late-life underweight conferred 39%, 31%, and 64% excess risk for cognitive impairment and dementia, while late-life overweight and obesity conferred 21% and 25% reduced risk.[27] In dose–response analysis in the same study, all-cause dementia, AD, and vascular dementia risk was significantly elevated when BMI in midlife surpassed 29, 30, and 32 kg/m^2. However, data on the effect of weight loss in dementia prevention is lacking. What we know from a meta-analysis (seven RCTs: 468 participants, 13 longitudinal studies: 551 participants) of overweight and obese adults without dementia is that a weight loss of 2 kg or more is associated with significant improvement in attention and memory.[28]

Physical Inactivity

Evidence from observational studies links physical inactivity with increased risk of dementia. Approximately, 1 in 15 cases of dementia may be attributable to physical inactivity defined by any criteria.[29] In an individual patient data meta-analysis (19 observational studies, 404,840 participants, mean baseline age 45.5 years, and mean follow-up 14.9 years), physical inactivity (during the 10-year period before the diagnosis of dementia) was associated with a 40% greater hazard of all-cause dementia and AD.[30] Numerous other studies have reported that midlife moderate-to-vigorous physical activity reduces the risk of dementia on follow-up.[31,32]

Based on multiple systematic reviews of RCTs[33-35] examining the effect of physical exercise on cognition, the World Health Organization (WHO)[36] recommends physical activity to adults with normal cognition (strong recommendation and moderate quality of evidence) and mild cognitive impairment (MCI) (conditional recommendation and low quality of evidence) to reduce the risk of cognitive decline. The recommendation includes at least 150 minutes of moderate-intensity aerobic physical activity throughout the week or at least 75 minutes of vigorous intensity aerobic physical activity throughout the week and muscle strengthening activities on 2 or more days per week. Physical activity includes recreational or leisure time physical activity, transportation (walking or cycling), occupational, household chores, play, games, sports, or planned exercise.

Smoking and Alcohol

As per literature, smokers have an increased risk of dementia and smoking cessation reduces this risk to that of nonsmokers. Current smokers have 30% excess risk for-all cause dementia, 40% for AD, and 38% for vascular dementia. For all-cause dementia, the risk increases by 34% for every 20 cigarettes smoked per day.[37] Exposure to second-hand smoke is also associated with greater memory deterioration. Alcohol is gaining increased recognition as an important risk factor for dementia, but the evidence is contradictory. The Lancet Commission of 2020 reported a RR of dementia associated with heavy drinking in midlife (>21 units or 168 g of alcohol weekly) of 1.18 (95% CI 1.06–1.31), compared to light drinking.[6] However, a recent individual patient data meta-analysis (15 prospective epidemiological cohort studies, 24,478 community-dwelling older adults aged over 60 years) found that the risk of dementia was 22% lower in occasional and light-to-moderate drinkers and 38% lower in moderate-to-heavy drinkers as compared to lifetime abstaining.[38] A previous systematic review and meta-analysis had also revealed that light-to-moderate drinking may decrease the risk of AD by 28% and all-cause dementia by 26%, whereas heavy drinking does not affect the risk.[39]

PSYCHOLOGICAL FACTORS

Depression

There is considerable research on the association of depression with dementia. Older literature considered late-life depression as a significant risk factor for all-cause dementia, but it is not clear if depression in later life is actually a prodrome of dementia resulting from dementia neuropathology and inflammation. A recent longitudinal study (10,189 UK men and women, aged 35–55 years, followed for 28 years) supported these findings and found that depressive symptoms emerged approximately a decade prior to dementia diagnosis.[40] Another study on 16,608 community dwelling dementia-free older adults followed for 6 years found that people in remission from adult-onset depression are not at greater risk of dementia, while adults with persistent depression were at greater risk of cognitive decline in older age.[41] While the abovementioned studies did not find a clear association between depression and an increased risk of dementia, another longitudinal study (246,499 Danish citizens) found a persistent association between dementia and depression diagnosed in early and middle life.[42] The question whether antidepressants are effective in ameliorating this increased risk remains open as the evidence is scarce. A study of 755 people with MCI and a history of depression found that >4 years of treatment with citalopram, a selective serotonin reuptake inhibitor, was associated with a delayed progression to clinically diagnosed AD.[43]

COGNITIVE RESERVE

Cognitive reserve refers to the preexisting cognitive processing approaches that help an individual to cope with pathologic changes that take place due to dementia-related pathologies. People with higher cognitive reserve are more resilient to brain damage and can maintain function despite pathology. Epidemiologic studies suggest that lifetime exposures, including educational and occupational attainment, and leisure activities in late life can increase this reserve.[44]

Education

Higher childhood education levels reduce the risk of dementia.[44] Although the impact of education is maximum during early life (as brain plasticity reaches plateau by adolescence), evidence suggests that engaging in activities that stimulate cognition such as reading, playing games, betting, etc. after 65 years of age reduces the odds of developing dementia.[45] Also, midlife activities such as travel, social outings, playing music, art, physical activity, reading, and speaking a second language help to maintain cognition.[46] Older age at retirement has been shown to be associated with faster cognitive decline.[44]

Occupation

Occupational factors also have an important effect on cognitive functions. A systematic review and meta-analysis (43 studies) reported that mental work conferred a 44% reduced risk for MCI.[47] High strain in occupation and a passive job lead to a 1.21- and 1.15-fold excess risk of cognitive decline, while higher work complexity conferred a 5% reduced risk.[47]

Social Contact

Engagement in social leisure activities such as meeting up with family or friends and having a large social network size and more social support have been associated with better cognitive performance and lower risk of developing dementia.[48] In a meta-analysis of 31 cohort and two case-control studies (2,370,452 participants) examining the association between social engagement or loneliness and dementia risk, it was found that people with poor social network and poor social support had 59% and 28% excess risk of developing dementia.[49] Long-term studies (≥10 years) have revealed that good social engagement is modestly protective and reduces the risk of dementia by 12%.[49] In midlife, marital status is an important contributor to social engagement. A systematic review and meta-analysis (812,047 people) found dementia risk to be elevated in lifelong single (RR 1.4; 95% CI 1.1–1.9) and widowed people (1.2, 1.0–1.4), compared with married people. This association was similar in different sociocultural settings.[50] Some studies have used a five-point scale for social contact based on marital status, exchanging support with family members, having contact with friends, participating in community groups and engaging in paid work, and found the score to be linearly associated with reduced dementia risk.[51]

Another systematic review and meta-analysis of 43 studies examined the neural substrates of social engagement and reported significant heterogeneity among the studies, with few studies assessing these factors in midlife. In some studies, cognitive and social activities were positively associated with total brain, global and cortical gray matter, and hippocampal volume, as well as white matter microstructural integrity.[48]

There is scarce evidence on effect of social interventions on dementia risk or cognition. As reported in a systematic review (low-quality RCTs, 576 adults, aged 60 years or more), people with normal cognition showed an improvement in global cognition and brain volume after social engagement in the form of facilitated meeting and discussion groups.[52]

MISCELLANEOUS FACTORS

There are several miscellaneous factors that have been implicated in the risk associations with dementia and are listed further.

Sensory Impairment

Sensory impairment plays an important role in the development of dementia through reduced cognitive stimulation. Midlife hearing loss had the highest PAF in the 2017 Lancet Commission Report (RR 1.9; 9–17 years follow-up, reverse causation bias less likely due to long follow-up period). Subsequently, studies have found 30% excess risk of dementia per 10 dB of hearing loss in midlife[53] and steeper temporal lobe volume loss including the medial temporal lobe.[54] Also, prospective studies with long follow-up periods have suggested that hearing aid use is protective.[55]

Vision loss due to age-related macular degeneration and glaucoma are also linked to AD. A meta-analysis of 14 prospective cohort studies (6,204,827 participants, 171,888 dementia patients) found that vision impairment was associated with 47% excess risk of dementia.[56]

Sleep

In the past few years, many prospective cohort studies have explored the longitudinal influence of sleep-related problems on incidence of cognitive disorders. In a meta-analysis of 51 cohort studies, insomnia, prolonged latency, sleep fragmentation, excessive time in bed, rapid eye movement sleep behavior disorder, and daytime dysfunction have been linked to higher risk of all-cause cognitive disorders. Sleep duration and cognitive dysfunction had a U-shaped relationship.[57] Apnea or obstructive sleep apnea syndrome have been shown to have an association with neuronal injury biomarkers in AD (phosphorylated-tau and total-tau).[58] Natural sleep is associated with increased interstitial solute clearance such as amyloid-beta.[6] Sleep dysfunction has also been suggested to increase amyloid-beta deposition in nondemented elderly. Also, sleep is a primary driver of glymphatic clearance.

Others

Midlife traumatic brain injury (all severities) is associated with a pooled RR of 1.84 (95% CI 1.54–2.20) for all-cause dementia.[6] Greater exposure to airborne pollutants in the form of particulate matter ($PM_{2.5}$), nitrogen dioxide, and carbon monoxide are all associated with increased risk of dementia.[59] Stressful life events that occur earlier in the lifespan, such as loss of a parent, psychological stress experienced in midlife, and extreme stress responses such as post-traumatic stress disorder, correlate with higher risk of dementia.[60] Serum cortisol and plasma adrenocorticotrophic hormone (ACTH) levels have been shown to associate with stressful life events in patients with cognitive impairment.[61]

Figures 1A and B summarize the weighted PAFs of the life course potentially modifiable risk factors of dementia globally[6] and in India.[7] PAF is the percentage reduction in new cases over a given time if a particular risk factor were completely eliminated. The attributable risk depends on both the prevalence of the risk factor and the strength of its association with the disease (RR).[10]

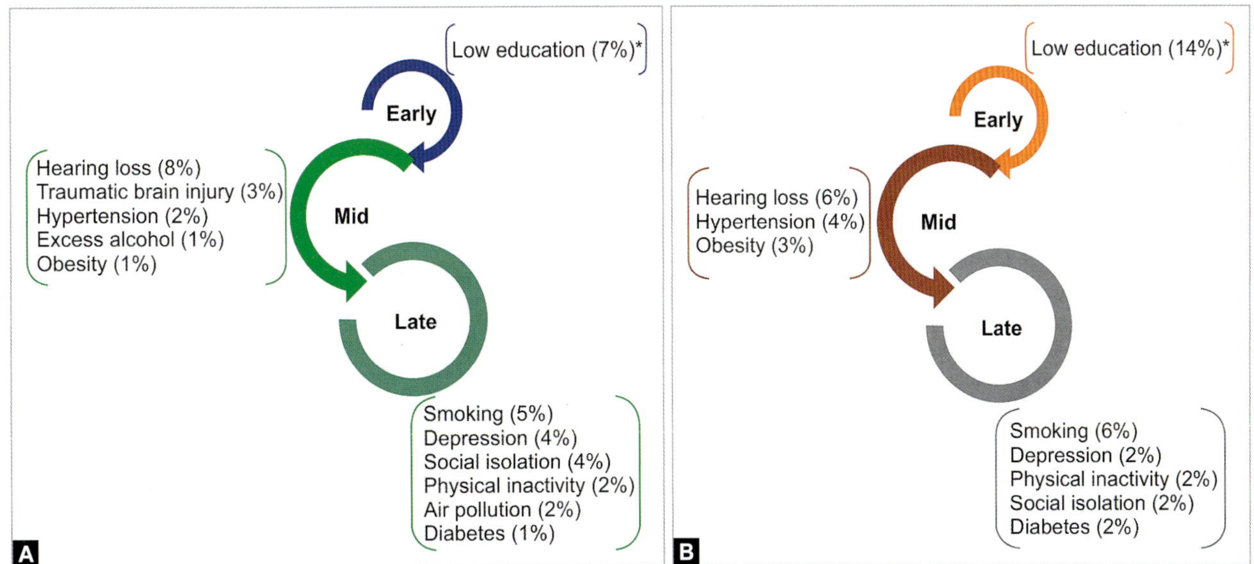

* Percentage reduction in prevalence of dementia if this risk factor is eliminated.

FIGS. 1A AND B: Population attributable fraction (PAF) of the life course potentially modifiable risk factors of dementia: (A) Globally and (B) from India.

INDIAN SCENARIO

The Global Burden of Disease Study (2016) estimated that 2.93 million people are affected with dementia in India.[62] The estimated figures in 2020 stand at 8.8 million individuals above 60 years of age.[2] The prevalence of vascular risk factors (hypertension, diabetes, dyslipidemia, obesity, and tobacco use) in India has increased substantially over the last few decades. Routine screening of vascular risk is not practiced, so data emanating from studies using self-reported measures grossly underestimates the prevalence of these risk factors. The overall PAF for dementia was higher in India (41%) than worldwide estimates and highest for low education in early life **(Figs. 1A and B)**.[7] There are emerging risk factors that still need evaluation, such as air pollution. Women in rural areas are exposed to high levels of air pollution due to solid fuel burning. Air pollution is becoming a colossal problem in urban areas as well. Studies have also delved on the role of nutritional factors, such as low levels of vitamin B12 and folic acid in the pathogenesis of degenerative dementia. Mansoori et al. reported that patients having folic acid < 8.45 ng/mL had 2.4 times higher odds of having AD and 2.1 times higher odds of having vascular dementia than patients having folic acid ≥ 8.45 ng/mL.[63]

RISK PREDICTION MODELS

A number of risk prediction models have been developed and some have been externally validated. More information is required on their generalizability, cost-effectiveness, and predictive value before they can be used in clinical practice. The Cardiovascular Risk Factors, Aging, and Dementia (CAIDE) risk score is one such example, which uses age, education, and gender along with the midlife risk factors of BMI, BP, cholesterol, smoking history, and physical activity.[64] This score predicts dementia risk in 20 years with moderate levels of accuracy [area under the curve (AUC) 0.77; 95% CI 0.71–0.83). The future is set to embrace the role of machine learning methods such as ensemble-based approaches and deep learning to predict future risk of dementia decades in advance and to assess the relative role of multiple risk factors.[65]

TRIALS OF MULTIMODAL INTERVENTION IN DEMENTIA PREVENTION

The Finnish Geriatric Intervention Study to Prevent Cognitive Impairment and Disability (FINGER)[66] was the first long-term study to investigate the efficacy of (2 years) multidomain lifestyle interventions (diet, exercise, cognitive training and vascular management, and intensive sessions over 2 years) among the older at-risk population (1,260 people with cardiovascular risk factors, aged 60–77 years) with the aim of prevention of cognitive decline, in comparison to controls who received standard health advice. The group receiving intervention improved in a composite measure of cognition ($d = 0.13$), on executive functions and processing speed but not memory. Based on this study, a worldwide network was formulated named WW-FINGERS to facilitate global multidomain dementia prevention trials.[67] A recent Cochrane review analyzed nine RCTs (18,452 participants) comparing multidomain intervention against usual care or sham intervention for dementia prevention. The review found no evidence that multidomain interventions can prevent incident dementia (only two studies reported incident dementia as an outcome), but there was a small improvement in cognitive functions assessed by a neuropsychological test battery in participants receiving the multidomain intervention. Interventions were diverse in terms of their components and intensity.[68] Another meta-analysis of 17 RCTs (effect of multidomain lifestyle interventions on outcomes of cognition or dementia risk) reported a small but significant effect of intervention on the risk of dementia [standardized mean difference (SMD) –0.11, 1,981 participants] and the cognitive composite score (SMD +0.10, 2,643 participants) but no effect on measures of global cognition.[69]

INTERACTION WITH GENETIC RISK

The apolipoprotein E ε4 variant (APOE ε4) is the major driver of the risk of AD in the general population. Studies from India have shown an association of this allele with both AD and vascular dementia.[70,71] In the FINGER trial, the beneficial effect of the lifestyle intervention was only observed in APOE ε4 carriers.[66] However, it is still not conclusive whether genetic risk modifies the influence of lifestyle on dementia. The UK Biobank Study did not find an association between lifestyle factors and polygenic risk score in relation to all-cause dementia risk.[72] However, there was a significant interaction between a composite of lifestyle and health factors and APOE/polygenic risk in relation to all-cause dementia in the Rotterdam Study.[73] Overall, more evidence is required to understand if targeted dementia prevention interventions have more benefit in people with higher genetic risk.

PRIMARY PREVENTION GUIDELINES

The UsAgainstAlzheimer's risk reduction workgroup has advocated 11 recommendations for individuals aged 45 years and older **(Fig. 2)** and urged the medical community to convert these recommendations into actionable strategies.[74] Most of these guidelines (except

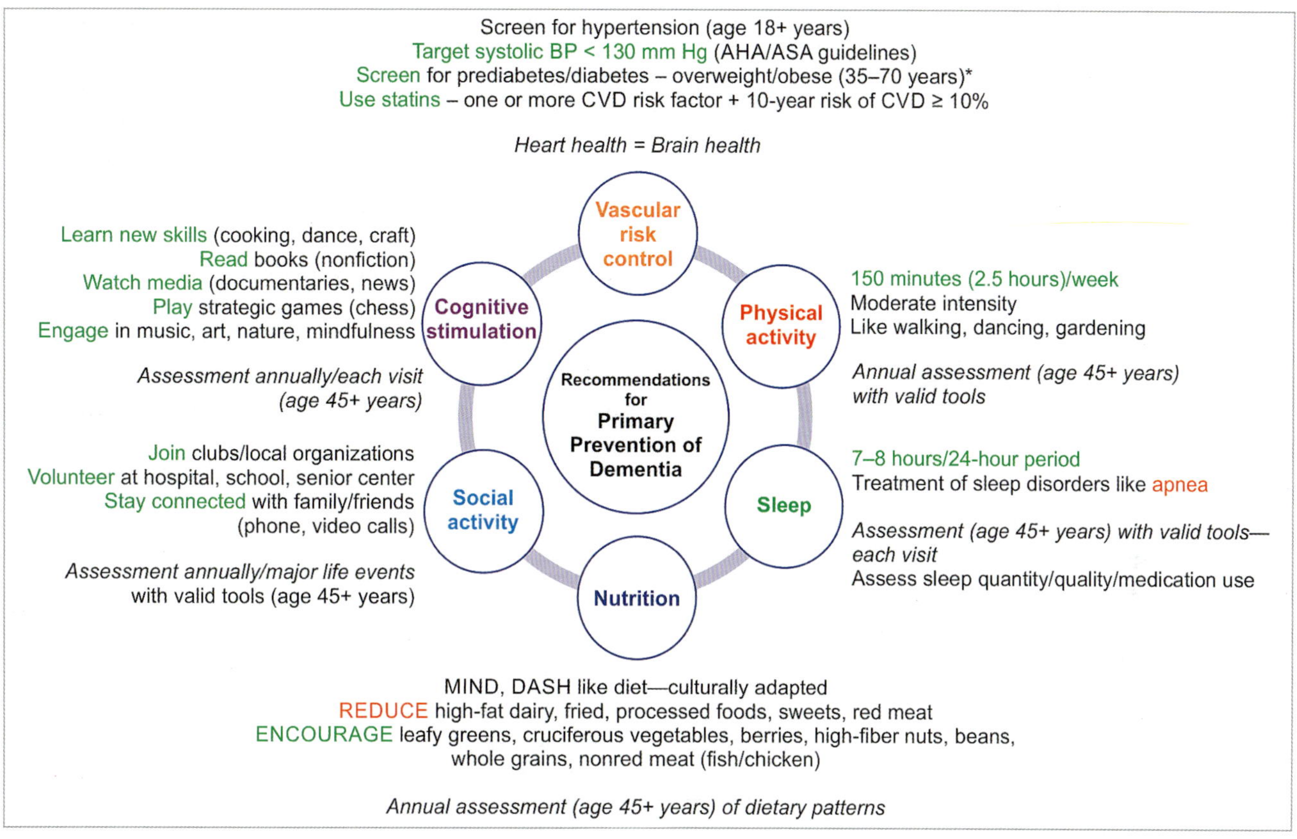

* May vary as per prevalence of risk factors, for example, in the Indian setting, it may be prudent to screen in age 30+ years, with or without obesity.

FIG. 2: Summary of recommendations for primary prevention of dementia.

(AHA: American Heart Association; ASA: American Stroke Association; BP: blood pressure; CVD: cardiovascular disease; MIND: Mediterranean–DASH Diet Intervention for Neurodegenerative Delay)

those for social activity or cognitive stimulation) are consistent with standard of care for patients with existing cardiovascular conditions. Walsh et al. have summarized the empirical, interventional evidence for population-level interventions to reduce or control each of the 12 modifiable life course risk factors for dementia identified by the Lancet Commission. The group identified that interventions such as removing primary school fees, plain packaging of tobacco products, cleaner fuel replacement programs for cooking stoves, and mandated provision of hearing protective equipment at noisy workplaces may have an effect at the population level.[75]

CONCLUSION

The major current challenges lie in the understanding of mechanisms that link various risk factors to dementia, to determine their causality (pathway or mediation analysis using large sample sizes, machine learning methods, and analyzing timing and trajectory of risk factors), analyzing multimodal data such as omics, histology, imaging, and clinical and digital information to unveil novel mechanistic insights. The ultimate goal will be to develop a person-specific approach leading to personalized preventative interventions for dementia prevention.

REFERENCES

1. Gustavsson A, Norton N, Fast T, Frölich L, Georges J, Holzapfel D, et al. Global estimates on the number of persons across the Alzheimer's disease continuum. Alzheimers Dement. 2023;19(2):658-70.
2. Lee J, Meijer E, Langa KM, Ganguli M, Varghese M, Banerjee J, et al. Prevalence of dementia in India: National and state estimates from a nationwide study. Alzheimers Dement. 2023;19(7):2898-912.
3. Pattanayak RD, Jena R, Tripathi M, Khandelwal SK. Assessment of burden in caregivers of Alzheimer's disease from India. Asian J Psychiatr. 2010;3(3):112-6.
4. Malapur PU, Kumar N, Khandelwal SK, Tripathi M. Cost of Illness of Major Neurocognitive Disorders in India. Neurol India. 2021;69(5):1265-8.
5. Kalaria RN, Maestre GE, Arizaga R, Friedland RP, Galasko D, Hall K, et al.; World Federation of Neurology Dementia

Research Group. Alzheimer's disease and vascular dementia in developing countries: prevalence, management, and risk factors. Lancet Neurol. 2008;7(9):812-26.

6. Livingston G, Huntley J, Sommerlad A, Ames D, Ballard C, Banerjee S, et al. Dementia prevention, intervention, and care: 2020 report of the Lancet Commission. Lancet. 2020; 396(10248):413-46.
7. Mukadam N, Sommerlad A, Huntley J, Livingston G. Population attributable fractions for risk factors for dementia in low-income and middle-income countries: an analysis using cross-sectional survey data. Lancet Glob Health. 2019;7(5):e596-603.
8. Tripathi M, Vibha D, Gupta P, Bhatia R, Srivastava MV, Vivekanandhan S, et al. Risk factors of dementia in North India: a case-control study. Aging Ment Health. 2012;16(2):228-35.
9. GBD 2019 Collaborators. Global mortality from dementia: Application of a new method and results from the Global Burden of Disease Study 2019. Alzheimers Dement (N Y). 2021; 7(1):e12200.
10. Livingston G, Sommerlad A, Orgeta V, Costafreda SG, Huntley J, Ames D, et al. Dementia prevention, intervention, and care. Lancet. 2017;390(10113):2673-734.
11. Hughes D, Judge C, Murphy R, Loughlin E, Costello M, Whiteley W, et al. Association of Blood Pressure Lowering with Incident Dementia or Cognitive Impairment: A Systematic Review and Meta-analysis. JAMA. 2020;323(19):1934-44.
12. Sierra C. Hypertension and the Risk of Dementia. Front Cardiovasc Med. 2020;7:5.
13. Lennon MJ, Lam BCP, Lipnicki DM, Crawford JD, Peters R, Schutte AE, et al. Use of Antihypertensives, Blood Pressure, and Estimated Risk of Dementia in Late Life: An Individual Participant Data Meta-analysis. JAMA Netw Open. 2023;6(9):e2333353.
14. van Dalen JW, Brayne C, Crane PK, Fratiglioni L, Larson EB, Lobo A, et al. Association of Systolic Blood Pressure with Dementia Risk and the Role of Age, U-Shaped Associations, and Mortality. JAMA Intern Med. 2022;182(2):142-52.
15. Rajan KB, Barnes LL, Wilson RS, Weuve J, McAninch EA, Evans DA. Blood pressure and risk of incident Alzheimer's disease dementia by antihypertensive medications and APOE ε4 allele. Ann Neurol. 2018;83(5):935-44.
16. Peters R, Xu Y, Fitzgerald O, Aung HL, Beckett N, Bulpitt C, et al.; Dementia rIsk REduCTion (DIRECT) collaboration. Blood pressure lowering and prevention of dementia: an individual patient data meta-analysis. Eur Heart J. 2022;43(48):4980-90.
17. Biessels GJ, Despa F. Cognitive decline and dementia in diabetes mellitus: mechanisms and clinical implications. Nat Rev Endocrinol. 2018;14(10):591-604.
18. Xue M, Xu W, Ou YN, Cao XP, Tan MS, Tan L, et al. Diabetes mellitus and risks of cognitive impairment and dementia: A systematic review and meta-analysis of 144 prospective studies. Ageing Res Rev. 2019;55:100944.
19. Chatterjee S, Peters SA, Woodward M, Mejia Arango S, Batty GD, Beckett N, et al. Type 2 Diabetes as a Risk Factor for Dementia in Women Compared with Men: A Pooled Analysis of 2.3 Million People Comprising More Than 100,000 Cases of Dementia. Diabetes Care. 2016;39(2):300-7.
20. Barbiellini Amidei C, Fayosse A, Dumurgier J, Machado-Fragua MD, Tabak AG, van Sloten T, et al. Association between Age at Diabetes Onset and Subsequent Risk of Dementia. JAMA. 2021;325(16):1640-9.
21. Areosa Sastre A, Vernooij RW, González-Colaço Harmand M, Martínez G. Effect of the treatment of Type 2 diabetes mellitus on the development of cognitive impairment and dementia. Cochrane Database Syst Rev. 2017;6(6):CD003804.
22. McMillan JM, Mele BS, Hogan DB, Leung AA. Impact of pharmacological treatment of diabetes mellitus on dementia risk: systematic review and meta-analysis. BMJ Open Diabetes Res Care. 2018;6(1):e000563.
23. Zhang JH, Zhang XY, Sun YQ, Lv RH, Chen M, Li M. Metformin use is associated with a reduced risk of cognitive impairment in adults with diabetes mellitus: A systematic review and meta-analysis. Front Neurosci. 2022;16:984559.
24. Kuate Defo A, Bakula V, Pisaturo A, Labos C, Wing SS, Daskalopoulou SS. Diabetes, antidiabetic medications and risk of dementia: A systematic umbrella review and meta-analysis. Diabetes Obes Metab. 2024;26(2):441-62.
25. Standards of Medical Care in Diabetes-2017: Summary of Revisions. Diabetes Care. 2017;40(Suppl 1):S4-5.
26. Albanese E, Launer LJ, Egger M, Prince MJ, Giannakopoulos P, Wolters FJ, et al. Body mass index in midlife and dementia: Systematic review and meta-regression analysis of 589,649 men and women followed in longitudinal studies. Alzheimers Dement (Amst). 2017;8:165-78.
27. Qu Y, Hu HY, Ou YN, Shen XN, Xu W, Wang ZT, et al. Association of body mass index with risk of cognitive impairment and dementia: A systematic review and meta-analysis of prospective studies. Neurosci Biobehav Rev. 2020;115:189-98.
28. Veronese N, Facchini S, Stubbs B, Luchini C, Solmi M, Manzato E, et al. Weight loss is associated with improvements in cognitive function among overweight and obese people: A systematic review and meta-analysis. Neurosci Biobehav Rev. 2017;72: 87-94.
29. Feter N, Leite JS, da Silva LS, Cassuriaga J, de Paula D, Lopes GW, et al. Systematic review and meta-analysis on population attributable fraction for physical inactivity to dementia. Alzheimers Dement. 2023;19(10):4688-704.
30. Kivimäki M, Singh-Manoux A, Pentti J, Sabia S, Nyberg ST, Alfredsson L, et al.; IPD-Work consortium. Physical inactivity, cardiometabolic disease, and risk of dementia: an individual-participant meta-analysis. BMJ. 2019;365:l1495.
31. Zotcheva E, Bergh S, Selbæk G, Krokstad S, Håberg AK, Strand BH, et al. Midlife Physical Activity, Psychological Distress, and Dementia Risk: The HUNT Study. J Alzheimers Dis. 2018;66(2):825-33.
32. Hörder H, Johansson L, Guo X, Grimby G, Kern S, Östling S, et al. Midlife cardiovascular fitness and dementia: A 44-year longitudinal population study in women. Neurology. 2018; 90(15):e1298-305.
33. Northey JM, Cherbuin N, Pumpa KL, Smee DJ, Rattray B. Exercise interventions for cognitive function in adults older than 50: a systematic review with meta-analysis. Br J Sports Med. 2018;52(3):154-60.
34. Song D, Yu DSF, Li PWC, Lei Y. The effectiveness of physical exercise on cognitive and psychological outcomes in individuals with mild cognitive impairment: A systematic review and meta-analysis. Int J Nurs Stud. 2018;79:155-64.
35. de Souto Barreto P, Demougeot L, Vellas B, Rolland Y. Exercise Training for Preventing Dementia, Mild Cognitive Impairment, and Clinically Meaningful Cognitive Decline: A Systematic Review and Meta-analysis. J Gerontol A Biol Sci Med Sci. 2018;73(11):1504-11.
36. WHO. Risk reduction of cognitive decline and dementia: WHO guidelines. Geneva: World Health Organization; 2019.

37. Hong G, Wang Y, Zhang Y, Guo JJ, Zhao Y. Smoking is associated with an increased risk of dementia: a meta-analysis of prospective cohort studies with investigation of potential effect modifiers. PLoS One. 2015;10(3):e0118333.
38. Mewton L, Visontay R, Hoy N, Lipnicki DM, Sunderland M, Lipton RB, et al.; Collaborators from the Cohort Studies of Memory in an International Consortium (COSMIC). The relationship between alcohol use and dementia in adults aged more than 60 years: a combined analysis of prospective, individual-participant data from 15 international studies. Addiction. 2023;118(3):412-24.
39. Ilomaki J, Jokanovic N, Tan EC, Lonnroos E. Alcohol Consumption, Dementia and Cognitive Decline: An Overview of Systematic Reviews. Curr Clin Pharmacol. 2015;10(3):204-12.
40. Singh-Manoux A, Dugravot A, Fournier A, Abell J, Ebmeier K, Kivimäki M, et al. Trajectories of Depressive Symptoms before Diagnosis of Dementia: A 28-Year Follow-up Study. JAMA Psychiatry. 2017;74(7):712-8.
41. Lee ATC, Fung AWT, Richards M, Chan WC, Chiu HFK, Lee RSY, et al. Risk of incident dementia varies with different onset and courses of depression. J Affect Disord. 2021;282:915-20.
42. Elser H, Horváth-Puhó E, Gradus JL, Smith ML, Lash TL, Glymour MM, et al. Association of Early-, Middle-, and Late-Life Depression with Incident Dementia in a Danish Cohort. JAMA Neurol. 2023;80(9):949-58.
43. Bartels C, Wagner M, Wolfsgruber S, Ehrenreich H, Schneider A; Alzheimer's Disease Neuroimaging Initiative. Impact of SSRI Therapy on Risk of Conversion from Mild Cognitive Impairment to Alzheimer's Dementia in Individuals with Previous Depression. Am J Psychiatry. 2018;175(3):232-41.
44. Stern Y. Cognitive reserve in ageing and Alzheimer's disease. Lancet Neurol. 2012;11(11):1006-12.
45. Lee ATC, Richards M, Chan WC, Chiu HFK, Lee RSY, Lam LCW. Association of Daily Intellectual Activities with Lower Risk of Incident Dementia among Older Chinese Adults. JAMA Psychiatry. 2018;75(7):697-703.
46. Chan D, Shafto M, Kievit R, Matthews F, Spink M, Valenzuela M, et al.; Cam-CAN. Lifestyle activities in mid-life contribute to cognitive reserve in late-life, independent of education, occupation, and late-life activities. Neurobiol Aging. 2018;70:180-3.
47. Huang LY, Hu HY, Wang ZT, Ma YH, Dong Q, Tan L, et al. Association of Occupational Factors and Dementia or Cognitive Impairment: A Systematic Review and Meta-analysis. J Alzheimers Dis. 2020;78(1):217-27.
48. Duffner LA, DeJong NR, Jansen JFA, Backes WH, de Vugt M, Deckers K, et al. Associations between social health factors, cognitive activity and neurostructural markers for brain health - A systematic literature review and meta-analysis. Ageing Res Rev. 2023;89:101986.
49. Penninkilampi R, Casey AN, Singh MF, Brodaty H. The Association between Social Engagement, Loneliness, and Risk of Dementia: A Systematic Review and Meta-analysis. J Alzheimers Dis. 2018;66(4):1619-33.
50. Sommerlad A, Ruegger J, Singh-Manoux A, Lewis G, Livingston G. Marriage and risk of dementia: systematic review and meta-analysis of observational studies. J Neurol Neurosurg Psychiatry. 2018;89(3):231-8.
51. Saito T, Murata C, Saito M, Takeda T, Kondo K. Influence of social relationship domains and their combinations on incident dementia: a prospective cohort study. J Epidemiol Community Health. 2018;72(1):7-12.
52. Kelly ME, Duff H, Kelly S, McHugh Power JE, Brennan S, Lawlor BA, et al. The impact of social activities, social networks, social support and social relationships on the cognitive functioning of healthy older adults: a systematic review. Syst Rev. 2017;6(1):259.
53. Loughrey DG, Kelly ME, Kelley GA, Brennan S, Lawlor BA. Association of Age-related Hearing Loss with Cognitive Function, Cognitive Impairment, and Dementia: A Systematic Review and Meta-analysis. JAMA Otolaryngol Head Neck Surg. 2018;144(2):115-26.
54. Armstrong NM, An Y, Doshi J, Erus G, Ferrucci L, Davatzikos C, et al. Association of Midlife Hearing Impairment with Late-Life Temporal Lobe Volume Loss. JAMA Otolaryngol Head Neck Surg. 2019;145(9):794-802.
55. Sarant JZ, Busby PA, Schembri AJ, Fowler C, Harris DC. ENHANCE: a comparative prospective longitudinal study of cognitive outcomes after 3 years of hearing aid use in older adults. Front Aging Neurosci. 2024;15:1302185.
56. Shang X, Zhu Z, Wang W, Ha J, He M. The Association between Vision Impairment and Incidence of Dementia and Cognitive Impairment: A Systematic Review and Meta-analysis. Ophthalmology. 2021;128(8):1135-49.
57. Xu W, Tan CC, Zou JJ, Cao XP, Tan L. Sleep problems and risk of all-cause cognitive decline or dementia: an updated systematic review and meta-analysis. J Neurol Neurosurg Psychiatry. 2020;91(3):236-44.
58. Kang J, Tian Z, Wei J, Mu Z, Liang J, Li M. Association between obstructive sleep apnea and Alzheimer's disease-related blood and cerebrospinal fluid biomarkers: A meta-analysis. J Clin Neurosci. 2022;102:87-94.
59. Peters R, Ee N, Peters J, Booth A, Mudway I, Anstey KJ. Air Pollution and Dementia: A Systematic Review. J Alzheimers Dis. 2019;70(s1):S145-63.
60. Luo J, Beam CR, Gatz M. Is Stress an Overlooked Risk Factor for Dementia? A Systematic Review from a Lifespan Developmental Perspective. Prev Sci. 2023;24(5):936-49.
61. Manoj S, Nehra A, Dalal K, Sagar R, Tripathi M. Association of Stressful Life Events with Dementia in North Indian Populations. Neurol India. 2021;69(5):1326-30.
62. GBD 2016 Neurology Collaborators. Global, regional, and national burden of neurological disorders, 1990-2016: a systematic analysis for the Global Burden of Disease Study 2016. Lancet Neurol. 2019;18(5):459-80.
63. Mansoori N, Tripathi M, Alam R, Luthra K, Sharma S, Lakshmy R, et al. Serum folic acid and RFC A80G polymorphism in Alzheimer's disease and vascular dementia. Am J Alzheimers Dis Other Demen. 2014;29(1):38-44.
64. Kivipelto M, Ngandu T, Laatikainen T, Winblad B, Soininen H, Tuomilehto J. Risk score for the prediction of dementia risk in 20 years among middle aged people: a longitudinal, population-based study. Lancet Neurol. 2006;5(9):735-41.
65. Newby D, Orgeta V, Marshall CR, Lourida I, Albertyn CP, Tamburin S, et al.; Deep Dementia Phenotyping (DEMON) Network. Artificial intelligence for dementia prevention. Alzheimers Dement. 2023;19(12):5952-69.
66. Ngandu T, Lehtisalo J, Solomon A, Levälahti E, Ahtiluoto S, Antikainen R, et al. A 2 year multidomain intervention of diet, exercise, cognitive training, and vascular risk monitoring versus control to prevent cognitive decline in at-risk elderly people (FINGER): a randomised controlled trial. Lancet. 2015;385(9984):2255-63.
67. Rosenberg A, Mangialasche F, Ngandu T, Solomon A, Kivipelto M. Multidomain Interventions to Prevent Cognitive

Impairment, Alzheimer's Disease, and Dementia: From FINGER to World-Wide FINGERS. J Prev Alzheimers Dis. 2020;7(1):29-36.

68. Hafdi M, Hoevenaar-Blom MP, Richard E. Multi-domain interventions for the prevention of dementia and cognitive decline. Cochrane Database Syst Rev. 2021;11(11):CD013572.
69. Meng X, Fang S, Zhang S, Li H, Ma D, Ye Y, et al. Multidomain lifestyle interventions for cognition and the risk of dementia: A systematic review and meta-analysis. Int J Nurs Stud. 2022; 130:104236.
70. Mansoori N, Tripathi M, Alam R, Luthra K, Ramakrishnan L, Parveen S, et al. IL-6-174 G/C and ApoE gene polymorphisms in Alzheimer's and vascular dementia patients attending the cognitive disorder clinic of the All India Institute of Medical Sciences, New Delhi. Dement Geriatr Cogn Disord. 2010;30(6):461-8.
71. Luthra K, Tripathi M, Grover R, Dwivedi M, Kumar A, Dey AB. Apolipoprotein E gene polymorphism in Indian patients with Alzheimer's disease and vascular dementia. Dement Geriatr Cogn Disord. 2004;17(3):132-5.
72. Lourida I, Hannon E, Littlejohns TJ, Langa KM, Hyppönen E, Kuzma E, et al. Association of Lifestyle and Genetic Risk with Incidence of Dementia. JAMA. 2019;322(5):430-7.
73. Licher S, Ahmad S, Karamujić-Čomić H, Voortman T, Leening MJG, Ikram MA, et al. Genetic predisposition, modifiable-risk-factor profile and long-term dementia risk in the general population. Nat Med. 2019;25(9):1364-9.
74. Sabbagh MN, Perez A, Holland TM, Boustani M, Peabody SR, Yaffe K, et al. Primary prevention recommendations to reduce the risk of cognitive decline. Alzheimers Dement. 2022;18(8): 1569-79.
75. Walsh S, Wallace L, Kuhn I, Mytton O, Lafortune L, Wills W, et al. Population-level interventions for the primary prevention of dementia: a complex evidence review. Lancet. 2023;402 (Suppl 1):S13.

CHAPTER

17

Imaging Biomarkers in Neurocognitive Disorders

Faheem Arshad, MM Samim, Howard J Rosen

ABSTRACT

The understanding of neurocognitive disorders has evolved from a clinical to a comprehensive biomarker-based approach with a special focus on imaging biomarkers. This has addressed the challenges posed by the subjective nature and variability of clinical phenotyping. Neurocognitive disorders are characterized by abnormalities at the molecular, synaptic, neuroanatomical, network, metabolic, and functional levels. Imaging biomarkers are pivotal in this context, offering insights into dementia pathophysiology, facilitating early diagnosis and disease monitoring, and potentially facilitating the development and assessment of treatments. The use of advanced imaging techniques such as structural, metabolic, functional, and molecular imaging is crucial for identifying respective changes in various neurocognitive disorders. More recent advances such as amyloid and tau imaging provide detailed visualization of amyloid plaques and tau protein accumulation in the brain, aiding in the diagnosis and monitoring of disease progression. Furthermore, advanced techniques such as arterial spin labeling and diffusion tensor imaging measure cerebral blood flow and white matter integrity, respectively. The integration of these advanced imaging modalities goes beyond diagnostics and disease monitoring, as they also hold promise in the realm of precision medicine, enabling the subtyping of various neurocognitive disorders and guiding therapeutic interventions in clinical trials by assessing treatment efficacy at the biological level.

Keywords: Neurocognitive disorders, Magnetic resonance imaging, Biomarkers, Dementia, Amyloid, Tau, Positron emission tomography.

INTRODUCTION

With the global burden of dementia reaching 57.4 million cases in 2019 and projected to rise to 152.8 million, constituting 19.1% of the total population by 2050, dementia is one of the most concerning public health challenges.[1] As clinical phenotyping faces challenges due to its subjective nature and the variability in assessments between experienced and novice clinicians,[2] there is a critical need to identify biomarkers that can detect dementia early or even preclinically, allowing for early intervention.[3] With the advent of biomarkers, there has been a change in the definition of dementia from clinical to biological based, including the assessment of amyloid deposition, tau accumulation, and neurodegeneration through various imaging modalities,[4,5] in addition to categorizing it based on autopsy-derived pathological subtypes.[5] With the emergence of landmark trials, the current impetus is to diagnose dementia as early and as accurately as possible to preserve the brain at an earlier stage and to become trial-ready and initiate therapy and rehabilitation, necessitating the need for robust imaging biomarkers.[6]

Brain imaging has evolved from pneumoencephalography to computed tomography in the 1970s, followed by structural and functional magnetic resonance imaging (fMRI) as a noninvasive modality to provide high-resolution images for diagnosing various neurocognitive disorders.[3] This evolution progressed further to study metabolic activity and abnormal protein deposition in the brain using more advanced techniques, such as 18-fluorodeoxyglucose (FDG) positron emission tomography (PET) and amyloid and tau PET,[7-9] underscoring the need for a biological definition of neurocognitive disorders. This advancement in imaging biomarkers has profound implications for early diagnosis and monitoring of disease progression, offering insights for research and development of treatment.

STRUCTURAL MAGNETIC RESONANCE IMAGING

Structural imaging is the most widely used and accessible technique and is recommended in diagnostic guidelines. It can exclude extra-axial pathologies such as chronic subdural hematoma, as well as intraparenchymal causes such as ventriculomegaly, idiopathic intracranial hypotension, and space-occupying lesions (SOLs). It also helps identify neurodegeneration through volume loss and atrophy in specific brain regions, along with vascular pathologies such as micro/macrohemorrhages, lacunes, infarcts, periventricular leukoaraiosis, and hemosiderosis.[10] Routinely employed sequences in structural imaging for dementia evaluation include coronal, axial, and sagittal T1-weighted, axial T2-weighted, and T2-weighted coronal sequences perpendicular to the long axis of the hippocampus and fluid-attenuated inversion recovery (FLAIR) sequences, as well as susceptibility-weighted imaging (SWI) and diffusion-weighted imaging (DWI)/ADC sequences. Patients should be scanned using 1.5T or 3.0T machines for optimal detection of brain atrophy in neurodegenerative diseases, with 3.0T scanners preferred for acquiring sequences such as SWI to enhance hemorrhage evaluation.

T1-weighted Image

Thin-slice T1-weighted images with multiplanar reconstruction were used to effectively identify regional atrophy, with coronal imaging essential for assessing the medial temporal lobe and hippocampal atrophy and sagittal imaging crucial for evaluating the precuneus and parietal lobe cortex **(Figs. 1A to C)**. Several semi-

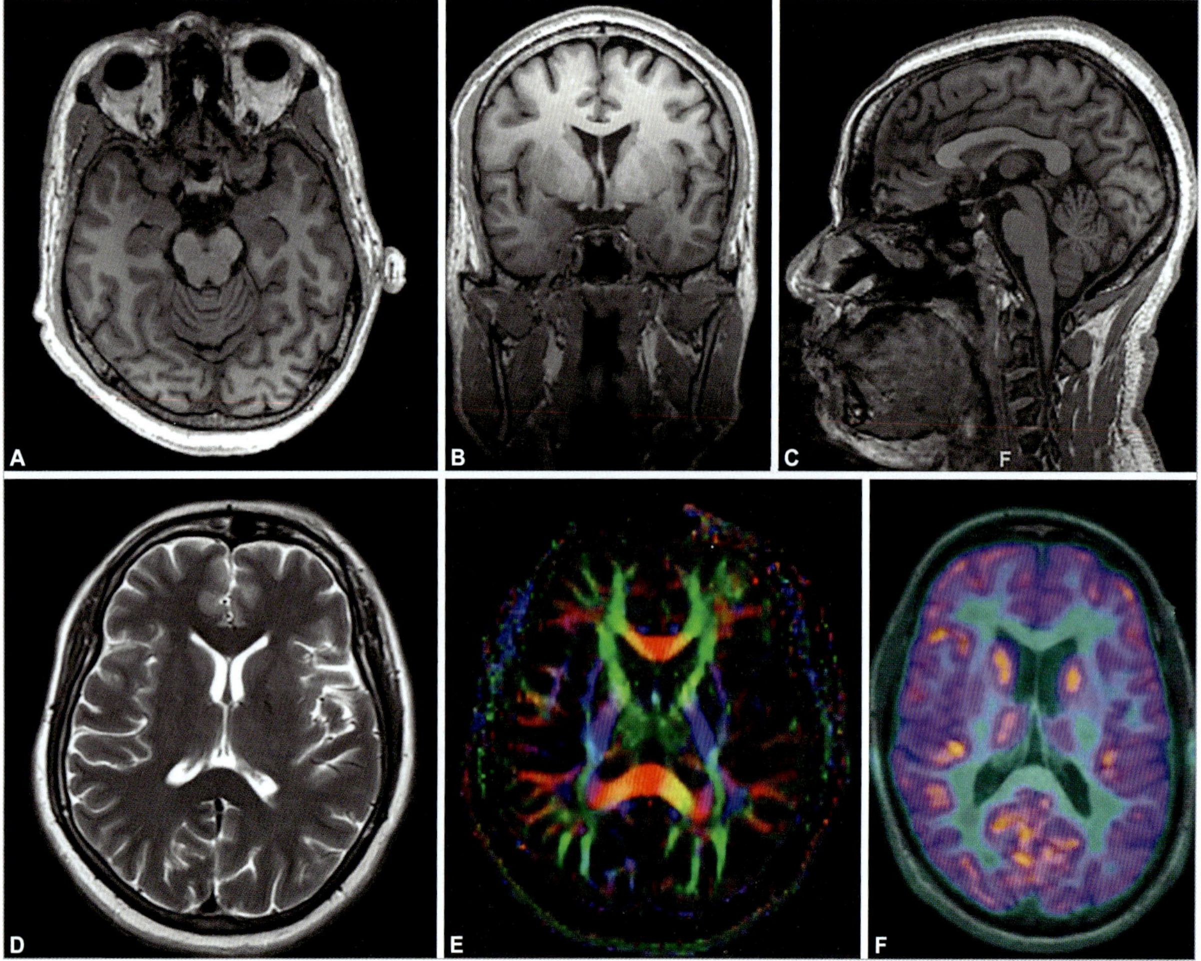

FIGS. 1A TO F: Normal magnetic resonance imaging (MRI) of brain: (A) Axial T1-weighted image; (B) T1-weighted coronal scan; (C) T1-weighted sagittal image; (D) T2-weighted scan; (E) diffusion tensor imaging (DTI) sequence; and (F) normal 18-fluorodeoxyglucose (FDG) positron emission tomography (PET) MRI—axial image.

TABLE 1: The Scheltens' scale for medial temporal atrophy (MTA).

Score	Width of		Height of hippocampal formation	Image
	Choroid fissure	Temporal horn		
0	Normal	Normal	Normal	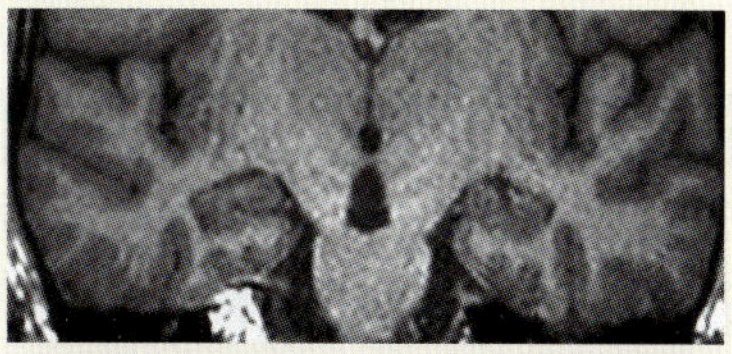
1	Slight widening (↑)	Normal	Normal	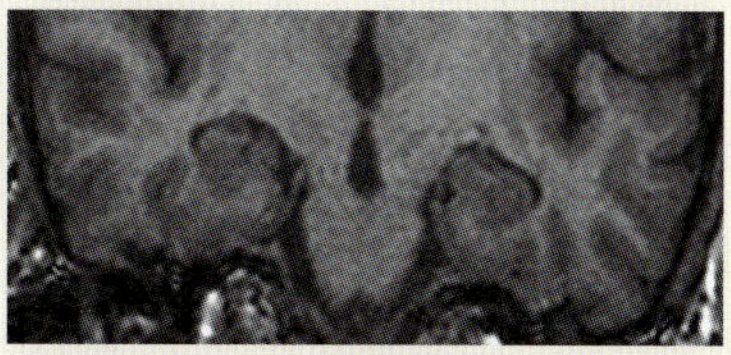
2	Moderate widening (↑↑)	Mild enlargement (↑)	Mild loss of hippocampal height (↓)	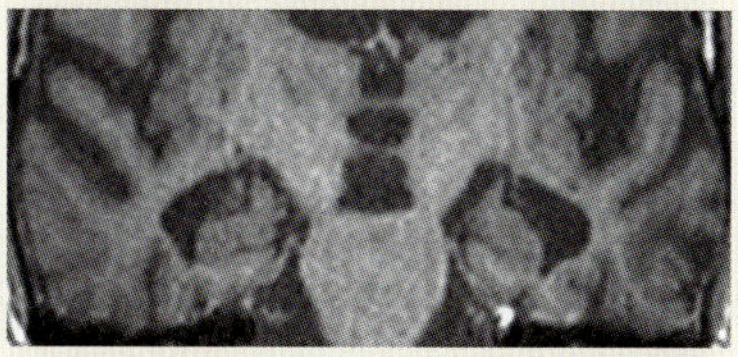
3	Marked widening (↑↑↑)	Moderate enlargement (↑↑)	Moderate loss (↓↓)	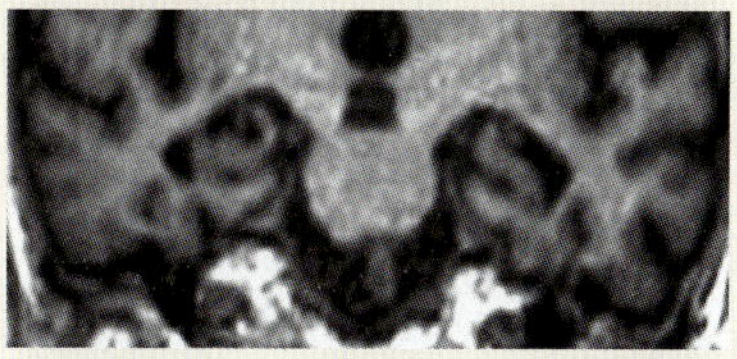
4	Marked widening (↑↑↑)	Marked enlargement (↑↑↑)	Marked atrophied and internal structure is lost (↓↓↓)	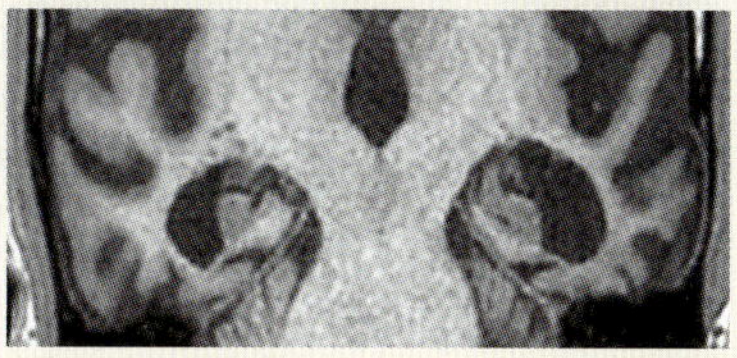

Abnormal score cutoff:

Age	*Score (abnormal, when)*
<65 years	≥1
65–74 years	≥1.5
75–84 years	≥2
>85 years	≥2

quantitative visual rating scales, such as Scheltens' Scale for medial temporal atrophy (MTA) **(Table 1)**, the entorhinal cortical atrophy (ERICA) score **(Table 2)**, the Koedam scale for parietal atrophy **(Table 3)**, global cortical atrophy (GCA), and the visual rating scale **(Table 4)**, can be applied to T1 images.[11-14]

Volumetric acquisitions typically employ a three-dimensional (3D) T1-weighted scan, such as T1 magnetization-prepared rapid gradient echo (MPRAGE) or radiofrequency-spoiled gradient recalled (SPGR) pulse sequence, depending on the manufacturer.[15] Voxel-based morphometry (VBM) analyses help in quantifying brain atrophy patterns in pathologically distinct dementias.[16] It standardizes each subject's image to a common space, allowing for the comparison of anatomical structures across subjects with a resolution of 1–2 cm. VBM identifies volume differences indicative of gray matter atrophy or changes in white matter density, facilitating the analysis of structural changes across the entire brain in various neurocognitive disorders.[17,18]

In addition, cortical thickness, determined using cortical-based morphometry, has also been shown to be a marker of various neurodegenerative disorders, such as Alzheimer's disease (AD) and frontotemporal dementia (FTD).[19] Both VBM and cortical-based morphometric imaging techniques are used as biomarkers in clinical trials targeting predementia stages.[20] Furthermore, longitudinal rates of atrophy monitor progression and can show treatment effects depending on the selected anatomical region.[21]

TABLE 2: Entorhinal cortical atrophy (ERICA) score assessment.

ERICA score	Grade of atrophy*	Detailed features	Images
0	Normal volume	None	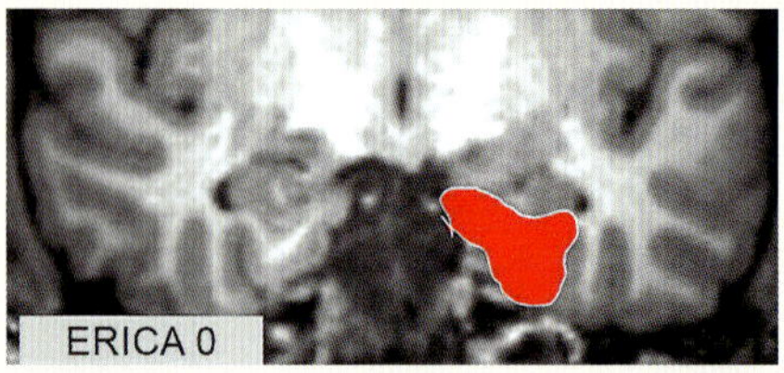 ERICA 0
1	Mild atrophy	Widening of the collateral sulcus	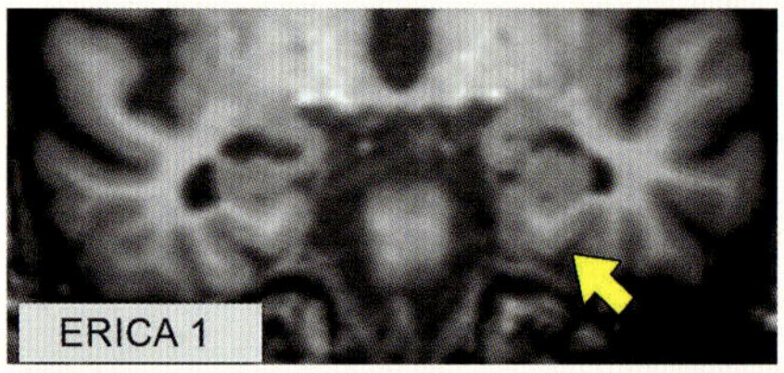 ERICA 1
2	Moderate atrophy	Elevation of the entorhinal cortex away from the adjacent cerebellar tentorium	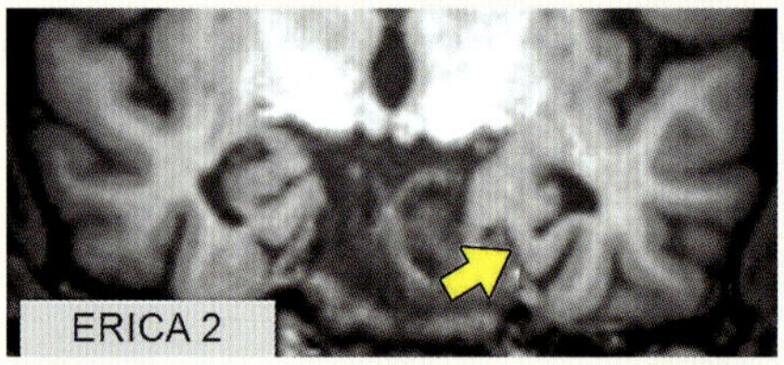 ERICA 2
3	Marked atrophy	Wide cleft between the entorhinal cortex and the adjacent cerebellar tentorium, presence of cerebrospinal fluid (CSF) termed the "tentorial cleft sign" (ERICA 2 or 3)	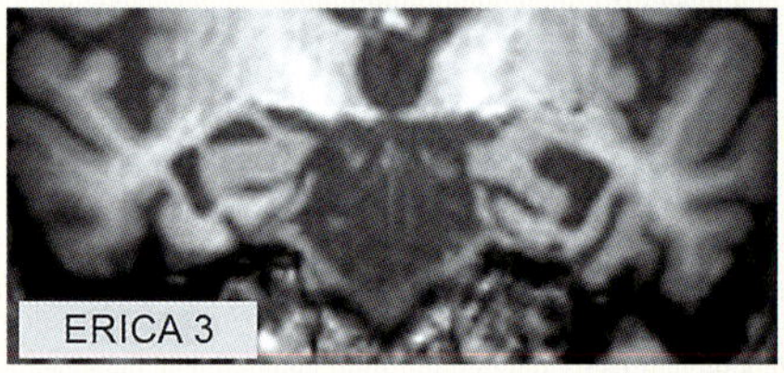 ERICA 3

*Refers to changes in the entorhinal cortex and parahippocampal gyrus.

TABLE 3: The Koedam scale for posterior atrophy.

Plane	Structure assessed	
Sagittal	Posterior cingulate sulcus, parieto-occipital sulcus, precuneus gyrus	
Coronal	Posterior cingulate sulcus, parietal gyrus	
Axial	Posterior cingulate sulcus, parietal lobes	
Koedam scale grade	**Description**	**Images**
Grade 0	Closed sulci, no gyral atrophy	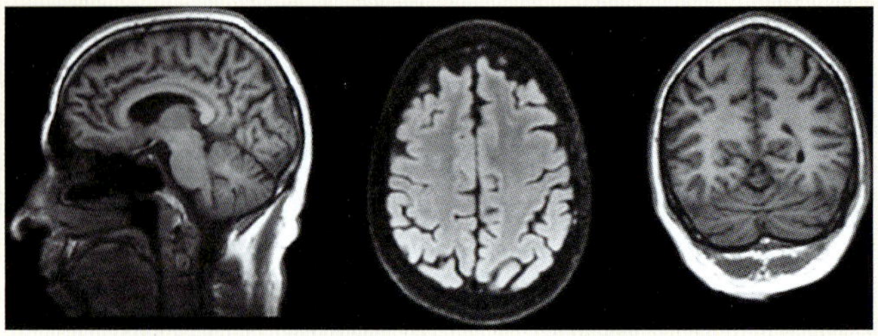

Continued

Continued

Koedam scale grade	Description	Images
Grade 1	Mild sulcal widening, mild gyral atrophy	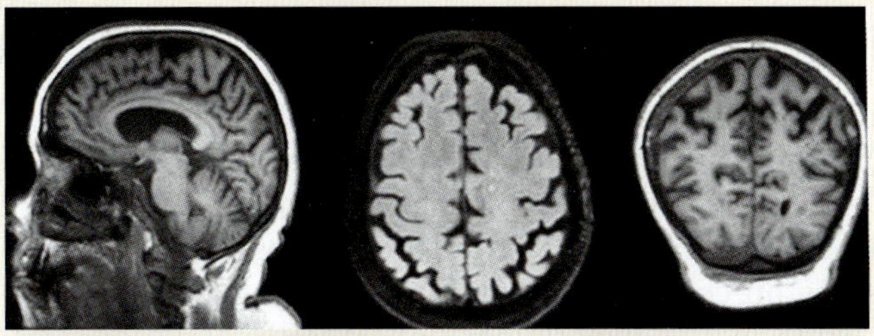
Grade 2	Substantial sulcal widening, substantial gyral atrophy	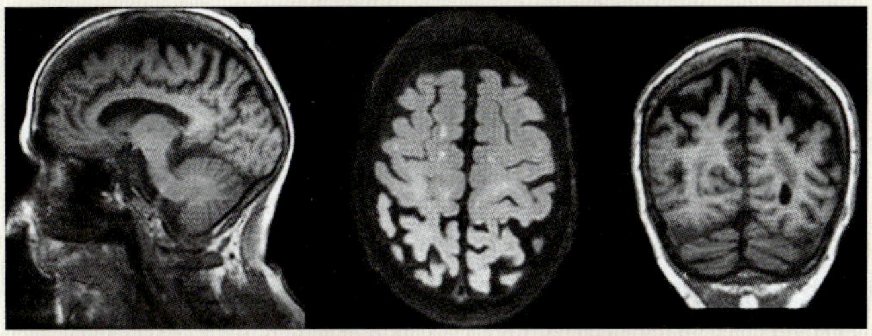
Grade 3	Marked sulcal widening, knife blade gyral atrophy	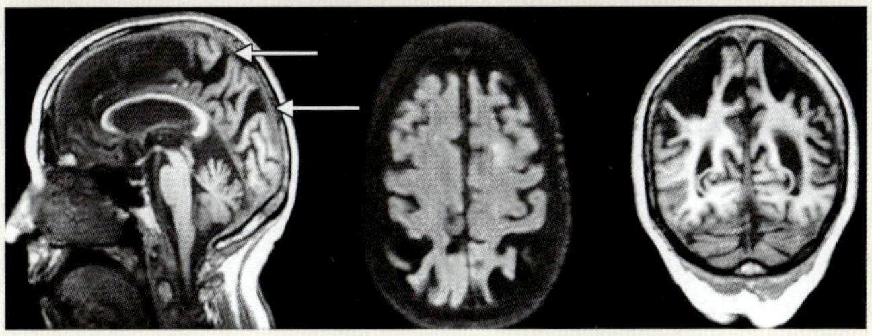

TABLE 4: Global cortical atrophy (GCA) scale assessment.

Region	Hemisphere	Score 0	Score 1	Score 2	Score 3
Sulcal dilatation	N/A	Normal volume	Opening of sulci	Volume loss of gyri	"Knife blade" atrophy
Frontal	Right and left	Normal volume/no ventricular enlargement	Opening of sulci/ mild ventricular enlargement	Volume loss of gyri/ moderate ventricular enlargement	"Knife blade" atrophy/ severe ventricular enlargement
Parieto-occipital	Right and left	Normal volume/no ventricular enlargement	Opening of sulci/ mild ventricular enlargement	Volume loss of gyri/ moderate ventricular enlargement	"Knife blade" atrophy/ severe ventricular enlargement
Temporal	Right and left	Normal volume/no ventricular enlargement	Opening of sulci/ mild ventricular enlargement	Volume loss of gyri/ moderate ventricular enlargement	"Knife blade" atrophy/ severe ventricular enlargement
Ventricular dilatation	Frontal	Normal volume/no ventricular enlargement	Mild ventricular enlargement	Moderate ventricular enlargement	Severe ventricular enlargement
Ventricular dilatation	Parieto-occipital	Normal volume/no ventricular enlargement	Mild ventricular enlargement	Moderate ventricular enlargement	Severe ventricular enlargement
Ventricular dilatation	Temporal	Normal volume/no ventricular enlargement	Mild ventricular enlargement	Moderate ventricular enlargement	Severe ventricular enlargement
Third ventricle	N/A	Normal volume/no ventricular enlargement	Mild ventricular enlargement	Moderate ventricular enlargement	Severe ventricular enlargement

Fluid-attenuated Inversion Recovery/T2 Magnetic Resonance Imaging

Axial T2-weighted sequences **(Fig. 1D)** are employed to detect gray and white matter signal abnormalities, including hippocampal and vascular changes, while 3D-FLAIR imaging is crucial for identifying edema, encephalomyelitis, and white matter changes, as well as assessing the impact of chronic hypertensive vascular disease on cognitive decline through the visualization of white matter hyperintensities (WMHs) or lesions. These lesions, which indicate underlying cerebral small vessel disease (CSVD), are graded using the Fazekas scale for severity and can predict brain atrophy.[15] Several algorithms are available to quantify white matter signal changes, including WMH segmentation packages such as the SPM lesion probability algorithm (LPA), SPM lesion growing algorithm (LGA), brain intensity abnormality classification algorithm (BIANCA), and half Gaussian mixture model (HGMM).[22]

Susceptibility-weighted Imaging/T2*

Susceptibility-weighted imaging is crucial for detecting neurodegenerative disorder indicators such as accelerated iron deposition and microhemorrhage and for differentiating cerebral microbleeds (CMBs) from calcifications using filtered phase SWAN. The location of microbleeds can often help in the diagnosis of underlying pathology; microbleeds associated with hypertension are found in deep brain regions, whereas amyloid-beta- (Aβ)-related microbleeds are more likely cortical. In addition, it is essential to monitor therapy-related amyloid-related imaging abnormalities (ARIAs) in clinical trials for AD.[23]

Diffusion-weighted Imaging/Apparent Diffusion Coefficient

Diffusion-weighted imaging analyzes the random motion of water molecules in the brain. The most important application of DWI is in Creutzfeldt-Jakob disease (CJD), where diffusion restriction is observed in the cerebral cortex called "cortical ribboning," often associated with the involvement of the basal ganglia with a sensitivity of 91% and specificity of 95%. Variant CJD (vCJD) shows diffusion restriction in the pulvinar region, with a sensitivity of 78% and specificity of 100%.[24,25] The ADC quantifies the diffusion of water molecules within tissues through magnetic resonance (MR) DWI, distinguishing true diffusion restriction [appearing dark on ADC and bright on diffusion coefficient (DWI)] from T2 shine through [appearing bright on diffusion coefficient (DWI) only].

FUNCTIONAL IMAGING

Resting State Functional Magnetic Resonance Imaging

Functional magnetic resonance imaging measures brain activity through sequences sensitive to hemoglobin oxygenation changes, with blood oxygenation level-dependent (BOLD) imaging being the standard technique during periods of relative rest, when no particular motor or cognitive activity is occurring. It leverages cerebral blood flow (CBF) differences to indicate regional brain activity. The brain regions that have correlated variation in their BOLD signal during this period are known as "resting state networks."[26] Different networks are affected in different neurodegenerative disorders and this is supported by patterns of atrophy and hypometabolism that closely correlate with the functional network identified using resting state fMRI (rsfMRI).[27]

Diffusion Tensor Imaging

Diffusion tensor imaging (DTI) helps in the quantification of microstructural properties of white matter tracts in the brain **(Fig. 1E)**. DTI measures isotropic and anisotropic diffusion in the brain, determining the type, orientation, and diffusion of molecules in different directions using a parameter called fractional anisotropy. In healthy white matter tracts, there is a high degree of anisotropic diffusion due to numerous neuronal axons traveling in the same direction. Diffusion measurements help identify tracts of interest in individuals, aiding in tractography. Although the majority of the pathology in neurodegenerative disorders occurs in gray matter, the role of white matter pathology is being recognized.[28]

METABOLIC IMAGING

Magnetic Resonance Spectroscopy

Magnetic resonance spectroscopy (MRS) is a noninvasive tool for assessing neurometabolite levels in the brain and is crucial for assessing brain functions. These metabolites include N-acetyl-aspartate (NAA), choline, creatine (Cr), lactate, and glutamate. NAA is a marker of neuronal integrity and has been reported to be lower in patients with AD than in healthy elderly subjects in the parietal gray matter and hippocampus.[29]

18F-fluorodeoxyglucose Positron Emission Tomography

Fluorodeoxyglucose-PET uses an 18F-fluoro-labeled glucose isotope to map metabolic activity in the brain, highlighting areas of metabolic patterns in brains that appear structurally normal **(Fig. 1F)**. To ensure accurate imaging, patient stimulation is minimized during scans, often through the use of eye covers to prevent cortical activation and maintain resting brain activity.

PERFUSION IMAGING

Arterial Spin Labeling

Arterial spin labeling (ASL) measures CBF by magnetically labeling blood water as an endogenous tracer at the tissue level. It can be used to quantify regional cerebral blood volumes. Different patterns of decreased ASL signals are associated with various types of dementia.[30]

Single-photon Emission Computed Tomography

Single-photon emission computed tomography (SPECT) employs radiotracers such as 123I-ioflupane and 99mTc-hexamethyl propylene amine oxime (HMPAO) to show distinct uptake patterns in various brain regions, allowing the tracking of cerebral perfusion and specificity for different dementia subtypes. SPECT is useful for distinguishing clinically diagnosed AD patients from age-matched controls and patients with vascular dementia (VaD), FTD, and dementia of Lewy body disease (DLBD). While FDG-PET has better sensitivity, SPECT has higher specificity in discriminating AD from normal aging.[31]

MOLECULAR IMAGING

Amyloid Positron Emission Tomography

Molecular imaging has revolutionized the visualization of pathology in vivo, including in the presymptomatic stages. Amyloid PET imaging tracers, such as 18F-florbetapir, 18F-florbetaben, and 18F-flutemetamol, are Food and Drug Administration (FDA) approved and reliably detect AD pathology across various disease stages. They bind to specific amyloid protein motifs and are closely correlated with postmortem amyloid deposition. Amyloid pathology typically begins in a diffuse regional pattern and progresses to the neocortex, with notable tracer uptake in the frontal, parietal, and lateral temporal cortices.[10] Positive amyloid PET scans show loss of gray/white matter distinction, while negative scans retain it.[10] These imaging patterns can predict cognitive decline in healthy individuals and those with mild cognitive impairment (MCI). However, the high sensitivity and lower specificity of amyloid PET for predicting MCI-to-AD conversion, along with concerns about cost and clinical overuse, have led to the development of appropriate-use criteria. These criteria recommend amyloid PET evaluation for individuals with unexplained MCI, atypical AD presentations, and early-onset dementia and are evaluated as endpoints in clinical trials.

Tau Positron Emission Tomography

Tau is the second protein associated with AD and is the focus of developing PET imaging tracers, i.e., flortaucipir. These tracers target specific motifs of phosphorylated-tau, such as tau paired helical filaments (PHFs) or neurofibrillary tangles (NFTs), and have been shown to correlate with AD severity and cognitive deficits in postmortem studies.[32,33]

All imaging modalities used in neurocognitive disorders have been summarized in **Table 5**.

IMAGING PATTERNS IN NEUROCOGNITIVE DISORDERS

Mild Cognitive Impairment

In healthy individuals and MCI, the degree and progression of medial temporal lobe atrophy are linked to the progression to dementia. Magnetic resonance imaging (MRI) findings of increased subcortical WMH and cortical infarction are also associated with MCI. A meta-analysis revealed that the prevalence of positive amyloid PET scans increases with age among individuals with normal cognition and is even greater in individuals with MCI. Apolipoprotein E (APOE) ε4 carriers are more likely to have a positive scan and are associated with greater rate of progression to dementia. A combination of a positive flutemetamol F-18-labeled PET scan, low hippocampal volumes on MRI, and cognitive status consistent with amnestic MCI is indicative of a high probability of progression to dementia. Additionally, individuals with abnormal PET results and impaired episodic memory are significantly more likely to convert to AD (11.7 times) than are those with normal results on both measures.[34]

Individuals with subjective cognitive decline (SCD), marked by self-reported cognitive issues despite normal test results and good insight, are three times more likely to develop MCI with AD-related biomarkers. Furthermore, 14% of those with normal cognitive function and SCD progress to dementia within 4 years of follow-up. SCD is also associated with elevated tau levels in the entorhinal cortex and a global increase in Aβ.[35]

Alzheimer's Disease

In AD, there is atrophy involving the temporoparietal regions, hippocampus, mesial temporal cortex, and precuneus while sparing the sensorimotor strip **(Fig. 2A)**. The "elephant sign" in T1/T2 coronal MR images results

TABLE 5: Imaging modalities used in neurocognitive disorders.

	Imaging modality	Indication
Structural imaging	T1 weighted	• Thin-slice T1-weighted images for identifying regional atrophy • Coronal T1-weighted imaging for quantitative analysis, especially for assessing atrophy in the MTL and hippocampal morphology • Sagittal T1-weighted imaging for evaluating the volume of the precuneus and parietal lobe cortex • Semiquantitative visual rating scales such as Scheltens' scale, ERICA, GCA, and the Koedam scale can be applied
	T2/FLAIR	• Axial T2-weighted and coronal T2-weighted sequences for identifying gray and white matter signal abnormalities, including hippocampal changes and vascular damage • 3D-FLAIR imaging for detecting edema, encephalomyelitis, and white matter changes • FLAIR images for assessing the role of chronic hypertensive vascular disease in cognitive decline and grading white matter hyperintensities using the Fazekas scale • Biomarkers within NABM in FLAIR MRI are linked to cognitive function
	SWI	• 3D SWAN or SWI for detecting accelerated iron deposition and microhemorrhages associated with neurodegenerative disorders • Filtered phase SWAN to differentiate CMBs from calcifications • SWI is essential for monitoring ARIA-H and detecting hemorrhagic lesions, stroke, cerebral amyloid angiopathy, venous anomalies, traumatic injuries, and neoplasms
	DWI/ADC	DWI sequence measures the random movement of water molecules to detect areas of restricted diffusion, indicating acute ischemia, tumors, inflammation, alcoholic encephalopathy, or changes in signaling linked to Creutzfeldt–Jakob disease
Functional imaging	rsfMRI	DMN includes posterior cingulate, inferior parietal, inferolateral, ventral anterior cingulate, and hippocampal regions—this network shows decreased connectivity in AD. Salience network includes the dorsal anterior cingulate and orbital frontoinsular regions and tracks with emotional measures that are involved in FTD
	DTI	DTI maps white matter microstructure, utilizing measures such as MD and FA to assess molecular displacement and directional diffusion
Perfusion imaging	ASL	• ASL MRI measures CBF by magnetically labeling blood water as an endogenous tracer • Patterns of brain hypoperfusion in ASL-MRI resemble those of hypometabolism in FDG-PET but with less accuracy for diagnosing dementia
	SPECT	• SPECT is a nuclear medicine imaging technique that merges scintigraphy with computed tomography, offering 3D, detailed visualizations of radionuclide distribution in the brain • In AD and vascular dementia, ioflupane SPECT shows normal uptake, while in DLB, it reveals a loss of uptake in the bilateral basal ganglia and in FTLD, the uptake is also normal
Metabolic imaging	MRS	• MRS is a noninvasive tool for assessing neurometabolite levels in the brain, crucial for brain functions • It utilizes proton resonance in magnetic fields, enhanced by high-field scanners and acquisition techniques such as STEAM, PRESS, MEGA-PRESS, LASER, and semi-LASER, to detect complex molecules like NAA, Cr, glutathione, glutamine, glutamate, and GABA
	FDG-PET	FDG-PET employs an 18-F-fluoro-labeled glucose isotope to detect metabolic changes in the brain, revealing early signs of neurodegenerative diseases before structural atrophy becomes apparent on MRI
Molecular imaging	Amyloid PET	Utilizes tracers such as 18F-florbetapir, 18F-florbetaben, and 18F-flutemetamol that bind to amyloid plaques, offering reliable detection of AD pathology at various stages. These tracers are employed to predict cognitive decline in presymptomatic individuals and those with mild cognitive impairment and are crucial for selecting patients for antiamyloid therapy and monitoring progression
	Tau-PET	Tau-PET tracers, such as flortaucipir, target phosphorylated-tau motifs in neurofibrillary tangles, correlating with AD severity and cognitive deficits, aiding in the diagnosis and staging of the disease

(3D: three dimensional; AD: Alzheimer's disease; ADC: apparent diffusion coefficient; ARIA-H: amyloid-related imaging abnormalities-hemorrhagic; ASL: arterial spin labeling; CBF: cerebral blood flow; CMBs: cerebral microbleeds; Cr: creatinine; DLB: dementia with Lewy bodies; DTI: diffusion tensor imaging; DWI: diffusion-weighted imaging; ERICA: entorhinal cortical atrophy score; FA: fractional anisotropy; FDG-PET: fluorodeoxyglucose positron emission tomography; FLAIR: fluid-attenuated inversion recovery; FTD: frontotemporal dementia; FTLD: frontotemporal lobar degeneration; GABA: gamma-aminobutyric acid; GCA: global cortical atrophy; MD: mean diffusivity; MRI: magnetic resonance imaging; MRS: magnetic resonance spectroscopy; MTA: medial temporal atrophy; MTL: medial temporal lobe; NAA: N-acetyl-aspartate; NABM: normal-appearing brain matter; rsfMRI: resting state functional MRI; SPECT: single-photon emission computed tomography; STEAM: stimulated echo acquisition mode; SWAN: susceptibility-weighted angiography; SWI: susceptibility-weighted imaging; VBM: voxel-based morphometry) from early atrophy of the medial temporal lobes, including the entorhinal cortex and hippocampus, resembling an elephant's trunk. Interestingly, in younger patients, brain atrophy may be more common in the parietal region, with less atrophy in the hippocampus.[10] Hippocampal volumetry using MRI can predict the progression from MCI to dementia.

Resting state fMRI studies have shown that the default mode network (DMN), which is normally active during rest, is disrupted early in the disease process, with decreased connectivity in the medial prefrontal cortex, inferior parietal lobule, posterior cingulate gyrus, hippocampal formation, and lateral temporal cortex. This decreased connectivity is independent of brain amyloidosis, especially in cognitively normal individuals with the APOE ε4 allele.[36]

Lower NAA or NAA/Cr ratios have been found in patients with AD than in MCI and controls, while myo-inositol (mI) and mI/Cr levels are generally greater in AD. Additionally, glutathione (GSH) is emerging as a differential biomarker, with metabolic changes in the posterior cingulate cortex (PCC) distinguishing patients with AD from MCI patients and healthy controls. Comparative studies indicate similar NAA/Cr reductions in patients with FTD and AD versus controls, yet with distinct spatial patterns—frontal decreases in FTD and posterior decreases in AD. Additionally, a lower NAA/Cr ratio has been reported in patients with Parkinson's disease (PD) dementia (PDD) than in patients with PD-MCI, PD and controls. One study linked high mI/Cr and low NAA/mI with increased amyloid deposition over time while another associated increased brain tau with decreased NAA/Cr and Glu/Cr in females.[37]

In the A/T/N model of AD, "N" represents neurodegeneration, which is evaluated using brain MRI to detect atrophy and FDG-PET to assess glucose hypometabolism.[5] FDG-PET imaging is particularly useful for early dementia detection and for distinguishing between different dementia subtypes by identifying specific patterns of hypometabolism before noticeable brain atrophy occurs. In AD, there is notable hypometabolism and/or hypoperfusion in the PCC and bilateral parietal areas, especially in the precuneus **(Figs. 2B and C)**. In contrast, ibupane SPECT generally shows normal uptake. Amyloid PET reveals widespread abnormal amyloid tracer uptake in the cortex, indicative of reduced gray-white matter differentiation, while tau PET detects abnormal tau protein accumulation that aligns with the Braak staging system. Imaging techniques such as amyloid and tau PET provide more precise insights into the molecular changes occurring in the brain.

Amyloid PET scans, using tracers like florbetapir, flutemetamol, and florbetaben, measure the amyloid burden in the brain and aids in diagnosing AD. A "negative" scan is indicated by nonspecific tracer retention throughout the white matter without cortical involvement, while a positive scan shows significant tracer retention in the medial and lateral temporal lobes, extending to frontal and parietal lobes. It can detect abnormalities up to 10 years before symptoms appear, but it is not exclusive to AD, as some healthy older adults also show amyloid deposits; thus, it is effective in ruling out AD.[38] In contrast, tau PET abnormalities are more closely linked to symptom onset, making it useful for confirming Alzheimer's disease. Positive results in both tau and amyloid PET scans in people without cognitive impairment indicate a greater risk of future cognitive decline.

Tau PET imaging mirrors the spread of NFTs indicative of AD, beginning in the entorhinal cortex and hippocampus and advancing through the inferior and lateral temporal regions to the parietal, occipital, and frontal cortices, in line with the Braak and Braak stages of tau deposition. High tracer retention in the mesial temporal lobe can be observed even in presymptomatic individuals, while those with MCI or AD exhibit tracer uptake in more extensive neocortical areas.

Alzheimer's Disease Variants

Posterior cortical atrophy (PCA) typically exhibits significant occipitoparietal or occipitotemporal atrophy, hypometabolism, or hypoperfusion on neuroimaging **(Figs. 2D to F)**. Patients with logopenic variant primary progressive aphasia (PPA) often present with left posterior perisylvian or parietal atrophy, with FDG-PET and SPECT highlighting corresponding hypometabolism or hypoperfusion. Amyloid PET imaging shows elevated signals in approximately 85% of logopenic variant patients, suggesting AD pathology, although it is not exclusively diagnostic due to mixed pathologies in some patients. The dysexecutive or frontal variant is characterized by more pronounced thinning in the frontoparietal cortical regions and typically follows a more rapid clinical progression.[39,40]

Limbic-predominant Age-related TDP-43 Encephalopathy

Limbic-predominant age-related TDP-43 encephalopathy (LATE) is a TDP-43 proteinopathy in older adults that often presents with hippocampal sclerosis characterized by atrophy and T2 prolongation in the hippocampus and temporal lobe white matter, along with a rostrocaudal pattern of volume loss that initially affects the amygdala, then the head of the hippocampus, and finally the body. This condition is distinct from AD by its restricted neuroanatomic distribution, absence of amyloid deposition, and more rapid hippocampal atrophy despite slower

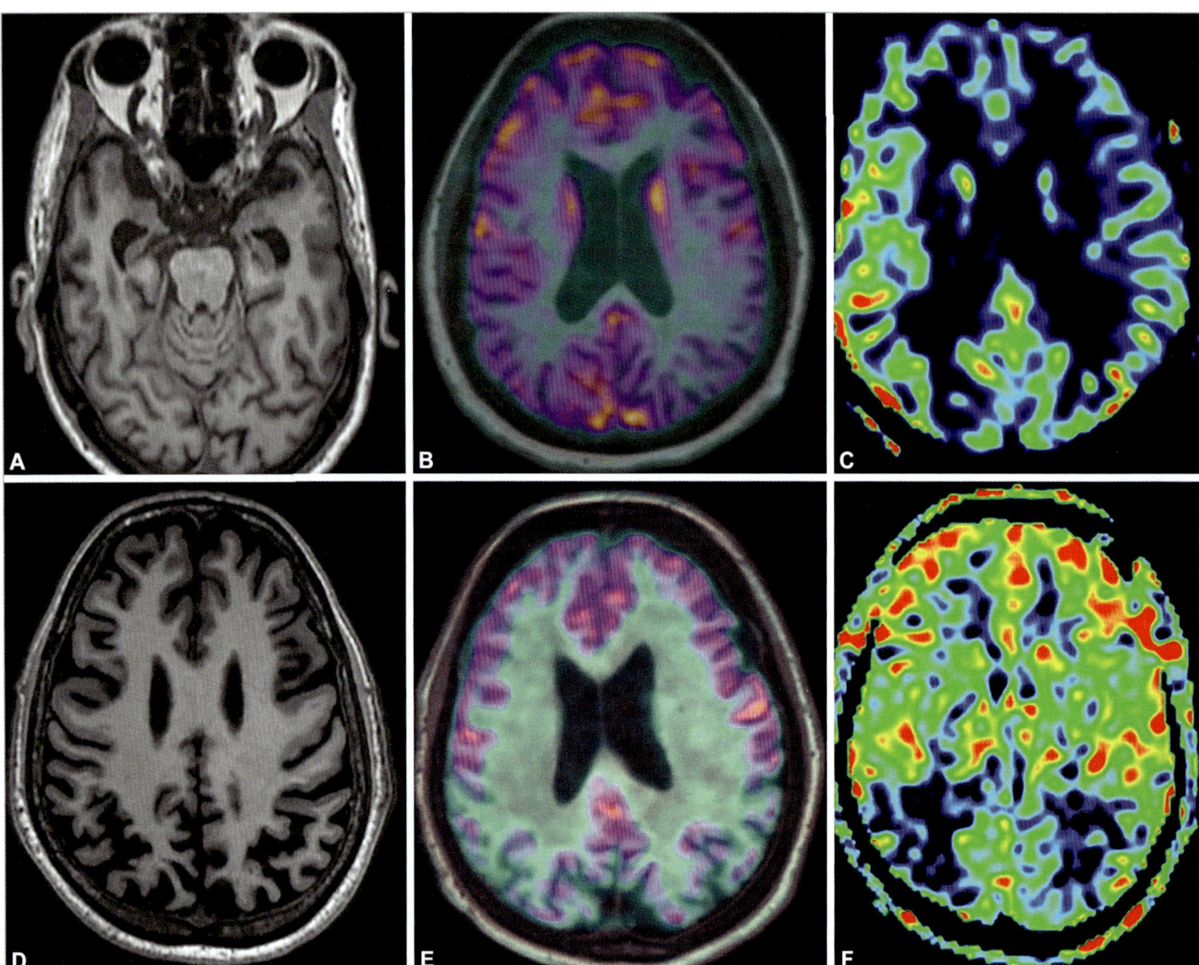

FIGS. 2A TO F: Imaging in Alzheimer's disease: (A) Axial T1-weighted scan shows bilateral medial temporal lobe atrophy. (B) Fluorodeoxyglucose (FDG) positron emission tomography (PET) magnetic resonance imaging (MRI) axial scan shows biparietal and posterior cingulate hypometabolism. (C) Arterial spin labeling (ASL) axial scan shows hypoperfusion in biparietal and posterior cingulate region. (D) T1-weighted axial scan shows posterior predominant atrophy suggestive of posterior cortical atrophy. (E) 18-FDG-PET MRI shows posterior-dominant cortical hypometabolism. (F) ASL scan shows hypoperfusion in posterior-dominant regions.

clinical decline, and it can be differentiated from AD by the absence of amyloid and/or tau on PET.[40]

Frontotemporal Dementia

In FTD, neuroimaging typically reveals anterior frontal and temporal lobe involvement, while the parietal lobes are relatively spared. Ioflupane SPECT generally shows normal uptake and amyloid PET often does not show abnormal uptake, although a positive result does not exclude FTD. The role of tau PET in FTD remains uncertain, as uptake appears to vary among different subtypes. Patients with behavioral variant FTD (bvFTD) exhibit atrophy, hypometabolism, or hypoperfusion in the anterior cingulate, prefrontal cortex, anterior temporal lobes, and limbic and subcortical regions **(Figs. 3A and B)**. In nonfluent variant PPA, neuroimaging reveals atrophy in the left posterior frontoinsular cortex, with SPECT or FDG-PET indicating hypoperfusion or hypometabolism in this region **(Figs. 3C and D)**. The semantic variant PPA is characterized by asymmetrical anterior temporal atrophy with more pronounced atrophy in the language-dominant hemisphere and corresponding hypoperfusion or hypometabolism **(Figs. 3E and F)**.

Vascular Dementia

Structural brain imaging is essential for identifying silent cerebrovascular disease and assessing the extent of damage that may contribute to cognitive decline. This includes a range of conditions such as multi-infarct dementia, subcortical ischemic vascular dementia, dementia related to strategic strokes, perfusion-related dementia, hemorrhagic stroke-related dementia,

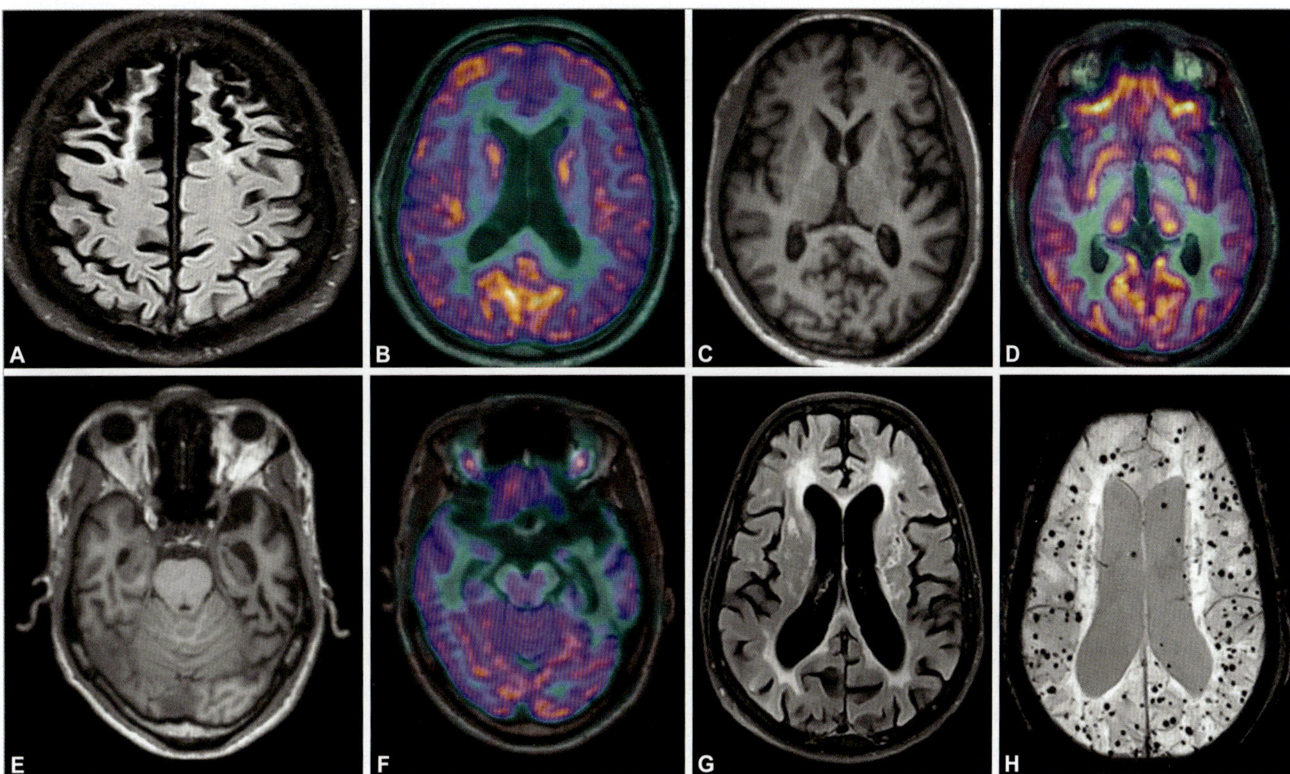

FIGS. 3A TO H: Imaging findings in frontotemporal dementia (FTD) spectrum disorders and vascular dementia: (A and B) T1 image and fluorodeoxyglucose positron emission tomography (FDG PET) showing atrophy in medial and lateral prefrontal and anterior cortex in behavioral variant FTD; (C and D) T1 image and FDG-PET scan depicts left frontoinsular atrophy and hypometabolism in progressive nonfluent aphasia; (E and F) axial T1 image and FDG-PET scan shows left anterior lateral temporal atrophy and hypometabolism in semantic dementia; (G) axial fluid-attenuated inversion recovery (FLAIR) image depicts small subcortical lacunar infarcts and diffuse white matter changes in small vessel disease; and (H) susceptibility-weighted image (SWI) shows microbleeds involving cortico-subcortical regions suggestive of blooming seen in cerebral amyloid angiopathy (CAA).

dementia associated with arteriopathies, and mixed dementia.[41,42] MRI sequences such as T2/FLAIR and SWI is favored over computed tomography (CT) for its greater sensitivity in detecting signs of CSVD, including microbleeds indicative of cerebral amyloid angiopathy (CAA) **(Figs. 3G and H)**. However, CT may be used if MRI is not available or contraindicated, although it is less likely to reveal a treatable cause of dementia not seen on MRI.

The Standards for Reporting Vascular Changes on Neuroimaging (STRIVE) criteria provide radiological definitions for brain changes due to CSVD.[43] Key signs include nonlacunar infarcts (larger than 15 mm or any size in the cortex), lacunes of presumed vascular origin (small, ≤15 mm infarcts in subcortical regions), WMH on MRI or hypodensities on CT, microbleeds (small areas of signal loss on SWI), superficial siderosis (linear hypointensity along the cortical surface on SWI), visible perivascular spaces, and accelerated brain atrophy associated with CSVD. État criblé, characterized by enlarged perivascular spaces in the basal ganglia and associated with confluent WMHs, serves as a significant marker of cerebrovascular disease. Similarly, strategic lacunes in the basal ganglia and thalami also act as potential indicators of vascular disease.[41]

Brain Imaging in Patients with Amyloid-related Imaging Abnormalities

Amyloid-related imaging abnormalities occur in approximately 40% of patients on high doses of aducanumab, especially those with the APOE ε4 allele. ARIA typically appears within the first eight doses and can manifest as edema (ARIA-E) or microhemorrhage (ARIA-H). ARIA-E is often asymptomatic but can cause symptoms such as fatigue and headache, while ARIA-H involves microhemorrhage and/or superficial siderosis. MRI monitoring is essential for detecting ARIA before treatment and at specific intervals using sequences such as FLAIR, T2, gradient echo (GRE) or SWI, and DWI.[44]

Dementia with Lewy Body

Dementia with Lewy body (DLB) is neuropathologically characterized by abnormal aggregation of α-synuclein and clinically characterized by executive and visuospatial dysfunction. Imaging shows more pronounced cortical atrophy than PDD patients **(Fig. 4A)**. SPECT and PET often show decreased overall perfusion and metabolism, particularly in the occipital areas. A notable feature of DLB is the preservation of posterior cingulate metabolism, known as the "cingulate island sign," which differs from that of AD **(Fig. 4B)**.[45] While occipital hypoperfusion is a potential diagnostic marker for DLB, MRI does not typically show occipital atrophy in these patients. A biomarker suggestive of DLB is ioflupane I 123, which labels the dopamine transporter in the nigrostriatal dopaminergic pathway on SPECT or PET. Reduced dopamine transporter uptake in the basal ganglia reflects abnormally low presynaptic dopamine typically observed in DLB, PD, multiple system atrophy (MSA), progressive supranuclear palsy (PSP), and corticobasal degeneration (CBD). This can be an indicative imaging biomarker for DLB when other clinical information is available.

Cardiac autonomic denervation, a feature of Lewy body disorders, can be assessed using 123-I-metaiodobenzylguanidine (MIBG) myocardial scintigraphy, which shows low uptake in DLB, indicating reduced sympathetic cardiac innervation.[46]

Corticobasal Syndrome

Imaging in corticobasal syndrome (CBS) shows asymmetric cortical atrophy, hypometabolism, and hypoperfusion, primarily affecting the frontoparietal regions encompassing the premotor, motor, and sensory association cortex, and typically develops contralateral to the more affected side of the body **(Fig. 4C)**. Asymmetrical perirolandic atrophy or hypometabolism on imaging supports a clinical diagnosis of CBS, although its absence does not exclude it. This is helpful in the disease course, when differentials may include other parkinsonism syndromes. T2-weighted images often show hyperintensity in the atrophic cortex and underlying white matter, with occasional minor signal hypointensity in the putamina and pallida.[34,47]

Progressive Supranuclear Palsy

In PSP-Richardson syndrome, there is generalized brain and brainstem atrophy, particularly in the midbrain, which leads to the "hummingbird sign" or "penguin silhouette" sign on midsagittal MR images, characterized by prominent midbrain atrophy with relatively preserved pons. Superior cerebellar peduncle atrophy is common in PSP and is correlated with disease duration. The "morning glory" flower sign indicates profound midbrain atrophy with concavity of the lateral margin of the midbrain tegmentum **(Figs. 4D and E)**.[48,49]

Positron emission tomography scans revealed decreased glucose metabolism in the midbrain as an early sign of PSP, with reduced metabolic activity in the caudate, putamen, and prefrontal cortex as the disease progressed. The "hypointense substantia nigra" (HSN) sign, visible on T1-weighted sequences, is a well-demarcated bilateral hypointensity of the medial aspect of the substantia nigra. On a sagittal plane, the HSN appears as a well-defined bilateral hypointense line with an oblique direction, resembling a crevice, known as the "midbrain crevice" sign. These are recent radiological signs described for PSP.[50]

Normal Pressure Hydrocephalus

Magnetic resonance imaging is the preferred imaging modality for normal pressure hydrocephalus (NPH), revealing characteristic features such as enlarged lateral and third ventricles, widened Sylvian fissures, ventriculomegaly [Evans index > 0.3 and anterior lateral ventricular index (ALVI) > 0.5], temporal horn widening (>6 mm not explained by hippocampal atrophy), an acute callosal angle (<90°) and disproportionately enlarged subarachnoid space hydrocephalus (DESH) **(Fig. 4F)**. The callosal angle is drawn at the posterior commissure on coronal images **(Fig. 4G)**. High signal abnormalities around the ventricles may indicate transependymal fluid egress or small vessel damage and can correlate with the extent of white matter disease, which may be associated with cognitive impairment and shunt response. An aqueduct flow void, suggesting increased cerebrospinal fluid (CSF) flow velocity, is frequently observed but lacks diagnostic value for shunt response.[39,51] A lack of hippocampal atrophy for ventriculomegaly in proportion to brain atrophy in the presence of clinical findings is supportive of NPH rather than AD, although these pathologies can coexist.[52]

Creutzfeldt–Jakob Disease

In sporadic CJD (sCJD), hyperintense signal changes are observed on DWI/ADC, FLAIR, and T2-weighted images. The cerebral cortex shows focal or diffuse, symmetric or asymmetric involvement of the superior frontal gyrus, superior parietal lobule, cingulate gyrus, and insular cortex, with sparing of the perirolandic cortex.[40] The basal ganglia also show symmetric or asymmetric involvement, particularly of the caudate head and putamen, with an anterior posterior gradient **(Figs. 4H and I)**. The "double

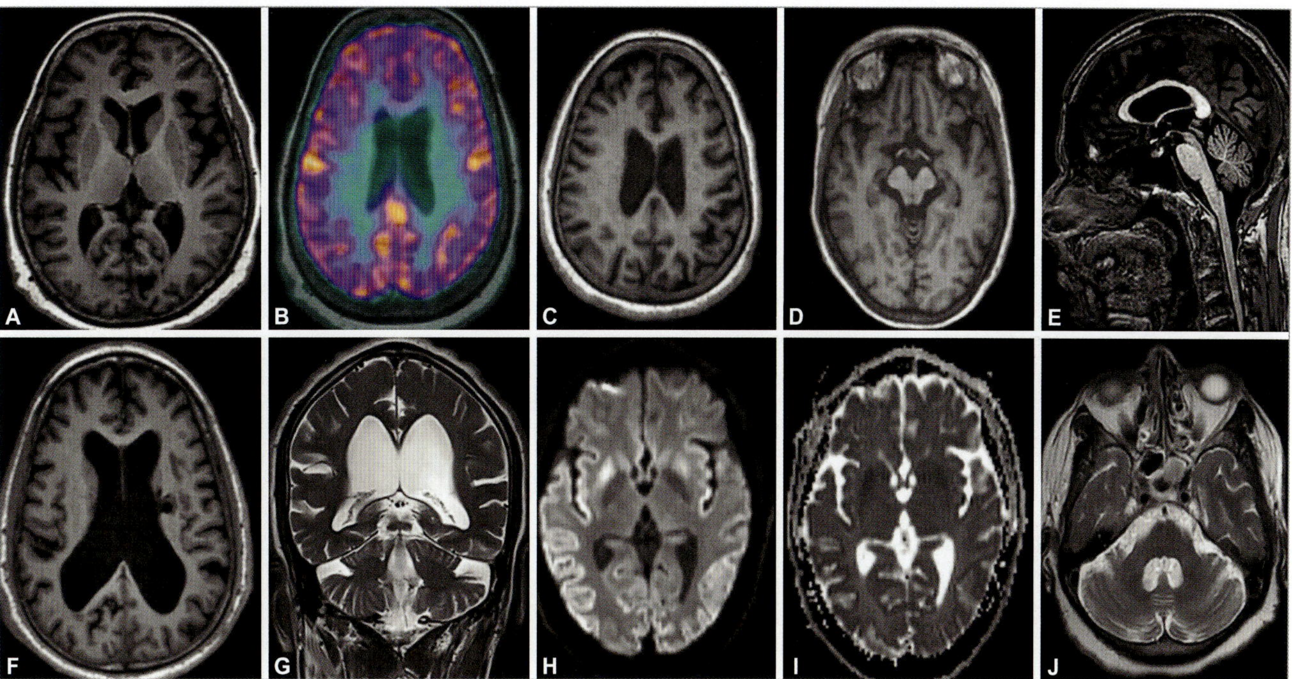

FIGS. 4A TO J: Imaging findings in different neurocognitive disorders: (A and B) Axial T1 magnetic resonance imaging (MRI) and fluorodeoxyglucose positron emission tomography (FDG-PET) depicts parieto-occipital atrophy and occipital hypometabolism with relative preservation of metabolism in posterior cingulate region also called "cingulate island" sign seen in Lewy body dementia. (C) T1 image shows left frontoparietal atrophy in corticobasal syndrome. (D) Axial T1 image depicts midbrain tegmentum atrophy with preservation of tectum and cerebral peduncles, called the "Mickey Mouse sign" or "morning glory sign." (E) Midsagittal T1-weighted MRI shows midbrain tegmental atrophy without pontine atrophy, associated with widening of interpeduncular cistern giving impression of head and body of a humming bird, called the "hummingbird sign" or the "penguin sign." (F) Axial T1-weighted image shows ventriculomegaly and disproportionately enlarged subarachnoid space hydrocephalus (DESH) seen in normal pressure hydrocephalus (NPH); (G) coronal MRI scan at the posterior commissure depicts acute callosal angle observed in NPH. (H and I) Diffusion-weighted image (DWI) and apparent diffusion coefficient (ADC) shows involvement of bilateral basal ganglia, insular cortex, and temporoparietal regions seen in Creutzfeldt–Jakob disease (CJD). (J) Axial T2-weighted image showing hyperintensity in form of a cross in the pontine region, called the "hot cross bun sign" due to selective degeneration of transverse pontocerebellar tracts and median pontine raphe nuclei.

hockey stick" or "pulvinar" sign, usually indicative of variant CJD (vCJD), can also appear in the mesial and dorsal thalami of some sporadic CJD patients, along with atypical MRI patterns such as DWI- and FLAIR-hyperintense signals and late-stage cerebellar atrophy.[40]

Other Neurocognitive Disorders: Multiple System Atrophy and Huntington's Disease

In MSA, imaging findings include atrophy of the putamen, pons, middle cerebellar peduncles, and cerebellum; T2 hypointensity in the posterior putamen; T2 hyperintensity in the lateral putaminal rim "putaminal rim sign"; and the "hot cross bun" sign (a hyperintense T2 signal in the shape of a cross within the pons) **(Fig. 4J)**. PET imaging may reveal regional glucose hypometabolism in the striatum, brainstem, and cerebellum, while SPECT imaging typically shows abnormal striatal dopamine transporter activity.[52]

In HD patients, axial MRI shows caudate atrophy with diminished head protrusion and "boxcarring" on T2/FLAIR sequences, which correlates with cognitive decline and abnormal caudate metabolism on PET.[53]

RECENT ADVANCES IN NEUROIMAGING BIOMARKERS

Advances in neuroimaging techniques for neurocognitive disorders are undergoing a revolution that is transforming neuroimaging research from merely describing changes in the brain to understanding what those changes mean. These emerging advances have been driven primarily by a need for biomarkers, leading to a better understanding of different neural mechanisms of pathology in vivo and ultimately to the evaluation of potential disease-modifying therapies for different neurocognitive disorders. The application of these advanced imaging techniques has the potential to uncover newer mechanisms involved in the pathogenesis of neurocognitive disorders **(Fig. 5)**.

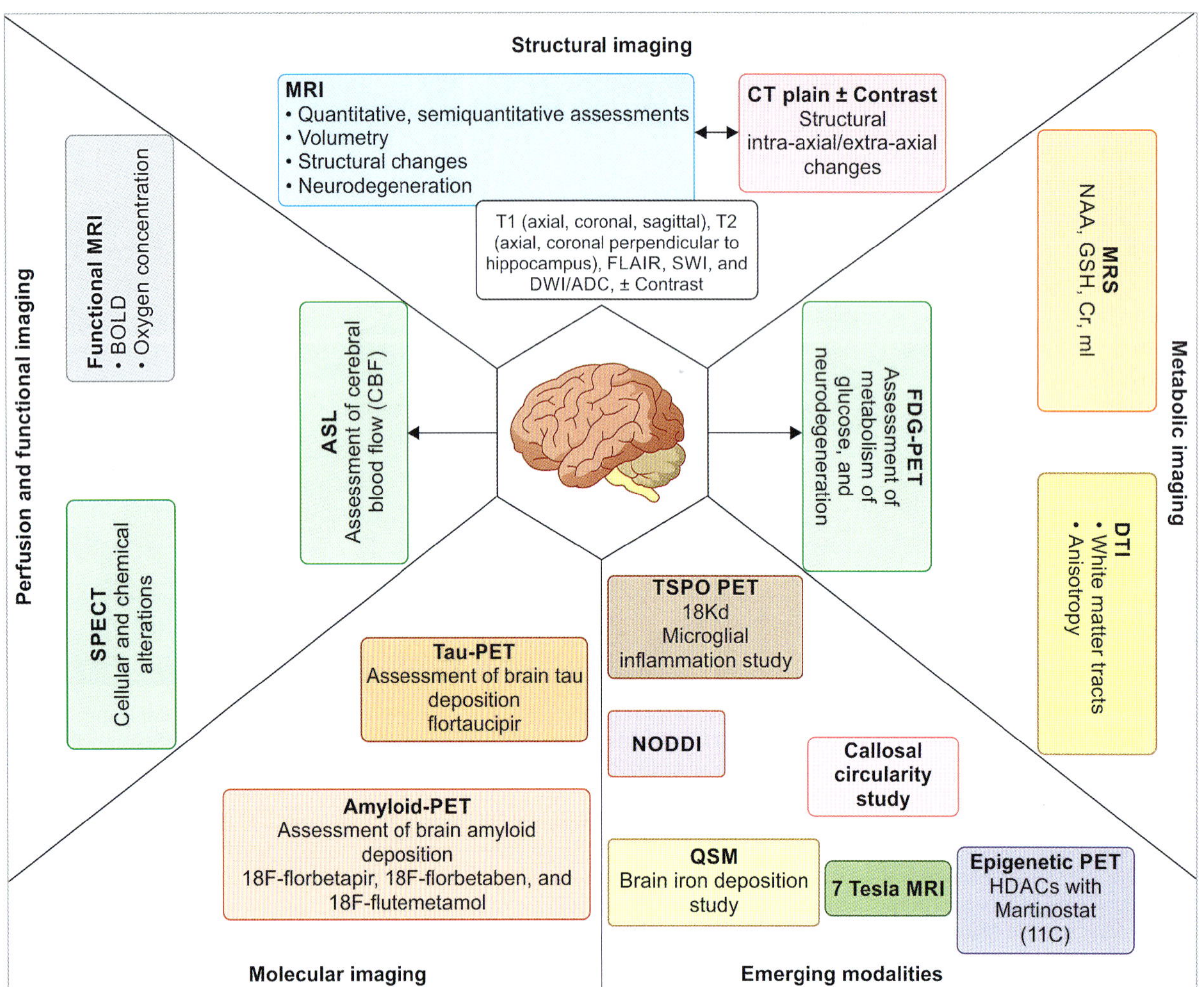

FIG. 5: Advanced imaging modalities used for different neurocognitive disorders.

(ADC: apparent diffusion coefficient; ASL: arterial spin labeling; BOLD: blood oxygenation level dependent; CBF: cerebral blood flow; Cr: creatinine; CT: computed tomography; DTI: diffusion tensor imaging; DWI: diffusion-weighted imaging; FLAIR: fluid-attenuated inversion recovery; GSH: glutathione; HDACs: histone deacetylases; ml: myo-inositol; MRI: magnetic resonance imaging; MRS: magnetic resonance spectroscopy; NAA: N-acetyl-aspartate; PET: positron emission tomography; SPECT: single-photon emission computed tomography; SWI: susceptibility-weighted imaging; TSPO: translocator protein; QSM: quantitative susceptibility mapping; NODDI: Neurite orientation dispersion and density imaging)

- *Translocator protein (TSPO) scan*: The 18 kDa TSPO, primarily located in the outer membrane of microglial mitochondria, is used as a PET target to quantify neuroinflammation in AD, with a focus on visualizing activated microglia through elevated TSPO expression.[37]
- *Quantitative susceptibility mapping (QSM)*: An advanced imaging technique that quantifies magnetic susceptibility, enabling the visualization of substances such as iron, hemosiderin, and deoxyhemoglobin in the brain and aiding in the evaluation of neurodegenerative diseases. In AD, QSM shows increased iron accumulation in deep gray matter, particularly in the hippocampus, amygdala, precuneus, and thalamus, which is associated with decreased cognitive function and correlates with amyloid plaque accumulation, serving as a potential biomarker for preclinical AD.[36]
- *Callosal circularity*: In 3D volumetric MR images, callosal atrophy in AD patients was assessed through the callosal area (CCA), circularity (CIR), corpus callosum index (CCI), and thickness profile, with reduced circularity in AD patients compared to MCI patients, and the CIR was correlated with CSF biomarkers (t-tau and p-tau) in MCI patients.[54]
- *Neurite orientation dispersion and density imaging (NODDI)*: DTI provides measures of the orientation dispersion index and neurite density index for detecting distinct microstructural features and alterations in regions associated with early atrophy in young-onset

AD patients have been found to be correlated with tau burden in animal models.

- *Higher magnetic field MRI*: Most MRI studies have been conducted using 1.5 and 3 Tesla scanners, but newer 7 Tesla MRI (7T) scanners offer higher resolution and have been used to measure hippocampal subfield volumes in AD, image the substantia nigra in PD, detect early stages of Aβ pathology (increased cortical phase) in AD, and improve sensitivity in detecting CMBs in vascular dementia; however, challenges with costs, operating complexity, and availability remain and the diagnostic superiority of 7T MRI for dementia over lower field strength MRI has yet to be established.[53]

CONCLUSION

Imaging plays a critical role in the diagnosis and management of dementia, offering insights into the heterogeneous nature of the disease and its potentially reversible etiologies. In addition, neuroimaging may also be used to predict future clinical courses in pre-symptomatic or mildly affected individuals, as well as longitudinal measures of disease progression. With ongoing therapeutic trials and emerging treatments, early detection through imaging is essential for effective treatment and rehabilitation in dementia care.

REFERENCES

1. GBD 2019 Dementia Forecasting Collaborators. Estimation of the global prevalence of dementia in 2019 and forecasted prevalence in 2050: an analysis for the Global Burden of Disease Study 2019. Lancet Public Health. 2022;7(2):e105-25.
2. Litvan I, Agid Y, Sastry N, Jankovic J, Wenning GK, Goetz CG, et al. What are the obstacles for an accurate clinical diagnosis of Pick's disease? A clinicopathologic study. Neurology. 1997;49(1):62-9.
3. Ahmed RM, Paterson RW, Warren JD, Zetterberg H, O'Brien JT, Fox NC, et al. Biomarkers in dementia: clinical utility and new directions. J Neurol Neurosurg Psychiatry. 2014;85(12): 1426-34.
4. Practice parameter for diagnosis and evaluation of dementia. (summary statement) Report of the Quality Standards Subcommittee of the American Academy of Neurology. Neurology. 1994;44(11):2203-6.
5. Jack CR, Bennett DA, Blennow K, Carrillo MC, Dunn B, Haeberlein SB, et al. NIA-AA Research Framework: Toward a biological definition of Alzheimer's disease. Alzheimers Dement. 2018; 14(4):535-62.
6. Cummings J. Anti-Amyloid Monoclonal Antibodies are Transformative Treatments that Redefine Alzheimer's Disease Therapeutics. Drugs. 2023;83(7):569.
7. Chouliaras L, O'Brien JT. The use of neuroimaging techniques in the early and differential diagnosis of dementia. Mol Psychiatry. 2023;28(10):4084-97.
8. Van Schependom J, Niemantsverdriet E, Smeets D, Engelborghs S. Callosal circularity as an early marker for Alzheimer's disease. Neuroimage Clin. 2018;19:516-26.
9. Clarke WT, Mougin O, Driver ID, Rua C, Morgan AT, Asghar M, et al. Multi-site harmonization of 7 tesla MRI neuroimaging protocols. Neuroimage. 2020;206:116335.
10. Haller S, Jäger HR, Vernooij MW, Barkhof F. Neuroimaging in Dementia: More than Typical Alzheimer Disease. Radiology. 2023;308(3):e230173.
11. Scheltens P, Launer LJ, Barkhof F, Weinstein HC, van Gool WA, et al. Visual assessment of medial temporal lobe atrophy on magnetic resonance imaging: Interobserver reliability. J Neurol. 1995;242(9):557-60.
12. Du AT, Schuff N, Amend D, Laakso MP, Hsu YY, Jagust WJ, et al. Magnetic resonance imaging of the entorhinal cortex and hippocampus in mild cognitive impairment and Alzheimer's disease. J Neurol Neurosurg Psychiatry. 2001;71(4):441-7.
13. Scheltens P, Pasquier F, Weerts JGE, Barkhof F, Leys D. Qualitative assessment of cerebral atrophy on MRI: inter- and intra-observer reproducibility in dementia and normal aging. Eur Neurol. 1997;37(2):95-9.
14. Wahlund LO, Barkhof F, Fazekas F, Bronge L, Augustin M, Sjögren M, et al. A new rating scale for age-related white matter changes applicable to MRI and CT. Stroke. 2001;32(6):1318-22.
15. Boccardi M, Sabattoli F, Laakso MP, Testa C, Rossi R, Beltramello A, et al. Frontotemporal dementia as a neural system disease. Neurobiol Aging. 2005;26(1):37-44.
16. Levy G, Louis ED, Mejia-Santana H, Côté L, Andrews H, Harris J, et al. Lack of familial aggregation of Parkinson disease and Alzheimer disease. Arch Neurol. 2004;61(8):1033-9.
17. Gilman S, Low PA, Quinn N, Albanese A, Ben-Shlomo Y, Fowler CJ, et al. Consensus statement on the diagnosis of multiple system atrophy. J Neurol Sci. 1999;163(1):94-8.
18. Boxer AL, Yu JT, Golbe LI, Litvan I, Lang AE, Höglinger GU. Advances in progressive supranuclear palsy: new diagnostic criteria, biomarkers, and therapeutic approaches. Lancet Neurol. 2017;16(7):552-63.
19. Tsuboi Y, Josephs KA, Boeve BF, Litvan I, Caselli RJ, Caviness JN, et al. Increased tau burden in the cortices of progressive supranuclear palsy presenting with corticobasal syndrome. Mov Disord. 2005;20(7):982-8.
20. Hoglinger GU, Respondek G, Stamelou M, Kurz C, Josephs KA, Lang AE, et al. Clinical diagnosis of progressive supranuclear palsy: the movement disorder society criteria. Mov Disord. 2017;32(6):853-64.
21. Armstrong MJ, Litvan I, Lang AE, Bak TH, Bhatia KP, Borroni B, et al. Criteria for the diagnosis of corticobasal degeneration. Neurology. 2013;80(5):496-503.
22. Chao LL, Buckley ST, Kornak J, Schuff N, Madison C, Yaffe K, et al. ASL perfusion MRI predicts cognitive decline and conversion from MCI to dementia. Alzheimer Dis Assoc Disord. 2010;24(1):19-27.
23. Kantarci K, Jack CR Jr, Xu YC, Campeau NG, O'Brien PC, Smith GE, et al. Regional metabolic patterns in mild cognitive impairment and Alzheimer's disease: A 1H MRS study. Neurology. 2000;55(2):210-7.

24. Douaud G, Smith S, Jenkinson M, Behrens T, Johansen-Berg H, Vickers J, et al. Anatomically related grey and white matter abnormalities in adolescent-onset schizophrenia. Brain. 2007;130(9):2375-86.
25. Filippi M, Rocca MA, Arnold DL, Bakshi R, Barkhof F, De Stefano N, et al. EFNS guidelines on the use of neuroimaging in the management of multiple sclerosis. Eur J Neurol. 2006;13(4):313-25.
26. Wattjes MP, Rovira A, Miller D, Yousry TA, Sormani MP, de Stefano MP, et al. Evidence-based guidelines: MAGNIMS consensus guidelines on the use of MRI in multiple sclerosis—establishing disease prognosis and monitoring patients. Nat Rev Neurol. 2015;11(10):597-606.
27. Filippi M, Rocca MA, Ciccarelli O, De Stefano N, Evangelou N, Kappos L, et al. MRI criteria for the diagnosis of multiple sclerosis: MAGNIMS consensus guidelines. Lancet Neurol. 2016;15(3): 292-303.
28. Polman CH, Reingold SC, Banwell B, Clanet M, Cohen JA, Filippi M, et al. Diagnostic criteria for multiple sclerosis: 2010 revisions to the McDonald criteria. Ann Neurol. 2011;69(2):292-302.
29. Thompson AJ, Banwell BL, Barkhof F, Carroll WM, Coetzee T, Comi G, et al. Diagnosis of multiple sclerosis: 2017 revisions of the McDonald criteria. Lancet Neurol. 2018;17(2):162-73.
30. Ciccarelli O, Cohen JA, Reingold SC, Weinshenker BG; International Conference on Spinal Cord Involvement and Imaging in Multiple Sclerosis and Neuromyelitis Optica Spectrum Disorders. Spinal cord involvement in multiple sclerosis and neuromyelitis optica spectrum disorders. Lancet Neurol. 2019;18(2):185-97.
31. Kappos L, Radue EW, O'Connor P, Polman C, Hohlfeld R, Calabresi P, et al. A placebo-controlled trial of oral fingolimod in relapsing multiple sclerosis. N Engl J Med. 2010;362(5):387-401.
32. Kappos L, Bar-Or A, Cree BAC, Fox RJ, Giovannoni G, Gold R, et al. Siponimod versus placebo in secondary progressive multiple sclerosis (EXPAND): a double-blind, randomised, phase 3 study. Lancet. 2018;391(10127):1263-73.
33. Hauser SL, Bar-Or A, Comi G, Giovannoni G, Hartung HP, Hemmer B, et al. Ocrelizumab versus interferon beta-1a in relapsing multiple sclerosis. N Engl J Med. 2017;376(3):221-34.
34. Wingerchuk DM, Lennon VA, Lucchinetti CF, Pittock SJ, Weinshenker BG. The spectrum of neuromyelitis optica. Lancet Neurol. 2007;6(9):805-15.
35. Wingerchuk DM, Banwell B, Bennett JL, Cabre P, Carroll W, Chitnis T, et al. International consensus diagnostic criteria for neuromyelitis optica spectrum disorders. Neurology. 2015;85(2): 177-89.
36. Jarius S, Ruprecht K, Wildemann B, Kuempfel T, Ringelstein M, Geis C, et al. Contrasting disease patterns in seropositive and seronegative neuromyelitis optica: A multicentre study of 175 patients. J Neuroinflammation. 2012;9:14.
37. Kim HJ, Paul F, Lana-Peixoto MA, Tenembaum S, Asgari N, Palace J, et al. MRI characteristics of neuromyelitis optica spectrum disorder: an international update. Neurology. 2015;84(11): 1165-73.
38. Wingerchuk DM, Lennon VA, Pittock SJ, Lucchinetti CF, Weinshenker BG. Revised diagnostic criteria for neuromyelitis optica. Neurology. 2006;66(10):1485-9.
39. Jarius S, Wildemann B, Paul F. Neuromyelitis optica: clinical features, immunopathogenesis and treatment. Clin Exp Immunol. 2014;176(2):149-64.
40. Jiao Y, Fryer JD, Lennon VA, Jenkins SM, Quek AM, Smith CY, et al. Updated estimate of AQP4-IgG serostatus and disability outcome in neuromyelitis optica. Neurology. 2013;81(14):1197-204.
41. Jacob A, McKeon A, Nakashima I, Sato DK, Elsone L, Fujihara K, et al. Current concept of neuromyelitis optica (NMO) and NMO spectrum disorders. J Neurol Neurosurg Psychiatry. 2013;84(8):922-30.
42. Melamed E, Levy M, Waters PJ, Sato DK, Bennett JL, John GR, et al. Update on biomarkers in neuromyelitis optica. Neurol Neuroimmunol Neuroinflamm. 2015;2(4):e134.
43. Mealy MA, Wingerchuk DM, Palace J, Greenberg BM, Levy M. Comparison of relapse and treatment failure rates among patients with neuromyelitis optica: Multicenter study of treatment efficacy. JAMA Neurol. 2014;71(3):324-30.
44. Misu T, Fujihara K, Kakita A, Konno H, Nakamura M, Watanabe S, et al. Loss of aquaporin 4 in lesions of neuromyelitis optica: distinction from multiple sclerosis. Brain. 2007;130(5):1224-34.
45. Pittock SJ, Lennon VA, de Seze J, Vermersch P, Homburger HA, Wingerchuk DM, et al. Neuromyelitis optica and non-organ-specific autoimmunity. Arch Neurol. 2008;65(10):78-83.
46. Sellner J, Boggild M, Clanet M, Hintzen RQ, Illes Z, Montalban X, et al. EFNS guidelines on diagnosis and management of neuromyelitis optica. Eur J Neurol. 2010;17(8):1019-32.
47. Wingerchuk DM, Lennon VA, Lucchinetti CF, Pittock SJ, Weinshenker BG. The spectrum of neuromyelitis optica. Lancet Neurol. 2007;6(9):805-15.
48. Lennon VA, Wingerchuk DM, Kryzer TJ, Pittock SJ, Lucchinetti CF, Fujihara K, et al. A serum autoantibody marker of neuromyelitis optica: distinction from multiple sclerosis. Lancet. 2004;364(9451):2106-12.
49. Sato DK, Callegaro D, Lana-Peixoto MA, Waters PJ, de Haidar Jorge FM, Takahashi T, et al. Distinction between MOG antibody-positive and AQP4 antibody-positive NMO spectrum disorders. Neurology. 2014;82(6):474-81.
50. Huda S, Whittam D, Bhojak M, Chamberlain J, Noonan C, Jacob A. Neuromyelitis optica spectrum disorders. Clin Med (Lond). 2019;19(2):169-76.
51. Stellmann JP, Krumbholz M, Friede T, Gahlen A, Borisow N, Fischer K, et al. Immunotherapies in neuromyelitis optica spectrum disorder: efficacy and predictors of response. J Neurol Neurosurg Psychiatry. 2017;88(8):639-47.
52. Wingerchuk DM, Weinshenker BG. Neuromyelitis optica: clinical predictors of a relapsing course and survival. Neurology. 2003;60(5):848-53.
53. Mealy MA, Kessler RA, Rimler Z, Reid A, Totonis L, Cutter G, et al. Mortality in neuromyelitis optica is strongly associated with African ancestry. Neurol Neuroimmunol Neuroinflamm. 2018;5(4):e468.
54. Hor JY, Asgari N, Nakashima I, Broadley SA, Leite MI, Kissani N, et al. Epidemiology of neuromyelitis optica spectrum disorder and its prevalence and incidence worldwide. Front Neurol. 2020;11:501.

CHAPTER 18

Caregiver Management in Dementia: Addressing Challenges and Providing Support

Saadiya Hurzuk, Najamus Saquib, Mani Tolety

ABSTRACT

Dementia presents multifaceted challenges for both patients and caregivers, impacting families and healthcare systems. Caregivers endure substantial burdens, including stress, depression, and financial strain, exacerbated by a lack of formal support services, leading to feelings of overwhelm and isolation. As dementia advances, the demand for assistance amplifies, placing additional responsibilities on caregivers and healthcare providers. In India, where approximately 8.8 million people over 60 years are affected by dementia, sociocultural dynamics significantly shape caregiving experiences. Cultural norms, particularly emphasizing family support for women, intersect with attitudes toward aging and dementia stigma, presenting unique challenges. Addressing these challenges requires culturally sensitive interventions and tailored support services, highlighting the urgency of comprehensive approaches to dementia care despite significant barriers to access and awareness. Services such as caregiver support groups, dementia day-care centers, and local Alzheimer's associations offer vital assistance and respite to dementia family caregivers, aiding in alleviating their burden and improving their quality of life.

Keywords: Dementia-caregiver, Informal caregiver, Unpaid care, Home-based care, Caregiver Support, Family caregiver, Caregiver-services, Dementia-India.

INTRODUCTION

Dementia, a complex, progressive, age-related neurological disease, is one of the most challenging, not only for those who have been diagnosed with dementia but also for their family caregivers and healthcare professionals. The impact of dementia extends beyond the individual to their caregivers, who bear a significant burden. Caregivers often experience stress, depression, and financial strain as they navigate the challenges of caring for a loved one with dementia. Generally, the lack of formal support services exacerbates their burden, leaving many caregivers feeling overwhelmed and isolated.

During the course of dementia, the need for assistance in the activities of daily living (ADLs) increases, and the burden of continuous care and an extensive need for support falls on both family caregivers and social and healthcare service providers. Caregivers experience a complex role, with added responsibilities, new tasks, and emotional and relational challenges that are expressed through distressing emotions and demands for interaction. The caregiver's role and burden is well known and include physical, psychological, social, and financial aspects.[1]

In India, an estimated 8.8 million people aged over 60 years have dementia; this number is expected to double by 2030.[2] In India, dementia caregiving is profoundly influenced by unique sociocultural factors. Family plays a central role in caregiving, with cultural norms emphasizing filial piety and intergenerational support. As a result, caregiving responsibilities often fall on family members, particularly women, who face challenges balancing caregiving with other responsibilities.[3] Predominantly, females continue to assume the role of caregivers.[4] Cultural attitudes toward ageing also impact caregiving, with reverence for elders shaping caregiving practices and decision-making. Additionally, stigma surrounding dementia can lead to social isolation for both caregivers and individuals with dementia.[5] These sociocultural aspects underscore the importance of culturally sensitive interventions and support services for dementia caregivers in India.[6]

FORMAL AND INFORMAL CAREGIVERS

There is no exact definition of a dementia caregiver; a dementia caregiver refers to any individual who provides care, assistance, or support to a person living with dementia. The responsibility of caregiving for a person with dementia typically falls on various family members or close acquaintances, including children, daughter-in-law, son-in-law, siblings, relatives, or friends.[7] Often, these individuals assume the caregiver role not out of choice, but rather due to circumstances, as there may not be many alternatives available. This caregiving duty is frequently undertaken without recognition or acknowledgment from society.

Dementia caregivers play a crucial role in supporting the daily needs, well-being, and quality of life of individuals with dementia.[8] Caregivers can be divided into two categories; formal caregivers, who are healthcare professionals or trained staff in institutional settings, and informal caregivers, such as family members or friends who provide unpaid care in home environments. Understanding the caregiver role in dementia entails recognizing both formal and informal caregivers, each facing distinct challenges yet requiring training in the management of persons living with dementia. Formal caregivers often possess specialized skills acquired through professional training and education in dementia care, enabling them to deliver structured persons living with dementia interventions and medical assistance.[9] In contrast, informal caregivers, lacking formal training, may grapple with unmet needs and insufficient knowledge regarding dementia management, leading to heightened caregiver burden and decreased quality of care for their relative with dementia. Informal caregivers require access to community-based support services offering psychoeducation, respite care, and skill-building workshops to enhance their caregiving abilities and mitigate caregiver stress.

However, it is notable that in India, structured formal caregiving programs are lacking, with the few available programs often insufficient and inaccessible. Many private agencies resort to recruiting individuals from disadvantaged backgrounds, who are often underpaid and inadequately trained for the demanding responsibilities of dementia care.

Families in India encountering formal attenders, or paid caregivers, or as locally known as "Attenders" often grapple with numerous challenges. Firstly, these formal caregivers frequently possess limited training and knowledge in dementia care, impacting the quality of support provided. Additionally, finding reliable and skilled caregivers can be a daunting task, exacerbating the already stressful caregiving journey. Financial constraints present another significant hurdle, as many families struggle to afford the services of trained/paid caregivers (formal caregivers). Moreover, the high rotation rates among formal caregivers contribute to a lack of continuity in caregiving, disrupting the essential routine and relationship-building process. This results in frequent change, as they depart in short durations, leading to discomfort for families and the person with dementia. Family caregivers must then recruit and train new attenders repeatedly, restarting the rapport-building process each time. For the person with dementia, this constant change can be challenging, causing confusion and reluctance to accept new person. Building rapport with each new (formal) caregiver takes time, making the adjustment period difficult for both the individual with dementia and the family caregiver.

These paid attendants often lack dementia training, which hampers their ability to recognize symptoms, understand behaviors, and implement therapeutic interventions beneficial for dementia care. Due to their frequent changing of formal caregivers, family caregivers face the arduous task of continually establishing trust, educating, and training each new caregiver about dementia symptoms and management strategies. This repetitive cycle not only strains the family caregiver but also compromises the quality of care provided to the person with dementia.

DEMENTIA CARE IN THE INDIAN CONTEXT

About 8.8 million individuals aged 60 years and above in India are affected by dementia;[2] in low- and middle-income countries (LMICs), like India, only one person out of ten ever receives any diagnosis, treatment, or care.[9] Dementia caregiving in India is a complex and challenging task, often undertaken by family members within their home environment. The lack of awareness and understanding about dementia in India often leads to delayed diagnosis and inadequate support for affected individuals and their caregivers.[5]

India's healthcare infrastructure faces significant limitations in providing comprehensive dementia care. Access to diagnostic facilities and treatment options for dementia remains limited, further complicating the care landscape.[3] There is a shortage of specialized healthcare professionals trained in dementia diagnosis and management, particularly in rural areas. Furthermore in India, the treatment gap for dementia, representing the disparity between the number of individuals requiring care for the condition and those receiving it, stands at approximately 90%, which hints that this population of dementia in India is mostly cared for in their own homes.[10] Out-of-pocket expenditure for dementia care in India imposes a significant financial burden on families, with an estimated INR 45,000/person/month in 2010,[3] a figure that has now more than doubled.

Generally, families prefer to care for elderly relatives at home rather than seek professional care, resulting in impacting the quality of life for both the person with dementia and family caregivers who provide care to them. In Indian culture, filial piety and family duty dictate caring for ageing relatives, including those with dementia, as a moral obligation, highlighting the central role of family support. As a result, caregiving responsibilities often fall on family members, particularly women, who may face challenges balancing caregiving with other responsibilities.

Cultural attitudes toward ageing also impact caregiving, with reverence for elders shaping caregiving practices and decision-making. Additionally, stigma surrounding dementia can lead to social isolation for both caregivers and individuals with dementia.[5] Ageing is revered in Indian culture, but dementia is often misunderstood or stigmatized. There is a tendency to attribute symptoms to ageing rather than recognize them as signs of a medical condition, leading to reluctance to seek help.

Extended familial involvement not only lightens the caregiving burden but also reinforces the cultural value of collective responsibility toward elders. However, the families are becoming increasingly nuclear, the aforementioned traditional family support systems are ceasing to exist. Hence, it exuberates the caregiver's burden. The lack of formal support services additionally increases their burden, leaving many caregivers feeling overwhelmed and isolated.[1]

Balancing modern healthcare with traditional caregiving in dementia care poses challenges due to cultural beliefs and generational shifts. Conflicts between traditional views on dementia and medical recommendations emphasize the importance of culturally sensitive approaches toward dementia care in society. Generational changes in caregiving dynamics emphasize the importance of embracing both modern and traditional practices for inclusive care.

CASE VIGNETTE

Mrs Pihu, a diligent woman in her early 40s, resides in an urban city, from an affluent family. She struggles with the challenging task of caring for her 70-year-old mother, who has dementia. Amidst her corporate job responsibilities, Mrs Pihu has transitioned to working from home. Mrs Pihu lives with her husband and teenage daughter, while her mother continues to reside separately in their old house after her husband's demise. With her brothers living abroad and visiting only briefly each year, the bulk of caregiving falls on Mrs Pihu's shoulders.

Balancing work, family, and caregiving leaves Mrs Pihu feeling emotionally drained and overwhelmed. Despite her mother's pension, financial limitations add to the strain. The expense of hiring formal caregivers is considerable, additionally, Mrs Pihu had to hire a maid for household chores and a cook for her mother, further stretching her financial resources and time. To ensure her mother's safety and well-being, she installed CCTV cameras in her mother's home, which also enabled her to supervise all the people who came to support her mother.

She has enrolled her mother in a dementia activity cum daycare, providing some respite, but she has to drop off and pick up her mother daily from the daycare. With little time for herself, Mrs Pihu sacrifices personal activities like jogging and socializing with friends. She seeks help in community resources like the local Alzheimer's association, where she receives caregiver support. However, finding time to reach out to professionals for additional help and self-care proves to be yet another challenge in her demanding schedule.

Dementia caregivers in India encounter numerous challenges that impact their physical, emotional, and socioeconomic well-being. Caregivers have reported that the process of caregiving has led them to face setbacks in their health, work, and social life (52%, 49%, and 62%, respectively).[11] Common challenges that they face are:

- *Limited awareness and stigma*: Often there is a lack of awareness and understanding about dementia, leading to stigma and discrimination against both the person with dementia and their caregivers.[5]
- *Financial strain*: Family caregivers often face financial constraints due to limited access to affordable healthcare services and lack of financial assistance or insurance coverage for dementia-related expenses.[12]
- *Limited access to resources*: In Indian, there is inadequate healthcare infrastructure and limited access to dementia-specific support services, including respite care, counseling, and caregiver training programs.
- *Caregiver burden*: Caregivers experience significant burden due to the demanding nature of caregiving tasks, lack of support networks, and social isolation.[13]

- *Physical and mental health impacts*: Dementia caregivers often experience poor physical health due to the strain of caregiving responsibilities, lack of rest, and inadequate self-care practices. Additionally, they are at increased risk of mental health issues, such as depression and anxiety.[14]
- *Gender disparities*: Caregiving responsibilities typically fall on women, exacerbating gender disparities in caregiving burden and limiting women's opportunities for education and employment.

In addition to the multifaceted challenges, caregivers often experience a loss of control over their own lives and self-identity. Constantly managing various roles and responsibilities, including familial duties and caring for a relative with dementia, can blur the boundaries between caregiver and individual, leading to a diminished sense of autonomy and selfhood. The caregiver's own needs and desires may take a backseat as they prioritize the needs of their loved one, resulting in a gradual loss of their identity and fulfilment.[15]

Another major challenge faced by family caregivers is educating themselves on dementia symptoms and how to manage the condition. Caregivers must learn about the various symptoms of dementia in different stages and understand effective management strategies. This includes grasping concepts such as communication techniques tailored to dementia, handling challenging behaviors associated with the condition, and familiarizing themselves with therapeutic interventions like cognitive stimulation, functional rehabilitation meaningful activities, and reminiscence therapy. After acquiring this knowledge, caregivers are tasked with either implementing these strategies themselves with individuals with dementia, which demands significant time and patience, or training paid caregivers. This training process involves caregivers imparting their knowledge and skills to formal caregivers or attendants, ensuring they are equipped to provide appropriate care. This additional responsibility adds to the caregiver's workload and requires ongoing effort to ensure consistency and effectiveness in care provision.

CAREGIVERS STRESS AND COPING SKILLS

Caregiver stress is a pervasive challenge that often accompanies the demanding role of caring for individuals with dementia. Family caregivers, in particular, experience heightened levels of stress due to the multifaceted nature of their responsibilities. The relentless demands of caregiving, coupled with the emotional strain of witnessing the progressive decline of their loved one, contribute to a profound sense of burden and overwhelm.

The constant vigilance required in managing the unpredictable symptoms of dementia, such as agitation, confusion, and wandering, further exacerbates caregiver stress. Additionally, the financial strain of covering the costs associated with dementia care, coupled with the disruption of personal and professional pursuits, compounds the caregiver's burden.

Many caregivers find themselves sacrificing their own needs and well-being to prioritize the care of their loved ones, leading to physical and emotional exhaustion over time.

Caregiver stress manifests in various ways, including physical symptoms such as fatigue, headaches, and sleep disturbances, as well as emotional symptoms such as anxiety, depression, and feelings of guilt. To cope with caregiver stress, caregivers need to prioritize self-care, seek social support, and set realistic expectations for themselves. Building a support network of friends, family, and community resources can provide invaluable assistance in managing caregiver stress. However, caregivers often face challenges in accessing support services, including limited availability of respite care and counseling options, as well as financial constraints that may hinder their ability to seek help.

Addressing caregiver burden necessitates prioritizing self-care, seeking social support, and setting realistic expectations. Caregivers need to cope with dementia patients by understanding the disease trajectory, managing behavioral and psychological symptoms, and implementing effective communication strategies. Additionally, caregivers must manage their stress through healthy coping mechanisms such as exercise, relaxation techniques, and seeking professional help when needed. By adopting these strategies, caregivers can better navigate the challenges of dementia care while preserving their well-being. This holistic approach not only supports the caregiver's mental and physical health but also enhances the quality of care provided to individuals with dementia, fostering a more sustainable and compassionate caregiving environment.

Respite care options for dementia include:

- *Day-care centers*: These facilities offer structured cognitive and meaningful activities, supervision, and socialization opportunities for individuals with dementia during the day, providing caregivers with a temporary break from caregiving duties.
- *Residential care/long-term care (LTC) facilities*: Some facilities specialize in providing long-term residential care for individuals with dementia, offering around-the-clock supervision, medical support, and assistance with daily activities.
- *Home-based care services*: These services may include home health aides, trained formal caregivers, or

nurses who provide temporary relief to family caregivers by assisting with caregiving responsibilities at home.

- *Support groups and counseling for family caregivers*: While not traditional respite care services, support groups and counseling sessions can offer emotional support and practical advice to caregivers, providing them with a reprieve from the challenges of caregiving.[16]

In India, cultural factors often pose challenges for family caregivers considering the use of day care and residential care facilities for individuals with dementia. Cultural norms emphasizing familial responsibility and intergenerational caregiving may deter families from seeking outside assistance, as caregiving is viewed as a familial duty rather than a service to be outsourced. The stigma associated with placing elders in institutionalized care settings can also discourage families from utilizing these services, as it may be perceived as abandonment or neglect of filial duties.[17] Many families face limited financial resources and may struggle to afford the costs associated with daycare or residential care for their loved ones with dementia. The high cost of care, coupled with the lack of financial assistance or insurance coverage, can make it difficult for families to afford these services, further perpetuating the reliance on informal caregiving arrangements within the family.[18]

Strengthening and empowering the caregivers with required strategies and coping mechanisms enhances the quality of life of the person with dementia. The biggest resource and support for caregiver management are the various Alzheimer's associations worldwide, like Alzheimer's and Related Disorder Society of India (ARDSI) and Alzheimer's Disease International (ADI). For example, ARDSI Hyderabad Deccan Chapter, a nonprofit organization for comprehensive Dementia care, offers extensive caregiver support services. Additionally, caregivers support group meetings for shared experiences and emotional support, counseling for navigating dementia care complexities, and educational resources for enhanced understanding of dementia and self-care, in regional and local languages. Online support systems through mail and caregiver meetings and caregiver meetings facilitate frequent access to support from dementia professionals, ensuring caregivers receive assistance from the comfort of their homes. Caregiver meetings held fortnightly in-person and virtually, facilitate for building a continuous partnership between healthcare professionals and family caregivers. ARDIS Hyderabad Deccan Chapter runs a day care and cognitive stimulation center, providing essential respite and support for people living with dementia and their caregivers. Furthermore, ARDSI Hyderabad Deccan chapter facilitates active regional WhatsApp support groups and a 24×7 telephonic helpline. Collaborative initiatives with ARDSI and ADI, such as Dementia Care Skills Training programs, provide tailored education and practical skills for effective dementia management.[19]

CONCLUSION

Addressing the multifaceted challenges faced by dementia caregivers requires a comprehensive approach that encompasses various interventions. Raising awareness, providing caregiver support, and improving access to resources are crucial components of this effort. Moreover, caregivers should actively seek professional support, lean on the assistance of family and friends, and develop strategies for self-care and respite. Every healthcare facility should have a caregiver support system in place to address the neglect caregivers may face. By prioritizing their well-being and seeking support, caregivers can better navigate the caregiving demands of dementia care.

REFERENCES

1. Dias A, Samuel R, Patel V, Prince M, Parameshwaran R, Krishnamoorthy ES. The impact associated with caring for a person with dementia: a report from the 10/66 Dementia Research Group's Indian network. Int J Geriatr Psychiatry. 2004;19(2):182-4.
2. Lee J, Meijer E, Langa KM, Ganguli M, Varghese M, Banerjee J, et al. Prevalence of dementia in India: National and state estimates from a nationwide study. Alzheimers Dement J Alzheimers Assoc. 2023;19(7):2898-912.
3. KS S, Jotheeswaran A, Girish N, Bharath S, Dias A, Pattabiraman M, et al. The Dementia India report: prevalence, impact, costs and services for Dementia: executive summary. Alzheimers Relat Disord Soc India. 2010:1-38.
4. Brinda EM, Rajkumar AP, Enemark U, Attermann J, Jacob K. Cost and burden of informal caregiving of dependent older people in a rural Indian community. BMC Health Serv Res. 2014;14:207.
5. Hurzuk S, Farina N, Pattabiraman M, Ramasamy N, Alladi S, Rajagopalan J, et al. Understanding, experiences and attitudes of dementia in India: A qualitative study. Dement Lond Engl. 2022;21(7):2288-306.
6. Garcia-Ptacek S, Dahlrup B, Edlund AK, Wijk H, Eriksdotter M. The caregiving phenomenon and caregiver participation in dementia. Scand J Caring Sci. 2019;33(2):255-65.
7. Gustafsson L, Asztalos Morell I, Johansson C, De S. Informal caregiving from the perspectives of older people living alone in India. Int J Older People Nurs. 2022;17(6):e12468.
8. World Health Organization. (2019). Risk reduction of cognitive decline and dementia: WHO guidelines. Geneva: World Health

Organization. [online] Available from https://www.who.int/publications/i/item/9789241550543 [Last accessed July, 2024].
9. Prince M, Ali GC, Guerchet M, Prina AM, Albanese E, Wu YT. Recent global trends in the prevalence and incidence of dementia, and survival with dementia. Alzheimers Res Ther. 2016;8(1):23.
10. Dias A, Patel V. Closing the treatment gap for dementia in India. Indian J Psychiatr. 2009;51(Suppl1):S93-7.
11. O'Connor D. (2019). World Alzheimer Report 2019: Attitudes to dementia. [online] Available from https://www.alzint.org/u/WorldAlzheimerReport2019.pdf [Last accessed July, 2024].
12. Alzheimer's Disease International. (2015). World Alzheimer Report 2015. The Global Impact of Dementia: An analysis of prevalence, incidence, cost and trends. [online] Available from https://www.alzint.org/u/WorldAlzheimerReport2015.pdf [Last accessed July, 2024].
13. Lamech N, Raghuraman S, Vaitheswaran S, Rangaswamy T. The support needs of family caregivers of persons with dementia in India: Implications for health services. Dementia. 2019;18(6):2230-43.
14. Basu I, Mukhopadhyay S, Maulik N. Family Caregiving in Dementia: Caregivers' Mental Health and Nature of Caregiving. Online J Anthropol. 2020;16(2):201.
15. Karner TX, Bobbitt-Zeher D. (2011). Losing Selves: Dementia Care as Disruption and Transformation. [online] Available from https://onlinelibrary.wiley.com/doi/abs/10.1525/si.2005.28.4.549 [Last accessed July, 2024].
16. Alladi S, Rajagopalan J, Hurzuk S, Pattabiraman M, Ramasamy N, Thomas PT, et al. (2022). The dementia care landscape in India: context, systems, policies and services. [online] Available from https://stride-dementia.org/desk-review/?country=india [Last accessed July, 2024].
17. Choi J, Ta Park V, Nguyen E, Jung A, Tsoh J. Understanding the caregiving experiences of Asian Indian, Chinese, Korean, and Vietnamese American family care partners of persons living with dementia. Aging Ment Health. 2024;28(3):473-81.
18. Prince M, Comas-Herrera A, Knapp M, Guerchet M, Karagiannidou M. (2016). World Alzheimer Report 2016. Improving healthcare for people living with dementia: Coverage, quality and costs now and in the future. [online] Available from https://www.alzint.org/u/WorldAlzheimerReport2016.pdf [Last accessed July, 2024].
19. Alzheimer's and Related Disorders Society of India - Hyderabad Chapter. Services: Daycare and Activity centre for persons with Dementia. [online] Available from https://www.ardsihyd.org/services.html [Last accessed July, 2024].

CHAPTER

19 Functional Rehabilitation in Dementia

Nirmal Surya, Porrselvi AP

ABSTRACT

Dementia poses a growing challenge in India, affecting millions and straining healthcare systems. Functional rehabilitation offers a beacon of hope, empowering individuals with dementia to maintain independence and improve quality of life. This chapter explores the various domains targeted in functional rehabilitation, including activities of daily living (ADLs), cognitive skills, and communication strategies.

Culturally appropriate interventions and addressing challenges like illiteracy and resource limitations are crucial for successful implementation in the Indian context. Family involvement is also a cornerstone of dementia care in India, and family-based rehabilitation approaches are explored. Telerehabilitation emerges as a promising solution to overcome geographical barriers and improve access to care. By acknowledging these considerations and harnessing the potential of functional rehabilitation, India can create a more supportive environment for individuals living with dementia.

Keywords: Dementia, Rehabilitation, Activities of daily living, Family, India.

INTRODUCTION

Dementia, a progressive neurodegenerative syndrome, disrupts cognitive function and daily life. Characterized by a gradual decline in memory, thinking, and behavior, dementia affects an individual's ability to perform activities of daily living (ADLs).[1] This decline significantly impacts independence and quality of life, posing a growing challenge for healthcare systems worldwide.

Functional rehabilitation emerges as a promising strategy to address these challenges. Encompassing a range of interventions, functional rehabilitation aims to improve an individual's capacity to perform everyday tasks and participate meaningfully in their environment.[2] Unlike treatments that focus on slowing disease progression, functional rehabilitation prioritizes maximizing remaining abilities and promoting independence. A core principle of functional rehabilitation is a person-centered, holistic approach that considers the individual's unique needs, strengths, and preferences.[3] This chapter explores the key domains of functional rehabilitation for dementia, with a focus on evidence-based implementation, measuring outcomes, and navigating challenges to ensure optimal care for individuals living with dementia.

DOMAINS OF FUNCTIONAL REHABILITATION

Functional rehabilitation for dementia targets various domains essential for daily living **(Table 1)**.

Activities of Daily Living

The ADLs are broadly categorized into basic ADLs (BADLs) and instrumental ADLs (IADLs). BADLs encompass fundamental self-care tasks like bathing, dressing, toileting, eating, and transferring.[4] IADLs involve more complex tasks necessary for independent living, such as managing finances, using transportation, and medication management.[5]

TABLE 1: Various domains of functional rehabilitation and common strategies used.

Domain	Description	Strategies
Activities of daily living (ADLs)	• *Basic ADLs (BADLs):* Bathing, dressing, toileting, eating, and transferring • *Instrumental ADLs (IADLs):* Managing finances, transportation, and medication management	• Assistive devices • Environmental modifications • Task breakdown/simplification
Cognitive rehabilitation	Targets memory, attention, and executive function	• Memory aids (calendars and planners) • Compensatory strategies (notes and routines) Attention/executive function training
Communication strategies	Maintains social connections and manages daily life	• Simple language and active listening • Addressing communication challenges (picture cards and gestures)

Strategies for supporting independence with ADLs include:

- *Assistive devices:* Utilizing tools like grab bars, dressing aids, and shower chairs can enhance safety and facilitate task completion.
- *Environmental modifications:* Adapting the living environment by widening doorways, installing ramps, and improving lighting can make daily activities less demanding.
- *Task breakdown and simplification:* Breaking down complex tasks into smaller, manageable steps can make them more achievable.

Cognitive Rehabilitation

Dementia affects various cognitive domains, with memory, attention, and executive function often showing the most significant decline.[2] Cognitive rehabilitation programs target these specific cognitive impairments with the aim of improving skills relevant to daily function.

- *Memory aids*: External memory aids like calendars, planners, and medication reminders can assist with memory retention and task completion.
- *Compensatory strategies:* Techniques like leaving notes, using routines, and placing frequently used items in designated locations can compensate for memory difficulties.
- *Attention and executive function training:* Computerized programs and targeted exercises can help improve sustained attention, planning, and problem-solving skills.

Communication Strategies

Effective communication is crucial for maintaining social connections and managing daily life for individuals with dementia. Rehabilitation strategies focus on:

- *Simple language:* Using clear, concise language, with short sentences and frequent repetition enhances comprehension.
- *Active listening:* Maintaining eye contact, offering verbal and nonverbal cues of attentiveness, and minimizing distractions foster effective communication.
- *Addressing communication challenges:* Techniques like using picture cards, gestures, and alternative communication methods can support individuals with aphasia or apraxia.

EVIDENCE-BASED IMPLEMENTATION OF FUNCTIONAL REHABILITATION PROGRAMS

Successful implementation of functional rehabilitation programs hinges on a comprehensive assessment process. This initial evaluation plays a critical role in identifying individual needs, strengths, and preferences, forming the foundation for a personalized rehabilitation plan.

Importance of Assessment to Identify Individual Needs and Goals

A thorough assessment serves several crucial purposes within functional rehabilitation for dementia.

- *Identifying cognitive and functional impairments*: Standardized assessments like the Mini-Mental State Examination (MMSE) and cognitive batteries can provide valuable insights into the individual's cognitive strengths and weaknesses across various domains such as memory, attention, and executive function.[6] Additionally, evaluations of ADLs using tools like the Lawton IADL scale[5] or the functional independence measure (FIM)[7] provide a baseline understanding of the individual's current level of independence in daily activities.
- *Identifying environmental and social factors:* The assessment process should extend beyond cognitive and functional abilities to encompass environmental and social factors that may impact the individual's daily life. This may involve a home assessment to

identify potential safety hazards or accessibility issues and discussions with caregivers to understand the individual's social support network and daily routines.

- *Determining goals and priorities:* Through a collaborative process involving individuals with dementia, their families, and healthcare professionals, the assessment findings are used to establish realistic and meaningful goals for rehabilitation. These goals should be tailored to the individual's specific needs and preferences, focusing on maximizing independence and improving participation in desired activities.

Role of the Rehabilitation Team

Functional rehabilitation for dementia necessitates a collaborative approach involving a multidisciplinary rehabilitation team. Each team member brings their unique expertise to comprehensively address the individual's needs.

- *Neurologists* diagnose and manage the underlying neurological condition causing dementia. They may also prescribe medications to manage specific symptoms.
- *Neuropsychiatrists* evaluate and treat neuropsychiatric symptoms of dementia, such as depression, anxiety, and psychosis.
- *Neuropsychologists* conduct neuropsychological assessments to understand the individual's cognitive strengths and weaknesses, which can inform rehabilitation strategies.
- *Urologists* may be involved in managing urinary incontinence, a common issue in dementia.
- *Geriatricians* possess specialized knowledge and experience in caring for older adults, including those with dementia. They can provide overall medical management and coordinate care with other specialists.
- *Occupational therapists (OTs)* assess and address difficulties with self-care tasks like bathing, dressing, and toileting. They work on improving the individual's ability to perform daily activities independently through strategies such as task simplification, environmental modifications, and the use of assistive devices.
- *Speech-language pathologists (SLPs)* evaluate and address communication challenges associated with dementia, such as aphasia or apraxia. They provide strategies for improving communication skills and fostering effective communication between the individual and their caregivers.
- *Physical therapists (PTs)* focus on improving physical strength, balance, and coordination, which are crucial for maintaining mobility and independence. They can also train individuals in safe transfer techniques and fall prevention strategies.
- *Social workers* assess social and environmental factors impacting the individual's well-being and connect them with community resources and support services.
- *Caregivers* play a vital role in the rehabilitation process. They provide crucial information during the assessment process and are instrumental in implementing rehabilitation strategies within the home environment.

The rehabilitation team works collaboratively to develop a comprehensive plan, ensuring all aspects of the individual's needs are addressed. Regular communication and coordination among team members is essential for a successful rehabilitation program.

Developing a Personalized Rehabilitation Program with Clear Goals and Interventions

Based on the assessment findings and established goals, a personalized rehabilitation program is developed. This program outlines specific interventions tailored to address the individual's identified needs. Here are some key aspects of an effective program:

- *Clear and measurable goals:* Goals should be specific, measurable, achievable, relevant, and time-bound (SMART).[8] For instance, a goal might be "to independently dress oneself within 15 minutes by utilizing a dressing aid".
- *Evidence-based interventions:* Interventions should be based on current research and best practices in dementia rehabilitation. Examples include memory aids, compensatory strategies for cognitive impairments, communication techniques, and physical exercise programs.
- *Individualized approach:* The program should be tailored to the individual's specific needs, preferences, and abilities. This ensures that interventions are meaningful and engaging for the person with dementia.
- *Progression and flexibility:* The program should be designed to allow for progression as the individual's skills improve. Additionally, the program should be flexible to adapt to changes in the individual's condition or circumstances.

Importance of Family and Caregiver Education and Training

Family and caregivers play an essential role in supporting the individual with dementia and ensuring the success of the rehabilitation program. By providing education and training, healthcare professionals can empower caregivers to effectively implement rehabilitation strategies within the home environment.

Education may include:

- *Understanding dementia:* Providing knowledge about the several types of dementia and the progression of the disease can help caregivers better understand the individual's challenges and respond effectively.
- *Communication strategies:* Training caregivers in effective communication techniques that consider the individual's cognitive impairments can foster more positive interactions and reduce frustration.
- *Rehabilitation techniques:* Providing instruction on the specific rehabilitation strategies outlined in the program empowers caregivers to support the individual with daily activities and promote independence.

Empowering caregivers with knowledge and skills not only enhances the effectiveness of the rehabilitation program but also contributes to their own well-being. Caregiver support groups can provide a valuable platform for caregivers to connect with others facing similar challenges, share experiences, and learn coping strategies for managing stress and emotional burden.[9]

The successful implementation of a functional rehabilitation program requires ongoing collaboration and communication between the rehabilitation team, the individual with dementia, and their family. Regular program reviews allow for adjustments to be made based on the individual's progress or changing needs, ensuring a dynamic and responsive approach to rehabilitation.

MEASURING OUTCOMES OF FUNCTIONAL REHABILITATION

Evaluating the effectiveness of functional rehabilitation programs is crucial for ensuring that they are meeting individual needs and optimizing care. This section explores various methods for measuring outcomes and the importance of ongoing evaluation.

Methods for Measuring Outcomes

A comprehensive approach to outcome measurement in functional rehabilitation uses a combination of objective and subjective measures.

- *Standardized assessments:* Standardized tools like the FIM and Lawton IADL scale provide objective, quantifiable data on an individual's performance in ADLs. These assessments can be administered at the beginning and throughout the rehabilitation program to track improvements in functional independence over time.
- *Performance-based assessments:* Direct observation of the individual performing daily activities within their natural environment provides valuable insights into their ability to complete tasks independently and identify areas requiring additional support. This can involve observing the individual with dementia during tasks like preparing a meal, bathing, or dressing.
- *Self-reported measures:* While individuals with dementia may face challenges in self-reporting, their perceptions of their own abilities and quality of life can be valuable indicators of program effectiveness. Simple self-report questionnaires can be adapted to gather information on factors such as perceived quality of life, independence, confidence in performing tasks, and overall well-being.
- *Caregiver reports:* Caregivers play a crucial role in providing information on the individual's performance in daily activities outside of formal therapy sessions. Caregiver reports can track changes in the individual's ability to complete tasks at home and identify areas where additional support may be needed.

Importance of Ongoing Evaluation

Regular evaluation of outcomes allows for adjustments to the rehabilitation program to be made based on the individual's progress or changing needs.

- *Monitoring progress:* Outcome data allows healthcare professionals to track changes in the individual's functional abilities over time. This data can be used to assess the effectiveness of current interventions and identify areas where the program may need to be modified.
- *Adapting interventions:* As the individual's condition progresses or their needs change, the rehabilitation program needs to adapt accordingly. Regular evaluation allows for timely adjustments to interventions, ensuring continued progress and optimal support.
- *Identifying new goals:* As the individual achieves established goals, new and more challenging goals can be set, maintaining a sense of motivation and engagement throughout the rehabilitation process.
- *Demonstrating effectiveness:* Outcome data can be used to demonstrate the effectiveness of the rehabilitation program and advocate for its continued implementation and potential expansion to benefit other individuals with dementia.

Beyond these objective measures, qualitative data from individuals with dementia themselves and their caregivers can offer valuable insights into the program's impact on their lives. Narrative reports or open-ended interviews can capture changes in well-being, emotional state, and overall satisfaction with daily life, providing a more holistic understanding of the program's impact.[2] It is crucial to discuss the appropriate follow-up schedule with the individual's healthcare provider that will be based on the specific needs of the individual like the severity of dementia, progression of the symptoms, and medical comorbidities to ensure optimal care and timely interventions.

CHALLENGES AND CONSIDERATIONS

While functional rehabilitation offers significant benefits for individuals with dementia, several challenges require careful consideration for successful implementation.

Challenges related to access and equity:

- *Illiteracy and language barriers:* Individuals with illiteracy or limited language proficiency may face difficulties understanding instructions or educational materials related to rehabilitation programs. Developing culturally and linguistically appropriate interventions, as well as utilizing alternative methods like visual aids and demonstrations can help overcome these barriers.
- *Poverty:* Financial limitations can restrict access to rehabilitation services. Programs with sliding fee scales, offering financial assistance, or exploring community resources can help bridge this gap and ensure affordability.
- *Distance from rehabilitation centers:* Limited access to transportation or the physical distance from rehabilitation centers can be a significant barrier for individuals with dementia and their caregivers. Telerehabilitation, mobile treatment units, or partnerships with local community centers can offer more accessible options.
- *Scarcity of trained professionals:* A shortage of trained professionals specializing in dementia rehabilitation can limit program availability. Strategies like training existing staff in basic rehabilitation techniques, utilizing telehealth to connect with specialists remotely, or advocating for increased investment in dementia-care workforce development are crucial to address this challenge.
- *Limited resources:* Functional rehabilitation programs can be resource-intensive, requiring trained professionals, specialized equipment, and dedicated time for therapy sessions. Limited access to these resources can hinder program availability and accessibility for individuals with dementia. Creative solutions might involve exploring telehealth options for remote therapy delivery, training existing staff in basic rehabilitation techniques, or advocating for increased funding for dementia-care services.
- *Lack of awareness:* Awareness of the benefits of functional rehabilitation for dementia may be limited among both healthcare professionals and the public. Increased education and dissemination of research findings highlighting the effectiveness of rehabilitation programs can encourage broader adoption and ensure individuals with dementia have access to these beneficial interventions.

Challenges related to dementia:

- *Heterogeneity of dementia:* Dementia encompasses a range of subtypes with varying presentations and trajectories. While functional rehabilitation offers significant benefits, the specific needs and interventions may vary depending on the type and severity of dementia. Rehabilitation programs should be tailored to address the specific challenges associated with each dementia subtype for optimal effectiveness.
- *Progressive nature of dementia:* Unlike many medical conditions, dementia is a progressive neurodegenerative disorder. This means cognitive and functional decline will continue over time. Functional rehabilitation interventions need to be adaptable, with goals and strategies adjusted as the individual's needs evolve.[3]
- *Behavioral and psychological symptoms of dementia (BPSD):* Encompassing symptoms like agitation, depression, and anxiety, these can significantly impact an individual's ability to participate in rehabilitation and cooperate with care.[10] Effective management of BPSD is essential for optimizing rehabilitation outcomes. This may involve medication management, nonpharmacological interventions like music therapy or aromatherapy, and addressing underlying causes such as pain or discomfort.

Individual challenges:

- *Motivation and preferences:* Individuals with dementia may experience reduced motivation or limited interest in participating in rehabilitation activities. Cognitive decline can also make it difficult for individuals to understand the purpose of rehabilitation or follow instructions. It is crucial to consider the individual's preferences and tailor interventions to be engaging and meaningful. Strategies such as breaking down tasks into smaller steps, providing positive reinforcement, and incorporating preferred activities can enhance motivation and participation.

- *Caregiver burden:* Caregivers play a vital role in supporting individuals with dementia and can experience significant physical, emotional, and financial burdens. Rehabilitation programs should consider the needs of caregivers and offer support systems to help them manage their own well-being. This may involve providing education on dementia management strategies, respite care services, or connecting caregivers with support groups.
- *Family involvement and support:* Family members play a critical role in supporting individuals with dementia throughout the rehabilitation process. However, integrating family members effectively requires addressing their own needs and challenges. Research suggests that family members may benefit from educational programs, support groups, and training in specific rehabilitation techniques.[9]
- *Family dynamics and relationships:* Preexisting family dynamics and relationships can influence the effectiveness of family-based rehabilitation interventions. It is crucial to consider these dynamics when designing programs and to provide support for navigating potential conflicts or emotional challenges.[11]

By acknowledging and addressing these challenges, healthcare professionals can create a supportive environment that fosters engagement in rehabilitation and maximizes the potential benefits for individuals with dementia. Family involvement and collaboration with medical professionals are crucial for the successful implementation of rehabilitation programs, ensuring optimal support for individuals with dementia throughout the course of the disease.

FUTURE DIRECTIONS

Functional rehabilitation is a rapidly evolving field with ongoing research exploring novel approaches and optimizing existing interventions. Several future directions hold promise for further enhancing the effectiveness of rehabilitation for individuals with dementia.

- *Integration of technology:* Technological advancements such as virtual reality (VR) and gamified interventions have the potential to make rehabilitation programs more engaging and accessible for individuals with dementia. VR simulations can provide a safe and controlled environment to practice daily activities, while gamified interventions can enhance motivation and reinforce learning through game mechanics.
- *Personalized medicine:* Advances in personalized medicine may allow for the development of individualized rehabilitation programs tailored to the specific genetic and biological profile of the person with dementia. This personalized approach could lead to more effective interventions and improved outcomes.
- *Focus on early intervention:* Early diagnosis of dementia allows for earlier intervention and potentially slows disease progression. Research exploring the benefits of initiating functional rehabilitation programs at the earliest stages of dementia is crucial for maximizing the potential for maintaining independence and quality of life.
- *Telerehabilitation:* The utilization of telecommunication technologies for remote delivery of rehabilitation services holds significant promise for individuals with dementia. Telerehabilitation can overcome geographical barriers, improve access to care, and provide flexibility for individuals who may struggle with transportation or fatigue. Additionally, telerehabilitation can offer opportunities for more frequent monitoring and intervention, potentially leading to improved outcomes, especially in a large country like India with a scarcity of trained professionals and resources.

CONCLUSION

Functional rehabilitation offers a valuable approach to supporting individuals with dementia in maintaining independence, improving quality of life, and maximizing their remaining abilities. Using an integrated multidisciplinary approach and early intervention that implements a person-centered, evidence-based approach incorporating targeted interventions across various domains of daily life, functional rehabilitation empowers individuals with dementia to live as meaningfully and independently as possible. Regular evaluation of program effectiveness ensures ongoing adaptation and optimization of interventions based on individual needs. While challenges exist, such as the progressive nature of dementia and limited resources, ongoing research and exploration of novel approaches hold promise for further refining and enhancing the effectiveness of functional rehabilitation programs. Functional rehabilitation, in conjunction with other supportive measures, empowers individuals with dementia to live with dignity and purpose throughout their journey with the disease.

REFERENCES

1. Alzheimer's Association. (2023). Alzheimer's disease facts and figures. [online] Available from https://www.alz.org/alzheimers-dementia/facts-figures [Last accessed July, 2024].
2. Lopez OL, Klunk WE, Mathis C, Coleman RL, Price J, Becker JT, et al. Amyloid, neurodegeneration, and small vessel disease as predictors of dementia in the oldest-old. Neurology. 2014;83(20):1804-11.
3. World Health Organization (WHO). (2021). Rehabilitation 2034: A vision for the future. World Health Organization.
4. Draper B, Low LF, Brodaty H. Integrated care for adults with dementia and other cognitive disorders. Int Rev Psychiatry. 2018;30(6):272-91.
5. Lawton MP, Brody EM. Instrumental activities of daily living scale (IADL scale). J Am Geriatr Soc. 1969;17(10):606-10.
6. Folstein MF, Folstein SE, McHugh PR. "Mini-mental state". A practical method for grading the cognitive state of patients for the clinician. J Psychiatr Res. 1975;12(3):189-92.
7. Granger CV. The emerging science of functional assessment: our tool for outcomes analysis. Arch Phys Med Rehabil. 1998;79(3):235-40.
8. Doran GT. There's a S.M.A.R.T. way to write management's goals and objectives. Management Review. 1981;70(11):35-6.
9. Häikiö K, Sagbakken M, Rugkåsa J. Family carers' involvement strategies in response to sub-optimal health services to older adults living with dementia - a qualitative study. BMC Geriatr. 2020;20(1):290.
10. Lyketsos CG, Lopez O, Jones B, Fitzpatrick AL, Breitner JCS, Steinberg M, et al. Neuropsychiatric symptoms of Alzheimer's disease: Part I. Consensus statement. Int J Geriatr Psychiatry. 2011;26(12):1165-73.
11. Teri L, Logsdon RG. The future of psychotherapy with older adults. Psychotherapy: Theory, Research, Practice, Training. 1992;29(1):81-7.

CHAPTER 20

Cognitive Stimulation Therapy and Environmental Modification in Patients with Cognitive Impairment

S Sandeep Kumar, Deenadayal Boopalan, Priya Treesa Thomas

ABSTRACT

Dementia is characterized by gradually progressive deterioration in one or more domains of cognition leading to impairment in activities of daily living. Noncognitive symptoms, especially neuropsychiatric symptoms such as aggression, depression, agitation, and wandering, are also associated with dementia, and are associated with rapid progression, increased hospitalization as well as significant caregiver burden. There are both pharmacological and nonpharmacological interventions available for improvement in cognition as well as reduction of neuropsychiatric symptoms. Among the nonpharmacological interventions cognitive stimulation therapy (CST) along with environmental medication are evidence-based interventions for the improvement of global cognition and also have a positive impact on neuropsychiatric symptoms.

Keywords: Neuropsychiatric symptoms, Daily living, Improvement.

INTRODUCTION

Dementia or major neurocognitive disorders as defined by Diagnostic and Statistical Manual of Mental Disorders, Fifth Edition (DSM-5) is a syndrome characterized by progressive impairment in one or more of the six cognitive domains leading to interference with independence in activities of daily living. Apart from neurocognitive impairment, dementia is also associated with various neuropsychiatric symptoms (NPS) previously known as behavioral and psychological symptoms of dementia (BPSD). These NPS are not only associated with poorer outcomes with increased morbidity and mortality but also associated with significant caregiver distress and burden leading to increased hospitalization and rapid progression of the disease.[1] The NPS can be classified into five subtypes:

1. *Cognitive/perceptual*: Delusion and hallucination
2. *Motor symptoms*: Pacing, wandering, repetitive behavior and movement, and physical aggression
3. *Verbal*: Yelling, calling out, repetitive speech, and verbal aggression
4. *Emotional*: Euphoria, depression, anxiety, apathy, and irritability
5. *Vegetative*: Disturbances in sleep and appetite

There are both biological (volume reduction of specific brain areas and neurotransmitter alteration) and nonbiological determinants (such as environmental factors and premorbid personality traits) for the development of these symptoms. The environmental factors that influence the development of NPS can be divided into three main categories: (1) Unmet needs, (2) behavioral/learning, and (3) patient-environment mismatch.[2] There are both pharmacological and nonpharmacological approaches for the management of NPS.

NONPHARMACOLOGICAL INTERVENTION

Nonpharmacological intervention (NPI) is a nonchemical-based, broad-spectrum approach focusing on improving or at least maintaining the cognitive function as well

BOX 1 Effect of nonpharmacological intervention (NPI) on cognition and neuropsychiatric symptoms.

- Cognitive impairment ⇄ Neuropsychiatric symptoms ⇄ Social isolation

↓

- Nonpharmacological intervention

↓

- Improve cognition ⇄ Behavioral and emotional stability ⇄ Social acceptance

as positively influencing the mood and behavior, so that the patient can maintain his/her independence while performing his/her activities of daily living.[3] This intervention not only targets the patient but also their caregivers, and physical and social environment and includes cognitive, behavioral as well as environmental interventions. The main goal of the nonpharmacological therapy is to break the vicious cycle of cognitive impairment, negative psychological reactions associated with cognitive impairment, and resulting social isolation **(Box 1)**.[4] There are various subtypes of NPIs:

- Cognitive intervention
- Stimulant-based interventions such as music therapy, reminiscence therapy, and validation therapy
- Social activity and interaction
- Environmental modification
- Caregiver-targeted intervention such as caregiver support group therapy and counseling

Theoretical Basis for Nonpharmacologic Therapy: Reserve and Neuroplasticity

Reserve

Region-specific brain atrophy and damage are attributed to the development of cognitive impairment in patients with dementia, but the severity of cognitive impairment does not always correspond to the degree of brain damage, i.e., patients with a similar degree of structural brain damage may not have the same degree of cognitive impairment. This discrepancy between the clinical manifestation and structural pathology can be explained by the concept of reserve.[5] It can be classified into passive brain reserve (BR) and active cognitive reserve (CR).

Brain Reserve

This reserve model represents the overall neurobiological substrate of the brain, i.e., specific for each person. It determines the level of threshold of brain damage that leads to the manifestation of cognitive impairment, i.e., a person with a larger brain with large reserves of neurons and synapses has a large capacity to tolerate brain damage. As it is predetermined and does not involve active adaptation, it is considered a passive entity. Brain reserve is determined by factors such as intracranial brain volumes, cortical thickness, number of neurons, and synapses. It is akin to the hardware of a computer.[6]

Cognitive Reserve

This reserve model represents the ability of an individual to adapt and cope with brain damage as efficiently as possible either by effective use of the available brain reserve or by recruiting compensatory strategies. At a physiological level, synaptic organization of recruiting existing or alternative brain networks is responsible for the manifestation of cognitive reserves. Proxies of CRs such as education level, intelligence quotient (IQ), and occupational complexity are indirect measures of an individual's CRs. Higher levels of CRs (high educational and occupational level) are associated with better cognitive performance than those with lower CRs at a given structural pathology and brain damage, i.e., persons with higher CR experience cognitive symptoms at an advanced stage of brain damage than those with lower CR. Mentally stimulating and leisure activities such as reading, writing, playing musical instruments, and socially engaging activities contribute to CRs as well as a reduction in the risk of developing dementia. In patients with similar levels of cognitive impairment, those with higher CR have higher burden of disease pathology than those with lower CR, indicating better coping mechanism to brain damage in patients with higher CR[7] **(Table 1)**.

Neuroplasticity

Neuroplasticity is the ability of our nervous system to modify/change itself by both structural and functional reorganization in response to internal and external

TABLE 1: Types of reserves.

Brain reserve	Cognitive reserve
• Passive structural reserve model • Akin to the hardware of a computer • It is a physical trait of an individual • Determined by intracranial volume, cortical thickness, and number of neurons and synapses	• Active reserve model • Akin to the software of a computer • It is the flexibility and adaptability of the brain to cope with brain damage efficiently by effective use of remaining brain reserve and recruiting of existing and alternative networks • It is determined by the level of education, professional complexities, and engagement in mentally stimulating leisure activities such as reading, calculation, and use of musical instruments

stimuli in order to adapt better to new environments. Two major mechanisms are included in neuroplasticity: (1) Structural neuroplasticity, which includes the formation of new synapses and modification of existing synapses in response to repetitive activities and adult neurogenesis; and (2) Functional reorganization in which changes occur in the functional properties of the neurons in response to learning and memory.[8]

Cognitive Interventions Based Nonpharmacological Intervention

Cognition-based intervention of nonpharmacological approach for management of dementia aims to improve or at least maintain cognition through sets of activities directed toward patients with mild-to-moderate cases of cognitive impairment. Clare et al. (2003) classified it into broadly three categories based on the pattern of response to targeted operations: (1) Cognitive stimulation, (2) cognitive training, (3) cognitive rehabilitation **(Box 2)**[9] **(Table 2)**.

BOX 2 Themes included in cognitive stimulation therapy (CST).

- Physical activities
- Use of childhood games and memories
- Word and number games including word association
- Calculation and money handling
- Sound and musical activities
- Creative activities
- Orientation to time and place
- Current affairs
- Categorization of objects
- Food
- Discussions focusing on opinion rather than facts
- Useful and household tips

COGNITIVE STIMULATION THERAPY

Definition: Cognitive stimulation therapy (CST) is an evidence-based NPI based on the concept of implicit learning, language stimulation, and strengthening of CR leading to general improvement in cognition and social function. The main focus of cognitive stimulation is intellectual and social stimulation through group or individual-based interactive activities and discussions, usually administered in multiple sessions.[10]

Principle and neurophysiological basis: The central basis for cognitive stimulation is based on the fact that lack of stimulating activities is associated with rapid decline in cognitive function in both normal aging and in dementia, i.e., *" use it or lose it"*. Neuroplasticity can be defined as the ability of our nervous system to adapt itself to intrinsic and extrinsic stimuli by both structural and functional reorganization. Cognitive-based intervention especially CST affects cognition by activating the neuroplasticity of nervous system and CR through repetitive and interactive activities.

The activities included in the CST are based on the concept of reality orientation (RO), reminiscence therapy (RT), validation therapy, and sensory motor and social activities.

- *RO:* Patients with cognitive impairment, mostly in the moderate stages of the disease, usually face difficulty in orientating themselves to time, place, and person leading to the development of significant distress. RO, first described by Taulbe and Foulson in 1966, focuses on orienting these patients to time, place, and person, thereby improving both cognitive functions as well as behavioral problems such as depression. The intervention can be administered in individual (24 hour informal RO) as well as in group settings (RO groups) and involves the use of external aids such as calendars, signs, and notice boards.

TABLE 2: Types of cognitive interventions.

Cognitive stimulation (CS)	Cognitive rehabilitation (CR)	Cognitive training (CT)
• Target of CS is overall improvement of global cognition rather than a specific domain • It consists of sets of activities administered to a group of patients in multiple sessions • It consists of activities related to reality orientation, reminiscence therapy, and other sensorimotor stimulating activities	• The focus of CR is to develop adequate personalized compensatory methods to overcome specific cognitive and functional disability • It consists of person-specific, individualized sessions focusing on activities of daily living • It mostly includes environmental modification, use of external aids, and emotional and cognitive adaptation	• The aim of CT is to develop specific aspects of cognition through use of repeated guided practices • It is administered in individuals or small groups with standardized procedures • It includes both computer-based and manual activities to improve specific cognitive skills

- *RT:* This approach of intervention includes recalling and discussing past events, memories, and experiences with the use of aids such as photographs, familiar items from the past, and use of memory boxes. It focuses on long-term memory ensuring active participation from the patients as remote memory is usually better preserved than recent memory. This therapy can be administered both individually and in a group. It has a positive effect on cognition, mood, and overall quality of life.
- *Validation therapy:* This approach is based on the communication strategy acknowledging the feeling expressed by the patient rather than the content. Often patients with cognitive impairment present with confusion due to unmet needs, feelings of loneliness, and boredom, and validation therapy focuses on the emotions that lead to confusion rather than the confusion itself. Validation therapy is effective in alleviating stress and reducing behavioral disturbances.

Intervention and Activities in Cognitive Stimulation Therapy

Cognitive stimulation therapy as an intervention was initially developed by Spector et al. (2003) in the United Kingdom (UK) and has been recognized by the National Institute for Health and Care Excellence (NICE), UK guidelines as an intervention for the management of cognitive symptoms in mild-to-moderate cases of dementia. It consists of 14 theme sessions administered over 7 weeks (2 sessions per week) usually conducted in a group of 5–7 patients with a similar stage of dementia. The theme activities in CST are based on principles of mental stimulation, language stimulation, person-centric, use of reminiscence as an aid, focusing on opinion rather than facts, using strategies for learning implicitly rather than explicit learning, involving each and every participant. and by building relationships.[4]

The list of activities included in CST are given in **Box 2.**

Effect of Cognitive Stimulation Therapy and Evidence

The improvement of cognition in CST is because of repetitive activity-induced improvement in central nervous system (CNS) connectivity, generation of new synapses, myelination of neural circuits, and overall neural structure recovery and reorganization underlying the cognitive functions. Even though CST targets global cognition, language, and memory, especially working memory domains are predominantly affected. It also has some positive effects on NPS, especially depression. 2011 World Alzheimer's Report recommends use of pharmacological therapy such as acetylcholinesterase inhibitors in combination with CST for mild-to-moderate dementia **(Table 3)**.[11-16]

Individualized CST (iCST): This intervention is an individualized, home-based approach that is designed to be fully or partially administered by the caregiver in the home setting and is based on the concept of "aging in place". The main principles of iCST are the same as that of group CST, i.e., mental stimulation, reminiscence, and RO through multiple fun-based activities. The caregiver in iCST can be the patient's spouse, family member, or friend. iCST is associated with improved cognitive functions such as immediate memory, attention, and problem-solving ability. It helps in delaying the institutionalization of persons with cognitive impairment and also improves communication and quality of relationship with their caregiver. As iCST is an individualized home-based intervention, it is suitable for people with cognitive impairment who are immobile or

TABLE 3: Evidence for the effectiveness of cognitive stimulation therapy (CST).

Study	Purpose	Result
Spector et al., 2003[11]	Test the hypothesis that CST improves cognition and quality of life in patients with dementia	Improvement than the control group in Mini–Mental State Examination (MMSE) and QoL-AD scale (quality of life in Alzheimer disease)
Knapp et al., 2006[12]	Investigate the cost-effectiveness of CST	More cost-effective than treatment as usual
Spector et al., 2010[13]	Effect of CST on a specific area of cognition	CST predominantly affects language function
Hall et al., 2013[14]	Effects of CST on cognitive domain	Memory, comprehension of syntax, and orientation are most impacted domain after CST
Yamanaka et al., 2013[15]	Develop Japanese version of CST (CST-J)	CST-J showed improvement in cognition, mood, and quality of life (QoL)
Silva et al., 2021[16]	A home-based individual cognitive stimulation program for older adults in cognitive impairment: A randomized controlled trial (RCT)	Individual cognitive stimulation therapy (iCST) implemented by caregivers showed promising results in improving the cognition of persons with cognitive impairment (PwCIs)

who have limited access to centers providing group CST sessions. It is also suitable for those patients who, because of their problem with communication, find group sessions difficult.[17]

ENVIRONMENTAL MODIFICATIONS

Functional rehabilitation of patients with cognitive impairment is a person-centered approach that is designed to help individuals with cognitive impairment to remain independent and engage in as meaningful activities as possible. It involves environmental modification that not only aims to improve safety but also helps to maintain "maximum performance potential" by making the home facilities easily accessible, thereby ensuring the patients with cognitive impairment to maintain their independence in doing activities of daily living as long as possible.

Environmental modification as an intervention is based on press-competence model (Lawton et al., 1973) according to which the environment places an increasing demand on the person with cognitive impairment as per their decline in competence, i.e., functional ability leading to the development of "maladaptive behaviors" which causes an increase in difficulty in performing their daily activities.[18] Applying this theory, environmental modification may help to maintain "maximum performance potential" and support independence in performing their daily activities.[19]

These environmental interventions which include home modifications (HMs), use of assistive devices, object modifications, task simplification, and modifications of ambience (light, temperature, and sound) and architectural layout as well as interior designing are important in supporting individuals with dementia in performing various daily activities and functions.[20] These activities include toileting, bathing, personal care, dressing, laundry, sleeping, cooking, dining (improving food and fluid intake), as well as interventions related to general safety and security, wandering, and assistance with perception, orientation, and memory.[20]

Available scientific evidence shows positive effects of environmental interventions on quality of life, behavior, and spatial/perceptual abilities.[19] Carrying out daily tasks may be particularly well supported by environmental interventions, given that they involve direct interaction with the external environment.

Based on the scientific evidence, few environmental interventions for daily activities and functions are given in **Table 4**.[19-23]

TABLE 4: Environmental interventions for daily activities and functions to support cognitively-impaired patients.[19-23]

Daily activity and functions	Environmental intervention
Toileting (Hoof et al., 2010)	• *To easily locate the toilet*: Place a red light at the restroom door, install a colored line on the floor leading to the restroom, affix a "restroom" sign on the door, and keep the access door open to enhance visibility • Illumination on the way to toilet/on corridor (from bedroom) • *To prevent fall*: Install grab bars, guardrails, toilet arm supports, and nonslip floor coverings near the toilet and washbasin • *To reduce confusion*: Remove waste baskets, hampers, and any other items that resemble toilet bowls
Bathing and personal care activities (Woodbridge et al., 2018)	• *To bath without caregiver*: Install reflective tape/strips and a padded transfer seat or fold-down wall seat in the shower, a bath seat or tub chair, grab bars on the rim of the tub and shower wall, nonslip material on the floor such as tiles or stickers, a chair in the bathroom, a grab bar in front of the sink, and a floor-to-ceiling safety pole • Replace towel racks with grab bars • Label taps hot and cold
Dressing (Hoof et al., 2010)	• *Dressing aids*: Sticks and stocking devices • *To avoid confusion*: Utilizing open shelves instead of drawers for clothing storage, incorporating two wardrobes—one prominently displayed and the other concealed—is a unique organizational approach • The overt wardrobe should contain only one or two sets of clothes, while the hidden one can accommodate the bulk of the wardrobe • Additionally, it is practical to segregate summer and winter attire into separate closets, as well as distinguish between day and night outfits
Doing laundry (Padilla et al., 2011)	Utilize steam irons equipped with automatic shutoff features for added safety during use. Ensure there is a comfortable chair available for convenience. Replace laundry baskets resembling toilet bowls with standard, nonresembling options. Implement measures to prevent the misuse of detergents and bleach. Opt for a top-loader washing machine to eliminate the need for bending over, and consider raising the machine for enhanced accessibility

Continued

Continued

Daily activity and functions	Environmental intervention
Doing laundry (Padilla et al., 2011)	Utilize steam irons equipped with automatic shutoff features for added safety during use. Ensure there is a comfortable chair available for convenience. Replace laundry baskets resembling toilet bowls with standard, nonresembling options. Implement measures to prevent the misuse of detergents and bleach. Opt for a top-loader washing machine to eliminate the need for bending over, and consider raising the machine for enhanced accessibility
Eating and drinking (Herke et al., 2018)	• To introduce a change of routine, consider utilizing furniture and decoration to alter the dining environment. Additionally, opt for tableware in high-contrast colors to enhance visibility and engagement during meals • Changing the context of mealtimes can involve adjustments to the ambience, such as modifying lighting, sound, smell, or temperature in the dining area • Another modification to consider is providing complementary food items that individuals with dementia can access during or between mealtimes, allowing them to enjoy snacks or refreshments as desired
Sleeping (Marquardt et al., 2014)	To prevent falls from the bed, consider lowering the bed and placing the mattress directly on the floor, ensuring it is near a secured window. Utilize beds equipped with trapeze devices, grab bars, bed railings, and bed handles for added safety. Additionally, install a wireless doorbell for easy communication

CONCLUSION

Even in the background of steady cognitive decline, patients with dementia retain the capacity to learn and enjoy a meaningful life by fulfilling all the societal roles with appropriate support and care. Nonpharmacological interventions such as CST and environmental modifications play a very important role predominantly by increasing the CR and neuroplasticity, thereby enabling the patients to lead an independent life as long as possible and form an essential arm besides pharmacological therapies in the management of cognitive impairment in patients with dementia.

REFERENCES

1. Sabates J, Chiu WH, Loi S, Lampit A, Gavelin HM, Chong T, et al. The associations between neuropsychiatric symptoms and cognition in people with dementia: A systematic review and meta-analysis. Neuropsychol Rev. 2024;34(2):581-97.
2. Kales HC, Gitlin LN, Lyketsos CG; Detroit Expert Panel on Assessment and Management of Neuropsychiatric Symptoms of Dementia. Management of neuropsychiatric symptoms of dementia in clinical settings: Recommendations from a multidisciplinary expert panel. J Am Geriatr Soc. 2014;62(4):762-9.
3. Berg-Weger M, Stewart DB. Non-pharmacologic interventions for persons with dementia. Mo Med. 2017;114(2):116-9.
4. Yates LA, Yates J, Orrell M, Spector A, Woods B (Eds). Cognitive Stimulation Therapy for Dementia: History, Evolution and Internationalism. London, UK: Routledge; 2017.
5. Pappalettera C, Carrarini C, Miraglia F, Vecchio F, Rossini PM. Cognitive resilience/reserve: Myth or reality? A review of definitions and measurement methods. Alzheimers Dement. 2024;20(5):3567-86.
6. Stern Y, Arenaza-Urquijo EM, Bartrés-Faz D, Belleville S, Cantilon M, Chetelat G, et al. Whitepaper: Defining and investigating cognitive reserve, brain reserve, and brain maintenance. Alzheimers Dement. 2020;16(9):1305-11.
7. Stern Y, Barnes CA, Grady C, Jones RN, Raz N. Brain reserve, cognitive reserve, compensation, and maintenance: Operationalization, validity, and mechanisms of cognitive resilience. Neurobiol Aging. 2019;83:124-9.
8. Puderbaugh M, Emmady PD. Neuroplasticity. In: StatPearls [Internet]. Treasure Island (FL): StatPearls Publishing; 2024. Available from http://www.ncbi.nlm.nih.gov/books/NBK557811/ [Last accessed July, 2024].
9. Clare L, Woods RT, Moniz Cook ED, Orrell M, Spector A. Cognitive rehabilitation and cognitive training for early-stage Alzheimer's disease and vascular dementia. Cochrane Database Syst Rev. 2003;(4):CD003260.
10. Rao GP, Sivakumar PT, Srivastava S, Sidana RC. Cognitive therapy and family intervention for patients with dementia and psychosis. Indian J Psychiatry. 2020;62(Suppl 2):S183-91.
11. Spector A, Thorgrimsen L, Woods B, Royan L, Davies S, Butterworth M, et al. Efficacy of an evidence-based cognitive stimulation therapy programme for people with dementia: Randomised controlled trial. Br J Psychiatry. 2003;183:248-54.
12. Knapp M, Thorgrimsen L, Patel A, Spector A, Hallam A, Woods B, et al. Cognitive stimulation therapy for people with dementia: Cost-effectiveness analysis. Br J Psychiatry. 2006;188:574-80.
13. Spector A, Orrell M, Woods B. Cognitive Stimulation Therapy (CST): Effects on different areas of cognitive function for people with dementia. Int J Geriatr Psychiatry. 2010;25(12):1253-8.
14. Hall L, Orrell M, Stott J, Spector A. Cognitive stimulation therapy (CST): Neuropsychological mechanisms of change. Int Psychogeriatr. 2013;25(3):479-89.
15. Yamanaka K, Kawano Y, Noguchi D, Nakaaki S, Watanabe N, Amano T, et al. Effects of cognitive stimulation therapy Japanese

version (CST-J) for people with dementia: A single-blind, controlled clinical trial. Aging Ment Health. 2013;17(5):579-86.

16. Silva R, Bobrowicz-Campos E, Santos-Costa P, Cruz AR, Apóstolo J. A home-based individual cognitive stimulation program for older adults with cognitive impairment: A randomized controlled trial. Front Psychol. 2021;12:741955.
17. Orrell M, Yates L, Burns A, Russell I, Woods RT, Hoare Z, et al. Individual cognitive stimulation therapy for dementia (iCST): Study protocol for a randomized controlled trial. Trials. 2012;13:172.
18. Lawton MP, Nahemow L. Ecology and the aging process. In: Eisdorfer C, Lawton MP (Eds). The psychology of adult development and aging. Washington, DC: American Psychological Association; 1973. pp. 619-74.
19. Woodbridge R, Sullivan MP, Harding E, Crutch S, Gilhooly KJ, Gilhooly M, et al. Use of the physical environment to support everyday activities for people with dementia: A systematic review. Dementia. 2018;17(5):533-72.
20. van Hoof J, Kort HS, van Waarde H, Blom MM. Environmental interventions and the design of homes for older adults with dementia: An overview. Am J Alzheimers Dis Other demen. 2010;25(3):202-32.
21. Padilla R. Effectiveness of environment-based interventions for people with Alzheimer's disease and related dementias. Am J Occup Ther. 2011;65(5):514-22.
22. Herke M, Fink A, Langer G, Wustmann T, Watzke S, Hanff AM, et al. Environmental and behavioural modifications for improving food and fluid. intake in people with dementia. Cochrane Database Syst Rev. 2018;2018(7):CD011542.
23. Marquardt G, Bueter K, Motzek T. Impact of the design of the built environment on people with dementia: An evidence-based review. HERD. 2014;8(1):127-57.

CHAPTER

21 Technology and Artificial Intelligence in Dementia

Christian Dansereau, Sinjan Ghosh

ABSTRACT

Artificial intelligence (AI) is transforming the landscape of dementia care and research. AI technologies, such as machine learning and deep learning, are being leveraged to improve early detection, diagnosis, and treatment of dementia. These systems can analyze vast amounts of data, including medical records, genetic information, and neuroimaging data, to identify patterns and biomarkers associated with the disease that might be missed by human clinicians.

Artificial intelligence algorithms are particularly adept at recognizing subtle cognitive decline through analysis of speech patterns, handwriting, and even everyday activities monitored through smart devices. This early detection is crucial, as it allows for timely interventions that can slow disease progression and improve quality of life.

In clinical settings, AI can support personalized treatment plans by predicting individual responses to various therapies, thus optimizing patient care. Additionally, AI-driven applications are aiding caregivers by providing real-time monitoring and alerts, helping to manage symptoms, and ensuring patient safety. The integration of AI in dementia care poses challenges, including ethical concerns related to privacy, data security, and the need for rigorous validation of AI tools to ensure their accuracy and reliability in diverse populations. Judicious AI tool selection and ethical application are essential.

Keywords: Technology, Artificial intelligence, Dementia, Alzheimer's disease, Cognitive impairment.

INTRODUCTION

Dementia is a progressive neurodegenerative disorder characterized by a decline in cognitive function, affecting memory, thought processing, behavior, and the consequent inability to perform everyday tasks. As the population ages, the prevalence of dementia is expected to increase, placing a significant burden on the global healthcare systems.[1] There is currently no curative treatment for dementia and available treatments only provide temporary relief of symptoms.

In recent years, the integration of technology and artificial intelligence (AI) into healthcare has revolutionized the landscape of dementia care. With the increasing prevalence of dementia worldwide, there is a growing need for innovative approaches to support individuals living with this condition and for their caregivers.

Before proceeding with this chapter, let us walk down the memory lane and peek into the history of AI and how it evolved over the years **(Table 1 and Fig. 1)**.

TABLE 1: Brief history of the inception and evolution of artificial intelligence (AI).

Year	History
1642	The first mechanical calculating machine was innovated by the French mathematician, Blaise Pascal
1950	Alan Turing, an English mathematician, introduced the "Turing Test" as a way of testing a machine's intelligence
1955	"Artificial Intelligence" was coined during a conference devoted to this topic
1956	Dartmouth Conference marked the birth of AI as a field of study

Continued

Continued

Year	History
1965	*ELIZA*, a natural language program was invented. It handled dialogs on any topic, similar to chatbots
	Evolution of the concept of natural language processing:
	Teaches computers to understand and use human language using techniques such as machine learning
1974	The "AI winter" began, marked by a decline in funding and interest in AI research, due to limited progress during this time
1980s	Edward Feigenbaum created expert systems which emulate decisions of human experts
	Concept of neural network:
	Machine learning models that simulate the brain learning to recognize patterns and make predictions via artificial neuron connections

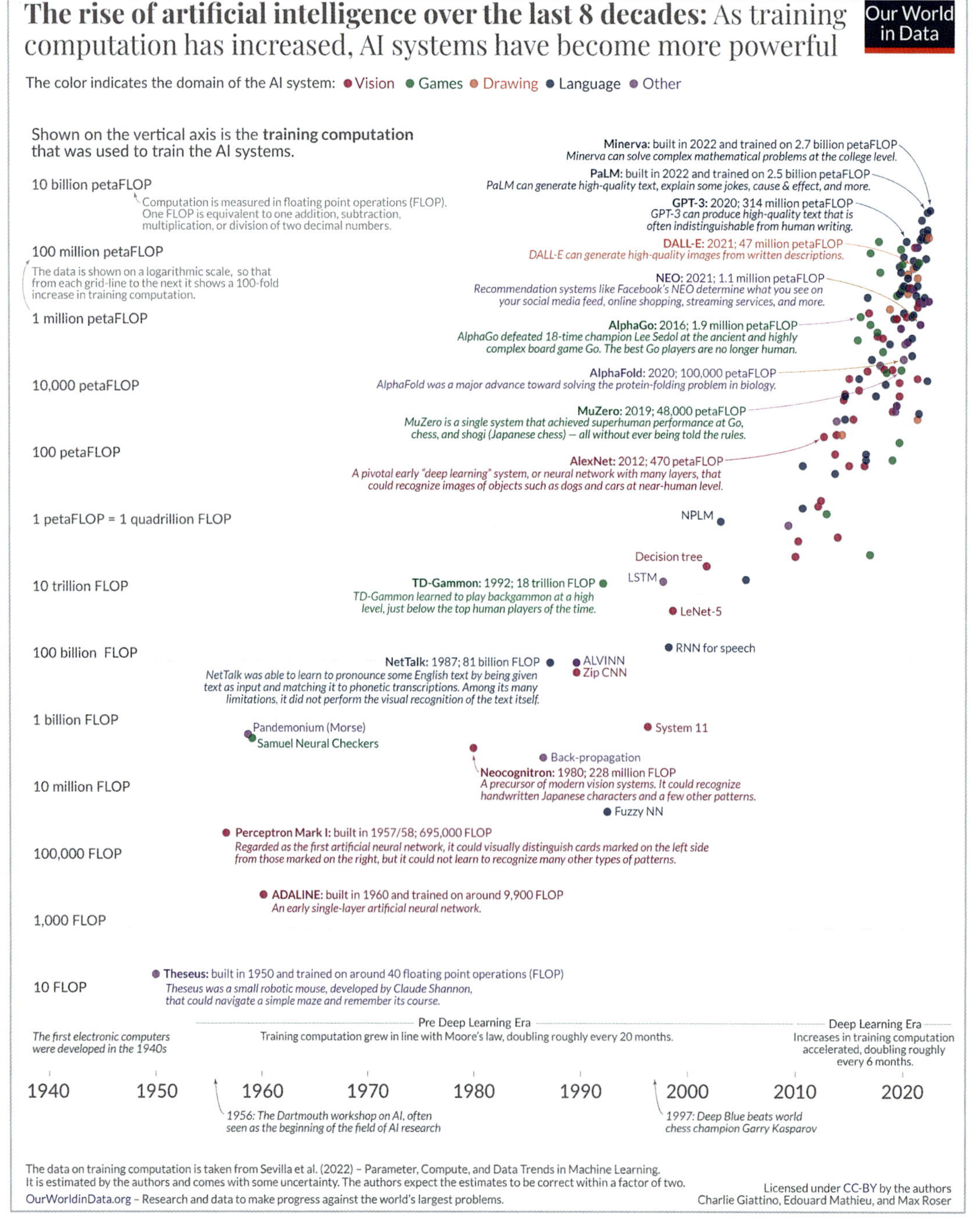

FIG. 1: The rise of artificial intelligence (AI) over the last eight decades: As training computation has increased, AI systems have become more powerful.

This chapter explores the role of technology and AI in the full spectrum of dementia care, highlighting their potential to enhance early detection, personalized treatment, and overall improvement in the quality of life for those affected by the diseases.

EARLY DIAGNOSIS AND PREDICTION

One of the key challenges in dementia care is the early detection of the disease. This is often due to the uncertainty in the diagnosis as a result of the high variability in the disease progression. AI technologies, such as machine learning (ML) algorithms, can analyze large amounts of data from medical records, imaging studies, and cognitive assessments to identify patterns and predictors of cognitive decline. By using AI to analyze these data, healthcare providers can detect early signs of dementia in patients who may not yet exhibit noticeable symptoms or very mild ones. This early diagnosis allows for timely interventions and treatment options that can slow the progression of the disease. If we consider Alzheimer's disease, the pathological changes may precede the full-blown clinical manifestations by 20–30 years, which provides a significant window of opportunity to diagnose and plan accordingly. The target should be the detection at the clinical stage of subjective cognitive decline or mild cognitive impairment (MCI).

Artificial intelligence can also be implemented to predict the likelihood of developing dementia in individuals at risk based on their genetic, lifestyle, and medical history. By analyzing these risk factors, AI algorithms can provide personalized recommendations for lifestyle modifications, preventive measures, and cognitive exercises to reduce the risk of developing dementia later in life. This predictive modeling can help individuals make informed decisions about their health and proactively manage their cognitive health.

Gait analysis could detect motoric cognitive risk (MCR), a predementia syndrome characterized by slow gait and cognitive complaints.[2,3] Gait speed when analyzed with the cognitive test results, using logistic regression and other statistical tests, help in determining the relation of MCR syndromes and brain volume. Motor control of hands, dexterity, and computer-assisted graphic drawings are alternative methods of discerning hand motor functions.[4]

Multiple studies have focused on speech and language as digital biomarkers for early detection of dementia.[5-8] Speech data are broadly divided into (1) acoustic features and (2) linguistic features.

- Acoustic features (deals with articulation)
  - Mel-frequency cepstral coefficients (MFCC)
  - Speech rate
  - Cepstral peak performance (CPP)
- Linguistic features (deals with content)
  - Vocabulary
  - Grammar
  - Syntax

COMPUTER-ASSISTED INTERPRETATION OF BRAIN SCANS

Artificial intelligence can be used in analyzing brain imaging scans, such as magnetic resonance imaging (MRI) and positron emission tomography (PET). These advanced imaging techniques can provide valuable insights into the structural and functional changes in the brain associated with dementia. AI algorithms can process and analyze these images to identify subtle abnormalities and complex patterns that may indicate the presence of the disease pathology, even before clinical symptoms manifest.[9-11] Two main AI methods applied in neuroimaging with dementia are as follows:

1. *ML techniques*: ML-based algorithms show promising results in various studies. With these techniques, it is difficult to discriminate early imaging changes of dementia. They require less data to train and often generalize well.
2. *Deep learning techniques*: It is more sensitive in detecting subtle imaging changes seen in the early stages of dementia. Three-dimensional (3D) neural network models are used in the detection of dementia. They are prone to more generalization problems and require orders of magnitude and more data compared to the classical ML approaches. The challenges are as follows:
   a. A huge amount of data is required for training or validation.
   b. The lack of interpretability in particular for deep learning models to understand which specific features of the scan are picked up by these models. However, some progress has been made on that front in recent years.

WEARABLE DEVICES AND SMARTPHONE APPLICATIONS

Another promising application of AI involves digital biomarkers derived from wearable devices and smartphone applications. These devices can track various parameters, such as gait, speech patterns, and social interactions, which can be indicative of cognitive decline. Combining AI methods and "smart environments" helps in formulating innovative digital biomarkers. AI algorithms can analyze this data in real time, providing continuous monitoring of an individual's cognitive function and alerting healthcare providers to any concerning changes.

Broadly, these are divided into ADL monitoring at home (real-world setting) or in a research laboratory, simulating real-life situations (scenario-based monitoring). This is an exciting and evolving area of research. Smart home environments may provide a completely new avenue in detection of dementia at a very early stage.[12,13]

Batista et al.[14] and Khodabandehloo et al.[15] set ambient sensors, Global Positioning System (GPS), and InfraRED and proximity sensors to detect the trajectory and wandering episode. They fed the data into ML accelerometers and gyroscope as wearable sensors.

NEW DISEASE-MODIFYING TREATMENTS IN ALZHEIMER'S: A PARADIGM SHIFT IN INTERVENTION

The development of new disease-modifying treatments in Alzheimer's represents a significant paradigm shift in the intervention strategies available to physicians. Traditionally, Alzheimer's has been treated with therapies that temporarily alleviate symptoms. However, recent advancements have led to the creation of treatments that target the underlying disease processes, such as the formation of amyloid plaques and tau protein tangles in the brain.

These treatments, including drugs such as monoclonal antibodies, work by reducing amyloid plaques or preventing tau proteins from tangling, thereby potentially slowing disease progression and improving cognitive function. The introduction of these therapies necessitates early intervention, as they are most effective in the initial stages of Alzheimer's disease. This shift requires physicians to adopt new treatment protocols, including regular monitoring of biomarkers and adjusting therapies based on patient responses.

While these treatments offer significant promise, they also present challenges. Side effects such as brain swelling and bleeding need careful management and the high costs pose accessibility issues. Continuous research is crucial to refine these treatments, enhance their efficacy, and reduce side effects. Future approaches may involve combination therapies that integrate disease-modifying treatments with lifestyle changes and other pharmacological interventions to maximize patient benefits.

The advent of disease-modifying treatments mark a transformative moment in Alzheimer's care, providing new hope for patients and necessitating a multidisciplinary approach that includes advanced diagnostics, personalized treatment plans, and comprehensive patient monitoring.[16]

PLASMA BIOMARKERS IN ALZHEIMER'S DISEASE

The use of plasma biomarkers in Alzheimer's disease represents a groundbreaking advance in early detection and monitoring. Plasma biomarkers are proteins or other substances found in blood that can indicate the presence of Alzheimer's disease. The most promising plasma biomarkers include amyloid-beta (Aβ) peptides, tau proteins, and neurofilament light chain (NfL).

Amyloid-beta peptides, particularly elevated levels of Aβ42 and changes in the Aβ42/Aβ40 ratio, serve as early indicators of amyloid plaque accumulation in the brain, a hallmark of Alzheimer's disease. Increased levels of phosphorylated tau (p-tau) in plasma correlate with neurofibrillary tangles, another characteristic feature of Alzheimer's pathology. Higher levels of NfL indicate neurodegeneration and neuronal injury, which are prevalent in Alzheimer's and other neurodegenerative diseases.

Plasma biomarkers offer numerous benefits. Unlike cerebrospinal fluid (CSF) testing and PET scans, plasma biomarker tests are minimally invasive, requiring only a blood sample. They enable the detection of Alzheimer's disease at an earlier stage, potentially before significant cognitive decline occurs. Regular blood tests can monitor changes in biomarker levels, helping to track disease progression and treatment response.

In clinical implementation, plasma biomarkers can be used for initial screening in at-risk populations, aiding in the early diagnosis of Alzheimer's. Biomarker levels can inform personalized treatment plans, indicating which therapies might be most effective for individual patients. Biomarkers are also valuable in clinical trials for assessing the efficacy of new treatments and understanding disease mechanisms.

However, challenges remain. There is a need for standardized testing protocols and validation across diverse populations to ensure accuracy and reliability. Implementing plasma biomarker testing in routine clinical practice requires education and training for healthcare providers. Additionally, making these tests affordable and accessible to a wide population is crucial for their widespread adoption.

Plasma biomarkers hold immense potential for transforming Alzheimer's disease management, offering a noninvasive, cost-effective, and efficient means of early detection, monitoring, and personalized treatment. As research continues to advance, these biomarkers may become a standard part of Alzheimer's care, significantly improving outcomes for patients.[16]

COMBINING MULTIMODAL DATA TO HAVE A HOLISTIC VIEW OF THE PATIENT

Combining multimodal data and biomarkers is crucial for obtaining a holistic view of the patient, particularly in complex diseases such as Alzheimer's. The complexity of the disease and the diversity of its manifestations mean that relying on a single test is insufficient. Alzheimer's disease affects multiple aspects of health, including cognitive function, physical health, and genetic predispositions.

Multimodal data integrates various types of information, such as biomarkers, genetic data, imaging results, clinical assessments, and lifestyle factors, providing a comprehensive profile of the patient. Biomarkers offer insights into specific pathological processes, but when combined with other data sources, they reveal a more complete picture of the disease's impact on the individual. This holistic approach allows for more accurate diagnosis, personalized treatment plans, and better monitoring of disease progression.

By viewing the patient as a whole, healthcare providers can address the multifaceted nature of Alzheimer's, tailoring interventions to meet the unique needs of each patient. This integrated perspective is essential for managing the disease effectively and improving patient outcomes, as it acknowledges the intricate interplay of factors contributing to the patient's overall health and disease progression.[17]

IMPROVING DRUG EFFICACY WITH A PRECISION MEDICINE APPROACH

The use of AI-driven predictive tools can revolutionize drug efficacy through precision medicine. These tools can analyze vast amounts of patient data to predict likely outcomes, enabling the identification of individuals who are more likely to respond positively to specific treatments. By targeting these likely responders, physicians can significantly increase the efficacy of treatments within this subgroup, ensuring that patients receive the most effective therapies tailored to their unique profiles.

Furthermore, as treatments are administered to a larger and more diverse pool of individuals, AI tools can help identify "super responders"—those who exhibit exceptional therapeutic responses. This data-driven approach allows for the refinement of treatment protocols and the development of highly personalized medical strategies. By continuously learning from real-world patient outcomes, AI enhances our understanding of treatment efficacy across diverse populations, ultimately leading to more precise and effective healthcare interventions.

BOX 1 Multimodal insight.

- Machine learning research integrates brain imaging with clinical data to predict disease progression in Alzheimer's disease (AD)
- Wearable technology like accelerometers and inertial measurement units (IMUs) can measure changes in gait, sleep, and physical activity in dementia
- Device-measured physical activity provides more objective measures and allows researchers to distinguish between different levels and intensities of activities
- Monitoring gait and physical activity over time can provide important information about disease progression
- Sleep markers, such as actigraphy, can reflect sleep disturbances in dementia and help adapt care provision
- Sensor devices, such as Global Positioning System (GPS)-enabled technologies, can monitor everyday mobility and function in real-life home environments
- "Life space behavior" measured through GPS tracking may inform disease progression in mild AD

Overall, integrating AI-driven predictive tools into precision medicine not only improves individual patient outcomes but also advances the field of personalized medicine, ensuring that treatments are both effective and tailored to the unique needs of each patient. This approach holds the promise of transforming drug development and therapeutic strategies, making healthcare more efficient and impactful **(Box 1)**.

MONITORING AND MANAGEMENT

Once a diagnosis of dementia is made, AI technologies can be used to monitor the progression of the disease and track changes in cognitive function over time. Wearable devices, such as smartwatches and fitness trackers, equipped with AI algorithms can collect data on physical activity, sleep patterns, and other health metrics to provide real-time monitoring of patients with dementia. This continuous monitoring allows caregivers and healthcare providers to identify subtle changes in behavior and cognition that may indicate disease progression or the onset of complications.

Artificial intelligence-powered virtual assistants, such as chatbots and voice-activated devices, can also provide support and reminders to individuals with dementia to help them manage daily tasks, medication schedules, and appointments. These virtual assistants can offer personalized assistance and guidance based on the patient's preferences and needs, enhancing their independence and quality of life. Additionally, AI-driven decision support systems can help healthcare providers make informed decisions about treatment options, care plans, and interventions for patients with dementia, optimizing their care and well-being.

Personalized Treatment and Intervention

Once dementia is diagnosed, personalized treatment plans are essential to address the unique needs and challenges of every individual. Technology and AI play a crucial role in tailoring interventions to the specific characteristics of the patient, thereby optimizing therapeutic outcomes. This precision medicine approach holds promise for improving treatment outcomes and reducing the burden of dementia on healthcare systems.

Virtual reality (VR) and augmented reality (AR) technologies have shown promise in cognitive rehabilitation programs by providing immersive environments for memory training, spatial navigation, and activities of daily living. These interactive experiences can stimulate cognitive functions, enhance neural plasticity, and improve overall cognitive functioning in individuals with dementia.

Providing information on the risk of a patient to progress to more advanced stages of the disease can be a valuable tool to manage patients and plan accordingly the care/intervention and resources appropriate for now and in the near future.

Remote Monitoring and Support

Caring for individuals with dementia often places a significant burden on family members and caregivers, leading to stress, burnout, and decreased quality of life. Technology offers solutions to alleviate these challenges by providing remote monitoring and support services.

Smart home technology equipped with sensors and smart devices can create a safe and supportive environment for individuals with dementia, detecting emergencies such as falls or wandering and alerting caregivers or emergency services promptly. Additionally, telemedicine platforms enable remote consultations with healthcare professionals, allowing caregivers to seek guidance and support without the need for frequent clinic visits.

Chatbots and virtual assistants equipped with natural language processing capabilities can provide personalized reminders, medication management, and emotional support to both individuals with dementia and their caregivers. These AI-powered companions offer companionship and engagement, reducing feelings of isolation and loneliness often experienced by those living with dementia[2,12] **(Fig. 2)**.

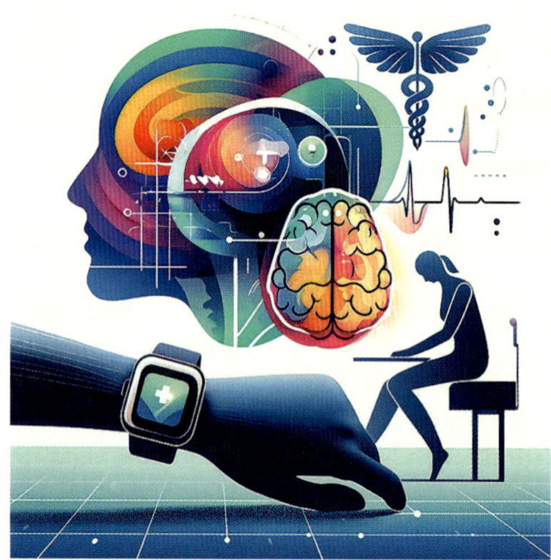

FIG. 2: Artificial intelligence (AI)-powered companions.

ETHICAL CONSIDERATIONS AND CHALLENGES

While the potential benefits of AI in dementia diagnosis and management are substantial, there are important ethical considerations and challenges that must be addressed. One of the key concerns is the protection of patient privacy and data security, particularly when utilizing sensitive healthcare information in AI algorithms. Robust data governance policies and encryption protocols are essential to safeguarding patient data and ensuring compliance with regulatory requirements.

Another ethical consideration is the potential for bias and discrimination in AI algorithms, which may perpetuate existing disparities in healthcare access and treatment outcomes. Biases can arise from the data used to train AI models, as well as from the design and implementation of the algorithms themselves. Healthcare providers and AI developers must carefully consider these issues and take proactive steps to mitigate biases and ensure the fair and equitable delivery of dementia care. Efforts to promote equitable access to technology and ensure cultural and linguistic sensitivity in digital health interventions are essential to address these disparities.

Additionally, there are challenges related to the implementation and integration of AI technologies into healthcare systems, including the need for specialized training for healthcare providers, regulatory approval processes, and reimbursement mechanisms.

WHO IS THE MASTER?

With the advent of AI and technology which is developing rapidly, alongside a lot of faith and reliance, controversies are surfacing too. There is also a lot of apprehension and skepticism about AI taking over human intelligence and resulting in the loss of jobs for people. Most of these AI solutions are aiming more at supporting and enabling healthcare professionals than replacing them. In the context of a lack of trained neurologists and dementia specialists, it will be important to empower them to make their work as effective as possible.

These hurdles must be overcome to maximize the benefits of AI in dementia care and ensure widespread adoption of these innovative solutions.

FUTURE PROSPECTS

- The inclusion of electronic health records (EHRs) in large-scale datasets is crucial for dementia research.
- Data sharing and harmonization are important for analyzing information across multiple sources and make datasets more representative of the diverse and general population.
- Natural language processing can be used to extract valuable insights from EHRs in mental healthcare.
- E-cohorts and remote testing can accelerate recruitment to dementia trials and improve assessment methods.
- Rapid data collection from diverse populations contribute to the understanding of dementia.
- Collaboration and engagement among clinicians, researchers, and the public are crucial for driving progress in digital health for dementia research.
- The use of prognostic information will help better manage care and provide timelier diagnostic and intervention for those patients.
- Brain-computer interface may be helpful in neurorehabilitation and management of advanced dementia.

LIMITATIONS

- The "black box" nature of AI/ML in healthcare creates complexity in clinical trust and responsibility for decision-making.
- *Generalizability of the predictive models*: Algorithms trained on one dataset may not effectively translate to diverse populations.
- The identification of risk factors in modeling may be influenced by a generalized "protective lifestyle" or reflect part of the disease process.
- Relatively small samples, covariance among risk factors, and marginal gains over established risk factors pose obstacles in ML applied to dementia.

CONCLUSION

Artificial intelligence holds great promise for transforming dementia care by facilitating early diagnosis, personalized interventions, and enhanced monitoring of patients with the disease. By harnessing the power of AI technologies, healthcare providers can improve the accuracy and efficiency of dementia diagnosis, predict the risk of cognitive decline, and support individuals with dementia in managing their symptoms and daily activities. As AI continues to evolve and advance, it is essential to integrate these technologies into dementia care practices to enhance the quality of life for patients and alleviate the burden on caregivers.

To realize the full potential of AI in dementia care, collaboration between healthcare providers, researchers, policymakers, and technology companies is essential, ensuring that these innovative solutions are ethically sound, effective, and accessible to all who need them. Technology and AI have the potential to usher in a new era of compassionate and effective dementia care. It is the wind of change and healthcare professionals should adapt to it. Judicious and ethical applications are the key. A spark or flame can light up the world or it may burn everything into ashes. The choice is ours.

REFERENCES

1. Livingston G, Huntley J, Sommerlad A, Ames D, Ballard C, Banerjee S, et al. Dementia prevention, intervention, and care: 2020 report of the Lancet Commission. Lancet. 2020;396(10248):413-46.
2. Li R, Wang X, Lawler K, Garg S, Bai Q, Alty J. Applications of artificial intelligence to aid early detection of dementia: A scoping review on current capabilities and future directions. J Biomed Inform. 2022;127:104030.
3. Beauchet O, Allali G, Annweiler C, Verghese J. Association of Motoric Cognitive Risk Syndrome With Brain Volumes: Results From the GAIT Study. J Gerontol A Biol Sci Med Sci. 2016;71(8):1081-8.
4. Sano Y, Yin Y, Mizuguchi T, Kandori A. Detection of Abnormal Segments in Finger Tapping Waveform using One-class SVM. Annu Int Conf IEEE Eng Med Biol Soc. 2019;2019:1378-81.
5. Mirheidari B, Blackburn D, Walker T, Venneri A, Reuber M, Christensen H. Detecting signs of dementia using word vector representations. Hyderabad, India: Interspeech; 2018. pp. 1893-97.
6. Luz S, de la Fuente S, Albert P. A method for analysis of patient speech in dialogue for dementia detection. Para-linguistic and Extra-Linguistic Data from People with Various Forms of Cognitive Impairment. Paris, France: European Language Resources Association (ELRA); 2018. pp. 35-42
7. Ujiro T, Tanaka H, Adachi H, Kazui H, Ikeda M, Kudo T, et al. Detection of dementia from responses to atypical questions asked by embodied conversational agents. Hyderabad, India: Interspeech; 2018. pp. 1691-5.
8. Chien YW, Hong SY, Cheah WT, Fu LC, Chang YL. An assessment system for Alzheimer's disease based on speech using a novel feature sequence design and recurrent neural network. Miyazaki, Japan: 2018 IEEE International Conference on Systems, Man, and Cybernetics (SMC); 2018. pp. 3289-94.
9. Yiğit A, Isik Z. Applying deep learning models to structural MRI for stage prediction of Alzheimer's disease. Turk J Elec Eng Comp Sci. 2020;28:196-210.

10. Iizuka T, Fukasawa M, Kameyama M. Deep-learning-based imaging-classification identified cingulate island sign in dementia with Lewy bodies. Sci Rep. 2019;9(1):1-9.
11. Bäckstrøm K, Nazari M, Yu-Hua Gu I, Jakola AS. An efficient 3D deep convolutional network for Alzheimer's disease diagnosis using MR images. 2018 IEEE 15th International Symposium on Biomedical Imaging (ISBI 2018). Washington DC, USA: IEEE; 2018. pp. 149-53.
12. Lyall DM, Kormilitzin A, Lancaster C, Sousa J, Petermann-Rocha F, Buckley C, et al. Artificial intelligence for dementia-Applied models and digital health. Alzheimers Dement. 2023;19(12):5872-84.
13. Tung JY, Rose RV, Gammada E, Lam I, Roy EA, Black SE, et al. Measuring life space in older adults with mild-to-moderate Alzheimer's disease using mobile phone GPS. Gerontology. 2014;60:154-62.
14. Batista E, Casino F, Solanas A. On wandering detection methods in context-aware scenarios. 2016 7th International Conference on Information, Intelligence, Systems & Applications (IISA). Catalonia, Spain: IEEE; 2016. pp. 1-6.
15. Khodabandehloo E, Riboni D. Collaborative trajectory mining in smart-homes to support early diagnosis of cognitive decline. IEEE Trans Emerg Topics Comput. 2020.
16. Cummings J. Anti-Amyloid Monoclonal Antibodies are Transformative Treatments that Redefine Alzheimer's Disease Therapeutics. Drugs. 2023;83(7):569-76.
17. Mc Ardle R, Del Din S, Donaghy P, Galna B, Thomas AJ, Rochester L. The Impact of Environment on Gait Assessment: Considerations from Real-World Gait Analysis in Dementia Subtypes. Sensors. 2021;21:813.

CHAPTER

22

Gadgets in Dementia

Ishwarya Thiruvuru, Ranganathan Lakshmi Narasimhan, Rithvik Ramesh

ABSTRACT

According to the World Health Organization (WHO), over 55 million people worldwide live with dementia, with more than 60% residing in low- and middle-income countries. Annually, nearly 10 million new cases arise. Dementia, an encompassing term, includes various neurodegenerative diseases, which cause a progressive decline in cognitive abilities. Dementia robs individuals of their independence and familiar routines, impacting their personal, professional, and caregiver lives. It starts with cognitive decline and escalates to the inability to carry out essential activities of daily living (ADLs). While dementia remains incurable, substantial support can be provided to both patients and caregivers. Encouragingly, technological advancements offer greater possibilities for those with dementia and their caregivers, promoting independence, improving quality of life, and alleviating caregiver burden. Technology, an evolving domain, holds the potential to enhance the quality of life for individuals with dementia and their caregivers, facilitating their ability to maintain residence within a community. Thus, using technologies for dementia provides many opportunities for considering various aspects of this disease as well can make lifestyle easier both for the patients and caregivers.

Keywords: Dementia, Assistive Technology, Domain-based gadgets, Living aids.

INTRODUCTION

Dementia, an encompassing term, includes various neurodegenerative diseases, which cause a progressive decline in cognitive abilities. It robs individuals of their independence and familiar routines, impacting their personal, professional, and caregiver lives.

Dementia starts with cognitive decline and escalates to the inability to carry out essential activities of daily living (ADLs).[1] Subsequently, it affects language, social behavior, and even motor functions. Individuals experiencing dementia may present a spectrum of symptoms, ranging from mild to severe, which may involve one of the following domains: Memory issues (such as short-term memory loss, characterized by misplacement of objects, forgetting to carry out important tasks, and becoming disengaged from conversations or TV programs and even forgetting to eat, drink, or take medication), executive dysfunction (like problems in money handling, planning and organizing events, and problem-solving), visuospatial (difficulty in navigating or locating items, getting lost), language and communication difficulties (difficulty in comprehending spoken or written language, or difficulty speaking), and even mental health concerns (such as anxiety, depression, confusion, and frustration). These symptoms can contribute to social isolation and loneliness, with "wandering" being a common occurrence. Additionally, living alone can pose specific risks, including falls, hypothermia, misuse of household appliances, accidents like fires, ingestion of harmful substances, and medication errors due to memory issues.[1]

The outcomes of dementia extend to individuals, families, societies, and nations, incurring substantial financial and human costs. According to the World Health Organization (WHO), over 55 million people worldwide live with dementia, with more than 60% residing in low- and middle-income countries. Annually, nearly 10 million new cases arise. While dementia remains incurable, substantial support can be provided to both patients and caregivers. Encouragingly, technological advancements offer greater possibilities for those with dementia and their caregivers, promoting independence, improving quality of life, and alleviating caregiver burden **(Fig. 1)**.

The gadgets for dementia can be discussed under or categorized into those used by the caregivers to improve quality of life or safety for the patients, or gadgets used by the patients with insight into their cognitive issues to improve quality of life **(Flowchart 1)**.

CAREGIVER GADGETS

Caregivers dedicate countless hours to providing care and ensuring the safety of their loved ones leading to stress, exhaustion, and feelings of isolation. Technology steps in, offering a new wave of gadgets specifically designed to empower caregivers. These tools are not a replacement for human connection but a vital support system, alleviating burdens and fostering a sense of control in managing dementia. They can be broadly watchful, and therefore require some direct attention from the caregiver or can be specifically tailored for the more common caregiver issues such as falls, wandering, and fire. The caregiver's responsibility is to ensure that the dementia patient does not get herself or himself into a dangerous situation within the house. Systems that have already been in place for a multitude of purposes can be repurposed to provide a watchful eye over the patients offering remote monitoring capabilities for caregivers.

- *Video monitoring cameras*: Video cameras can be used as security cameras to monitor patients in general, motion-activated camera detects and alters the caregivers. It can also be combined with audio as two-way audio cameras with two-way communication allow caregivers to check in visually and to help the patients verbally by offering reassurance/instructions. These devices learn the patient's daily routines to detect any deviations and alert family members accordingly. With integrated artificial intelligence (AI) and machine learning, they promptly notify support services if any issues arise.[2]
- *Motion detection devices*: These devices consistently relay alerts to caregivers, ensuring family members stay updated. Some advanced devices take proactive measures by issuing reminders upon activation of the alarm. For example, a pressure mat positioned at a kitchen entrance/exit can prompt a dementia patient to switch off the gas stove upon leaving the kitchen. Such reminders play a crucial role in averting potential disasters and minimizing losses.[3]
- *Sensors*: Sensors in doors and windows are security devices that can be particularly useful for dementia

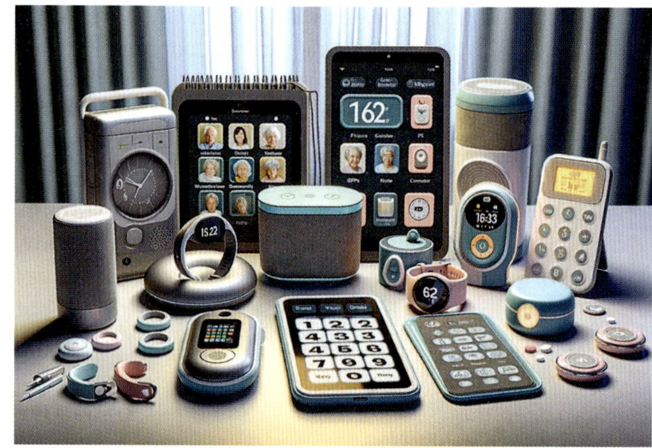

FIG. 1: Various gadgets designed for patients with dementia, including a digital calendar clock, wearable GPS tracker, smart speaker, picture phone, medication dispenser, and motion sensor night light. Image created with the assistance of DALL-E, an AI model by OpenAI.

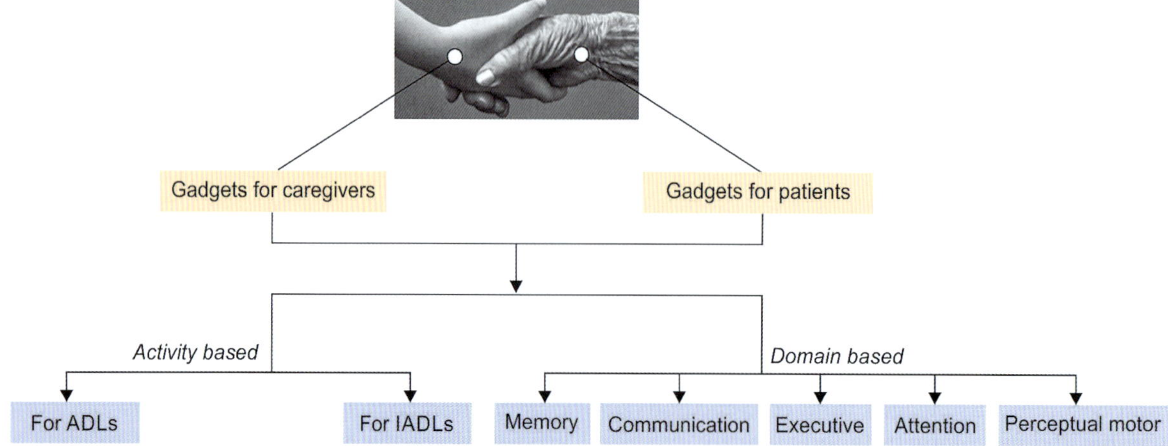

FLOWCHART 1: Categorization of gadgets available for dementia.
(ADLs: activities of daily living; IADLs: instrumental activities of daily living)

patients who are prone to wandering. These sensors detect unauthorized opening and closing of doors. With AI support, sensors can detect climate change like strong winds or rains, and alert the patient to close windows. Smoke and fire sensors can alert people about potential fire or smoke if detected. In addition to an alarm, these detectors have flashing strobe lights that can also be used that provide a visual warning for those who are hard of hearing or have difficulty processing the audio alert.

- *Fall detection and alert systems*: Falls can be very dangerous for seniors, and those with dementia are at especially high risk due to factors such as impaired balance, gait difficulties, and confusion. Wearable devices are available to detect falls and send alerts to caregivers, allowing for prompt medical attention and reducing the risk of injury. These are some specific issues faced commonly by patients unable to take preventive measures or take care of themselves. Fall detection sensors, when worn on the wrist or clipped onto clothing, can detect sudden changes in movement and trigger an alert if a fall is suspected. The device can automatically connect to a monitoring center where trained professionals can assess the situation and send help if needed. Similarly, sensors can be placed in specific areas of concern, like the bathroom or bedroom to detect falls. Fall detection mats are a type of home-monitoring system specifically designed to detect falls without requiring a wearable device. These mats are typically placed on the floor in areas where a person with dementia is at high risk of falling, such as the bathroom, bedroom, or living room. They can also identify if the patient lies on them for an extended period. When the mat senses a sudden change in pressure consistent with a fall, it will trigger an alarm or send a notification to a monitoring station.[4]
- *Wandering prevention and tracking devices*: Wandering is a very common symptom of dementia, posing a significant safety risk. Gadgets to help locate individuals or alert when the patient passes a predefined boundary are available.
- *GPS trackers*: Worn on a wristband or incorporated into a necklace, these devices transmit GPS location data, allowing caregivers to track the individual if they wander. Small electronic tags resembling RFID chips are available. These tags enable caregivers and family members to locate the individual should they embark on a solo excursion. Many of these tags come with companion Android or iOS applications, facilitating precise tracking of the patient's whereabouts.[5]
- *Smart home technology*: When configured with geofencing capabilities, smart home systems can send alerts if an individual with dementia leaves a designated safe zone.

Patient Gadgets

The patient gadgets have been categorized into domain-based usefulness in **Table 1**.[6] Some of the devices have been elaborated here.

Visual Clocks

Visual clocks can be a helpful tool for dementia patients who are struggling with telling time or understanding the concept of time altogether. Traditional analogy clocks can become confusing due to the abstract nature of their representation of time, making it difficult for those with cognitive impairments to interpret. Visual clocks display the time digitally in large, easy-to-read numbers and may also include features like day of the week, month, and year. Some models even incorporate additional visual cues such as color-coded sections or symbols to represent

TABLE 1: Domain-based dementia devices.[6]

Domain	Device (example)
Memory	• Digital clocks and calendars • Medication dispensers with alarms • Labeling systems • Preprogramed dispensers • Medication reminder apps • Digital photo frames • Reminiscence therapy tablets
Executive	• Simplified tablets with task management apps • Smart appliances like timed coffee maker to reduce decision-making • Automatic bill pay services • Pomodoro timers
Visuospatial	• High-contrast assistive devices • Magnifying devices • Adaptive utensils and plates • Motion-activated and smart floor mats-activated lighting • Talking compasses
Language and communication	• Augmentative and alternative communication (AAC) devices like picture communication boards, speech generating devices, and eye-gaze technology • Speech recognition software • Video chat applications
Gadgets to manage cognitive dysfunction	Immersive virtual reality or augmented reality

different times of day (e.g., morning, afternoon, and evening) or important events (e.g., medication reminders and appointments). By providing a clear and easily understandable representation of time, visual clocks can help reduce confusion, anxiety, and challenging behaviors in individuals with dementia and Alzheimer's disease. They can also help promote independence and maintain a sense of routine and structure in their daily lives. Additionally, caregivers and family members can use visual clocks as tools for communication and planning, helping to enhance the quality of life for both the individual with dementia and their caregivers.

Medication Dispensers

Medication dispensers can hold a supply of medications along with assisting individuals in taking their medication at the right time. They typically offer storage compartments for tablets, and configurable settings for dosage times allowing them to dispense at the correct timings. A prerecorded message from the device would be played as a reminder to alert the patient, and if neglected would alert the caregivers. These are powered by sources such as batteries. Hence, the total benefits would be improved medication adherence by making it easier to remember to take medications, also reduced risk of medication errors (wrong dose or wrong timing) and finally increased independence when trying to manage to be independent.

Robotic Technology

Robotic technology offers a promising new approach to dementia care. As technology continues to develop, robots have the potential to play a significant role in improving the quality of life for dementia patients and their caregivers.[7] Robots used for dementia patients are social assistive robots (SAR), reminder robots, and monitoring robots. The SAR robots are designed to interact with patients, providing companionship and emotional support. They can engage in conversations, play games, sing songs, or simply offer a friendly presence. Some robots are even designed to look cuddly and pet-like. The reminder robots can be programed to remind patients about taking medications, meals, or scheduled activities. They can also provide helpful prompts throughout the day, like gentle suggestions to drink water or go for a walk. Monitoring robots can monitor a patient's activity levels and well-being, sending alerts to caregivers if something seems amiss. This can provide peace of mind for caregivers and potentially detect health issues early on. The AAL Project eWare was initiated to develop intelligent robots designed to support dementia patients in their daily activities, such as cleaning, eating, and mobility. These innovative devices were intended not only to enhance physical mobility and cognitive capabilities but also to promote sustainable caregiving practices. Another key objective was to alleviate caregiver distress, affording them more leisure time for other tasks. One such creation was ReMind, a fusion of James (a nursing robot) and a tablet computer. MI-Tale facilitated meaningful intergenerational conversations for elderly patients. Leveraging music therapy, the robot proved beneficial in enhancing cognitive functions among dementia patients. Moreover, it guided patients through exercises and stimulated memory recall using music. Integration of the Keosity biography app enabled patients to revisit memories and cherished moments.[8] These robots reduce anxiety and loneliness, increase independence, and improve caregivers' support. However, the major downside lies in the considerable costs associated with these robots, making acquisition and maintenance expensive. Despite their utility, these caregiving robots still fall short of fully replacing human caregivers due to their limited functionalities.[9]

Hearing and Vision Aids

Older individuals with dementia may experience a decline in cognitive abilities, gradually impacting their hearing and vision. Hearing and vision loss can significantly worsen their confusion and disorientation. Fortunately, various hearing and visual aids can improve their quality of life. Consequently, tasks like operating a standard remote control become challenging for some patients. To facilitate independent interaction with video screens, specialized Braille remote controls are provided. Moreover, Braille signage in caregiving facilities' elevators enables users to navigate independently. For hearing, standard hearing aids can amplify sounds, making it easier for dementia patients to follow conversations and stay engaged with their surroundings. This can lead to better cognitive function, reduced anxiety, and improved overall well-being.[10]

Telecare

The Falkirk Mobile Emergency Care Service (MECS), offered through the council's housing and social work service, exemplifies a mainstream provision. The MECS passive alarm system is tailored for individuals with dementia, designed to enhance their sense of security through the installation of equipment that autonomously triggers assistance in case of home hazards.[11] This initiative has been providing support for more than a decade.

The scheme uses individual dispersed alarms, which can detect one or more of the following:

- Gas escapes
- Smoke
- The outside door opening
- Extreme temperatures (heat)
- Flood

The process operates through an activated device triggering a call to a response center. Subsequently, a computer presents tailored instructions regarding the appropriate response to the call. Options include contacting emergency services, reaching out to a designated carer or relative, or, in the absence of available contacts, dispatching a warden from the MECS response service.[12]

CHALLENGES AND CONSIDERATIONS

While gadgets can provide significant benefits to individuals with dementia, some challenges and considerations need to be addressed. One challenge is ensuring that the technology is user-friendly and accessible for people with cognitive impairments. Simple interfaces and clear instructions are essential to ensure that individuals can use these gadgets effectively. Another consideration is privacy and security. Wearable devices and monitoring systems often collect personal data, and it is important to ensure that this data is protected and used ethically.[13] Caregivers and family members should carefully research and select gadgets that prioritize user privacy. Lastly, the cost of these gadgets can be a barrier for some families. While technology can offer valuable support, not all individuals may have access to the financial resources needed to invest in these tools. Policymakers and healthcare providers should work together to ensure that individuals with dementia have access to affordable and effective technological support.

CONCLUSION

Technology, an evolving domain, holds the potential to enhance the quality of life for individuals with dementia and their caregivers, facilitating their ability to maintain residence within a community. To realize this potential, it is imperative to confront barriers to technology adoption, such as the necessity for collaborative efforts across multiple agencies and the heightened promotion of technology within the healthcare and social care sectors. Ethical considerations should be actively engaged, thoroughly considered, and effectively addressed. Thus, using technologies for dementia provides many opportunities for considering various aspects of this disease as well can make lifestyle easier both for the patients and the caregivers.

REFERENCES

1. Marshall M. State of the Art in Dementia Care. London: Centre for Policy on Ageing.
2. Chen D, Bharucha AJ, Wactlar HD. Intelligent video monitoring to improve safety of older persons. In: 2007 29th Annual International Conference of the IEEE Engineering in Medicine and Biology Society; 2007. pp. 3814-17.
3. Ray PP, Dash D, De D. A systematic review and implementation of IoT-based pervasive sensor-enabled tracking system for dementia patients. J Med Syst. 2019;43:1-21.
4. Pragnell M, Moore R, Spence L (Eds). The Market Potential for Smart Homes. York: York Publishing Services; 2000.
5. FISK M. Elderly people and independent living: the implications of SMART house technologies. In: Proceedings of British Society of Gerontology Annual Conference. 1996.
6. Products For Alzheimer's. [online] Available from https://www.alzstore.com/shop-alzheimers-store-s/2054.htm [Last accessed July, 2024].
7. Cash M. Assistive technology and people with dementia. Rev Clin Gerontol. 2003;13(4):313-9.
8. Woolham J, Frisby B. Technology how technology can help people feel safe at home. J Dementia Care. 2002;10(2):27-8.
9. Tang P, Curry R, Gann D (Eds). Telecare: New ideas for care and support@ home. Policy Press; 2000.
10. Moyle W. The promise of technology in the future of dementia care. Nat Rev Neurol. 2019;15(6):353-9.
11. Porteus J, Brownsell S (Eds). Using Telecare: Exploring Technologies for Independent Living for Older People. Kidlington, UK: Anchor Trust. 2000.
12. Porteus J (Ed). Assistive Technology and Telecare: Forging Solutions for Independent Living. Bristol: Policy Press; 2003.
13. Marshall PA, Rotimi C. Ethical challenges in community-based research. Am J Med Sci. 2001;322(5):241-5.

Index

Page numbers followed by *b* refer to box, *f* refer to figure, *fc* refer to flowchart, and *t* refer to table.

A

B

C